Therapeutic Activity Intervention with the Elderly:

Foundations & Practices

Therapeutic Activity Intervention with the Elderly:

Foundations & Practices

by

Barbara A. Hawkins, Re.D.

Marti E. May, M.S.

Nancy Brattain Rogers, Ph.D.

Venture Publishing, Inc.
State College, Pennsylvania

Production Manager: Richard Yocum
Design, Layout, and Graphics: Diane K. Bierly
Manuscript editing: Diane K. Bierly
Additional Editing: Katherine Young, Richard Yocum and Michele L. Barbin
Cover Design: Sandra Sikorski Design, 1996
Cover Photo: © Cheryl Maeder/FPG International Corp.

Library of Congress Catalogue Card Number 96-60329
ISBN 0-910251-81-9

This text is dedicated to Janice Hawkins, Becky Rothhaas, Eva May, and Fred Hancock—we love you all dearly. . . .

Contents

Foreword

It is a well-accepted fact that American society is aging. Most individuals are aware that the over-65 age group is the fastest growing segment of the American population. At the turn of the twentieth century, over 3 million Americans were 65 or over, but this figure has swelled to over 25 million at present. As the baby boom generation matures, it is projected to grow to over 65 million by the year 2050. Age demographers have forecast that by the middle of the next century one out of every five Americans, over 20% of the population, will be 65 years or older. While the impact of societal aging is unclear, at least one expert has predicted that it "will change every facet of our society in the coming years" (Dychtwald and Flower, 1989, p. 1). Is America ready to face the challenges associated with its graying?

One challenge that is already being faced concerns the health needs of older Americans. Although contemporary older Americans are generally much healthier compared with those from previous generations, a recent report issued by the U.S. Bipartisan Commission on Comprehensive Health Care projected that the number of individuals 65 or over who require long-term healthcare will grow from the current 6 million to more than 12 million by 2030. Because it is true that the use of health services increases with age, one consequence of societal aging is that the demand for services which help to maintain and/or improve the health of seniors will continue to grow in the forthcoming years.

One form of health service that has increasingly received attention for its preventive as well as therapeutic qualities is organized activity/recreation services. Indeed, the federal government's consumer oriented publication, *How to Select a Nursing Home* (U.S. Department of Health and Human Services: Health Care Financing Administration, 1980) recommends that the activity program at prospective facilities should be among the most important items evaluated by consumers prior to selecting a nursing home.

The importance of organized leisure services also was recognized in conjunction with the Nursing Home Reform Amendments of 1987. In the process of developing interpretive guidelines to be used for Medicare/Medicaid certification, the Office of Business, Research and Analysis (OBRA) included the following requirement:

> F255—The facility must provide for an ongoing program of activities designed to meet, in accordance with the comprehensive assessment of the interests and the physical, mental, and psychosocial well-being of each resident. (OBRA, 1987)

It is with this information in mind that one can begin to appreciate the significance of *Therapeutic Activity Intervention with the Elderly: Foundations & Practices.* While numerous texts exist that are designed to investigate philosophical and theoretical issues concerning leisure and aging, this book takes the logical next step. The authors have developed a detailed and practical analysis of the process of activity intervention and its role and function with older citizens. The strategies discussed cover the entire health spectrum from preventive services offered to the well elderly at the one end to therapeutic intervention for the most infirm at the other extreme. This book will help fill a recognizable void in the aging and leisure literature base, and it will be of use to a wide variety of activity service providers as well as to individuals who are receiving training in an effort to enter this professional field.

I applaud the effort of the authors in developing this most important text. It will prove to be a valuable addition to the libraries of all activity professionals who work with older Americans.

Richard MacNeil, Professor
University of Iowa
Iowa City, Iowa
July 18, 1995

References

Dychtwald, K., & Flower, K. (1989). *Age wave: The challenges and opportunities of an aging America.* Los Angeles, CA: Jeremy P. Tarcher, Inc.

Office of Business, Research and Analysis. (1987). *Interpretive guidelines: Skilled nursing facilities and intermediate care facilities.* Washington, DC: U.S. Government Printing Office.

U.S. Department of Health and Human Services: Health Care Financing Administration. (1980). *How to select a nursing home.* Washington, DC: U.S. Government Printing Office.

Preface

This book is a response to the need for pedagogical materials in the education of professionals who will provide activity programs and interventions to older adults in a variety of service settings. The authors, through their experience in providing basic college instruction in this area, have found no single source that can effectively meet their needs in the classroom or in the field. Thus, we hope that college students as well as activity specialists who work in senior centers, adult daycare, skilled nursing facilities, and in rehabilitation centers that serve older adults, will find this text to be a helpful resource.

The book has been written to cover a broad range of topics. Foundation information about aging and the elderly is presented in the first two units. Readers will be introduced to current demographic information and issues concerning the aging adult population. Unit II guides the reader through a basic introduction to normal aging processes, as well as common illnesses, diseases, and disabilities that affect older persons. After completing these two units, the reader will have a basic understanding of the elderly population.

Units III and IV provide entry-level information about therapeutic intervention which uses activities as the primary treatment modality. Professional practice topics such as assessment and program planning are covered, as well as special considerations when serving older adults. The reader is provided with introductory information about motivation, control, and environmental design considerations. Specific interventions are described in Unit IV spanning the areas of leisure education, physical activity and health promotion, cognitive activity interventions, and psychosocial activities. The last unit pertains to documentation and evaluation, ethical considerations and standards of practice, and future trends affecting therapeutic activity intervention.

Each chapter has been prepared to aid in the learning process whether it be in the classroom or through in-service education. Learning objectives, key words, and comprehension questions are provided to enhance the focus of the reader to the most important points of the chapter. A glossary of key terms is also provided at the end of the book.

Writing a book like this one poses certain challenges. While we were particularly interested in covering the wide range of material that we feel is necessary in introducing both gerontology studies as well as preparation for activity programming, we also hoped to provide sufficient detail to make the book useful beyond the classroom situation. We hope that the book can be a resource to activity specialists as they are planning and implementing intervention programs. In this regard, we may have omitted some important details for the sake of breadth and inclusiveness. We hope that the possibility of omission is minimal, and we hasten to advise practicing activity specialists to develop additional resource materials to assist them in their practice.

With any labor of love, such as writing a textbook, there are many hands that assisted in the process. We would like to thank Geof Godbey for encouraging us to write the book and keeping the faith that it eventually would be finished. We also thank our families, friends and colleagues for putting up with our obsession about finishing "the book." Above all, we thank all the older adults who have been our mentors in learning about the richness that long life can bring to those who embrace the journey with optimism and enthusiasm.

BAH, MEM, NBR

Unit I

Introduction

The delivery of therapeutic activities to older adults requires a thorough knowledge of the needs and desires of individuals who are elderly. The aim of this text is to provide information that will assist the reader in developing an understanding of the elderly and how activity intervention may be used to reach treatment and rehabilitation goals. The book introduces professionals, caregivers, and students to basic concepts dealing with the normal aging process as well as to illnesses and diseases common among older people for the purpose of enabling the readers to be better prepared to provide appropriate activities for older persons.

Unit I provides the reader with an introduction to the population and healthcare services for older adults. Chapter 1 begins the text with background information about the elderly population including demographic characteristics and population diversity considerations. Chapter 2 provides an overview of the need for healthcare services by older adults. The chapter distinguishes between chronic and acute diseases, and it describes the process of impairment that leads to disablement among older persons. The chapter concludes with information pertaining to current trends that are influencing healthcare and activity intervention for older adults.

Key Terms

Age Discrimination
    Employment Act
Chronological Age
Dependency Ratio
Feminization of Poverty
Functional Age
Life Expectancy

Near Poor
Older Adults
Oldest Old
Old Old
Poverty Level
Young Old

Learning Objectives

1. Describe general characteristics of the older adult population including age, gender, marital status, educational status, living arrangements, income, employment status, poverty, and geographic distribution.
2. Discuss common misconceptions and stereotypes concerning older adults.
3. Discuss practice of age discrimination.
4. Describe the growth trends in the size of the older population.
5. Identify demographic trends as they relate to gender, ethnicity, and impairment.
6. Define the term feminization of poverty and describe how it relates to older women.
7. Explain the difference between functional age and chronological age.
8. Discuss how demographic characteristics, age differences, and diversity affect the utilization of formal services.
9. Describe cultural differences among different ethnic groups in the older population.

Chapter 1

The Population: Demographic Characteristics and Diversity Considerations

Introduction

The purpose of this chapter is to familiarize the reader with demographic trends within the older adult population. These trends are described in relation to geographic distribution, living arrangements, income, poverty, employment, education, and utilization of formal services. The older population is a diverse population in many ways. Diversity is discussed in terms of age differences, gender, and ethnic group throughout the chapter. Frequently, older adults are referred to as a single demographic group. However, there are distinct differences between the functional abilities of age groups within the older population.

Ethnic diversity is also common among the older population. Ethnic groups differ markedly in terms of poverty, geographic distribution, life expectancy, family roles, and other demographic characteristics. Gender differences are more evident among older people, especially in the greater numbers of older, widowed women who are living in poverty. The chapter concludes with a discussion of future implications for the delivery of services to the elderly. Questions regarding who will pay for the costs of an aging society are critical issues for policymakers to address. A number of difficult ethical and economic issues will face society in the near future as healthcare and social service systems prepare to serve the growing older adult population.

Demographic Trends

The ever-increasing number of older adults in the population has become the focus of the media, the healthcare industry, and the academic community. Older adults, persons 65 years of age or older, currently comprise almost 13% of the population in the United States (AARP, 1995). This percentage translates to 33.2 million people. The increase in the older population since the turn of the century has been remarkable. In 1900 there were only 3.1 million older adults in the United States who comprised 4.1% of the population. Today the older population is 10 times that size. The growth in the last decade alone has been significant. Since 1980, the older population has grown by 6.1 million, a 24% increase. During the same decade, the under-age-65 population only grew by 9%. The population of adults over the age of 85 has increased at the highest rate. This group is 28 times larger than it was in 1900 (AARP, 1995).

The recent increase in the size of the older adult population is attributable to a variety of factors including lower infant mortality rates, medical advances that produced vaccines or cures for infectious diseases, treatment for chronic conditions, lifestyle changes, and improved public sanitation (AARP, 1995; Neugarten and Neugarten, 1991). This population growth is also accompanied by an increase in life expectancy. The life expectancy for a child born in 1993 is 75.5 years (AARP, 1995).

Life expectancy is defined as the average number of years a person born in a particular year can be expected to live. On average, women outlive men by a margin of approximately seven years (Hayslip and Panek, 1993). Women born in 1993 can expect to live to nearly 79 years of age. The life expectancy for men born in 1993 is approximately 72 years of age. Adults who survive to the age of 65 can expect to live an additional 17.3 years (AARP, 1995). Women can expect to live 18.9 more years, and men can expect to live 15.3 more years. Table 1.1 summarizes selected demographic characteristics of the older population organized by age brackets of five year increments.

Geographic Distribution

Not surprisingly, the majority of older adults live in the most heavily populated states (AARP, 1995). California leads all states with over 3 million older adults. Nearly 2.5 million older adults reside in Florida, the state with the second highest percentage of older adults (18.3%). Pennsylvania, Texas, Illinois, Ohio, Michigan, and New Jersey each claim over 1 million older adults.

With the exceptions of Pennsylvania and Florida, the states with the largest populations of older adults are not the states where older adults represent the highest percentage of the population. The populations of Florida, Pennsylvania, Iowa, Rhode Island, and West Virginia are composed of more than 15% older adults. Arkansas, South Dakota, North Dakota, Nebraska, and Missouri each have populations of over 14% older adults. In many of these states the high percentage of older adults is attributed to the flight of younger persons seeking work in other states.

The majority of older adults live in metropolitan areas. Of the 74% of older adults in urban areas, 30% live in the central city and 44% live in the suburbs

Table 1.1

Selected Demographic Characteristics of Older Adults According to Age

Age Category	Percent
Age 65 to 69 Years	
Women	55
Married	70
Living Alone	21
Claiming Good Health	75
In Labor Force	20
Under Poverty Level	8
Age 70 to 74 Years	
Women	57
Married	61
Living Alone	29
Claiming Good Health	68
In Labor Force	10
Under Poverty Level	11
Age 75 to 79 Years	
Women	62
Married	50
Living Alone	37
Claiming Good Health	66
In Labor Force	10
Under Poverty Level	14
Age 80 to 84 Years	
Women	64
Married	40
Living Alone	44
Claiming Good Health	63
In Labor Force	N.A.
Under Poverty Level	17
Age 85 Years and Older	
Women	67[a]
Married	24
Living Alone	50
Claiming Good Health	63
In Labor Force	N.A.
Under Poverty Level	17

[a](noninstitutionalized)

Note: Developed from information contained in Pol, May, & Hartranft, 1992.

(AARP, 1995). Older adults within ethnic minority groups are especially likely to live in the inner city. Only 29% of Caucasian older adults live in the inner city, compared to 55% of older African-American and 53% of older Hispanic adults (U.S. Bureau of the Census, 1989). Unfortunately, the older adults in the central cities carry the greatest burden in terms of poverty, crime, lack of adequate housing, and other social problems.

Older adults in rural areas, especially African Americans, generally have lower incomes and poorer health than do those in urban areas. This situation may be due, in part, to reduced availability of social services, healthcare services, and transportation. Rural elderly also are less likely to live close to their children. Evidence does indicate, however, that older adults in small communities interact more frequently with friends and neighbors (Schooler, 1975).

In spite of the popular myth which portrays older adults as lonely people abandoned by their children, the majority of older adults have regular contact with their family members. For the past 30 years, around 75% of older adults have lived within 25 miles of adult children (Crispell and Frey, 1993). Furthermore, research indicates that older adults who are not in the geographic proximity of their children maintain regular contact through letters, phone calls, and visits (Kornhober and Woodward, 1981).

Living Arrangements

The majority of older adults (68%) live with a spouse or other family members (AARP, 1995). However, the number of older adults living alone has grown recently. Older persons living alone account for 40% of all single-person households (Crispell and Frey, 1993). Only 5% of older adults currently reside in nursing homes or other long-term care facilities (AARP, 1995).

Housing arrangements differ significantly by gender due to women's increased life expectancy. Women are far more likely than men to live alone in old age. Eighty percent of older adults living alone are women (Crispell and Frey, 1993), and 42% of older women live alone, while only 41% live with a spouse (AARP, 1995). In contrast, 75% of older men live with a spouse, and only 19% live alone.

Older adults are more likely than other age groups to own their homes and be free of mortgages. An estimated 70% of older heads of households own their homes. Of this group, 82% do not have a mortgage.

Income

The majority of older adults have low to middle incomes. Family households headed by older adults average $26,512 per year. Households comprised of older adults living alone or with someone other than relatives are more likely to have low incomes (AARP, 1995). The average income of this group is $11,504. Although these averages are lower than the national average, it is important to keep in mind that older adults frequently have fewer expenses than younger adults (Crispell and Frey, 1993). Mortgages, childcare, college tuition, and similar major expenses typically are not present in older households. However, as the need for healthcare increases in these households, lower incomes may certainly become a problem for many older adults. The average older adult annually accumulates $5,360 in personal healthcare expenditures (AARP, 1995). Of that amount, 40% is not covered by insurance or Medicare. The costs that are left over and must be paid by the client can amount to between 10% and 25% of his or her yearly income.

While most older adults do not have large incomes, there is a significant number of affluent older households (Crispell and Frey, 1993). In 1989, 11% of older households had incomes greater than $50,000, and 4% had incomes of over $75,000.

Social security provides 40% of all income to the older adult population (AARP, 1995). It is important for adults to plan for retirement and not to rely on Social Security as their only means of support. The intention of the Social Security program is not to serve as a substitute for a pension or retirement fund. Consequently, older adults who plan on living only on Social Security may not be able to avoid poverty. Other important sources of income for older adults include pensions, work, and income from assets (AARP, 1995).

Poverty

Poverty affects older adults about the same as it does younger adults. Approximately 11.7% of the older population is living under the poverty level set by the federal government, compared to 11.9% of the population between the ages of 18 and 64. Poverty rates should be viewed with skepticism, however, since they do not indicate the high percentage of older adults whose incomes are only slightly higher than the poverty level. An estimated 7% of older adults live between the poverty level and 125% of this level (AARP, 1995). These individuals are often referred to as the *near poor*.

Gender and ethnic group are correlated with poverty. While only 10% of older Caucasians are poor, 23% of older Hispanics and 27% of older African Americans have incomes under the poverty level (AARP, 1995). The rate of poverty is higher for older women at 15% than it is for older men at 7%. An estimated 45% of older women live within 150% of the poverty level (Renzetti and Curran, 1992). Older black women appear to be at the greatest risk for living in poverty. Of black women over the age of 75, 62% live in poverty.

The *feminization of poverty* is a term used by sociologists to describe how society locks many women into poverty through social institutions and economic structure. Older women are at greatest risk for poverty if they are widowed, divorced, or never married. Most older women have not worked enough consecutive years to receive substantial pension or social security benefits. Many women are not eligible for any pension benefits of their own. Widows' benefits from most pensions typically are reduced to as much as 50% of what their husband was receiving (Hartman, 1990).

Employment

Only 12% of older adults are involved in the labor force (AARP, 1995). Labor force participation drops steadily during the late 50s and early 60s. While 74% of people in the 50 to 54 age group are in the labor force, only 44% of people ranging in age from 60 to 64 work outside the home. The rate drops to less than 10% in the 70 to 74 age group. Approximately half of older workers work part time (Pol, May, and Hartranft, 1992).

Age discrimination is a problem for many older workers. Many employers and younger workers believe that older workers are:

(a) less productive than their younger counterparts,
(b) unable to change,
(c) slow to perform and train, and
(d) diminished in their abilities to perform mentally and physically (Hayslip and Panek, 1993).

In order to combat age discrimination, the Age Discrimination Employment Act was passed in 1967. This legislation includes measures that restrict employers from (a) failing to hire a person because of age, (b) discharging an employee because of age, or (c) discriminating in pay because of age. Unfortunately some employers, including the federal government, are exempt from this legislation although federal reform in 1995 may change this situation.

Education

The median level of education in the older population is 12.2 years (AARP, 1995). Approximately 58% of older adults have completed high school and 13% have completed four or more years of college. These levels have risen steadily in the past two decades.

Adult education programs provide important opportunities for older adults to continue to grow intellectually. Each year, over 500,000 older adults enroll in adult education classes (Ferrini and Ferrini, 1993). This number is expected to grow as community and adult education programs continue to develop the growing senior market.

Utilization of Formal Services

In spite of common myths, most older adults do not place a heavy financial burden on society. Generally, the healthcare costs and low incomes of older adults do not place financial demands on public assistance and formal service programs until the age of 85 (Ferrini and Ferrini, 1993). The vast majority of care provided to older adults is given by the family (Older Women's League, 1989). Most families choose to utilize formal care services only when informal sources can no longer meet the needs of their disabled relative (Aronson, 1992). Over 50% of older adults with functional limitations related to activities of daily living or instrumental activities of daily living receive no formal services and rely solely on informal help (AARP, 1995).

Diversity in the Older Population

Age Differences

Although the older population is often stereotyped as a homogeneous group, nothing could be further from the truth. Differences in ability to function cognitively, socially, and physically may be more evident in this age group than any other. The wide range of differences in the older population has led many service providers and researchers to divide the older population into subgroups based on age. The 65 to 74 age group is frequently referred to as the *young old*. The *old old* are those who fall into the 75 to 84 age group. Individuals who are above 85 years of age are referred to as the *oldest old*. There are 10.3 million older adults between the ages of 75 and 85. The remaining older population, those over the age of 85, number 3.2 million.

Oldest Old

The over-85 age group is in greatest need of health and social services. As their numbers continue to grow, they will be of primary concern to healthcare and social policy planners, in spite of remaining a relatively small percentage of the total older population (Neugarten and Neugarten, 1991). Service providers who work with the oldest old understand that longevity and good health do not always go hand-in-hand. Chronic conditions lead to functional limitations and disability with much greater frequency in the oldest old population. As estimated, 45% of the oldest old require assistance with basic activities, compared to 9% of adults between the ages of 65 and 69. On a more positive note, 63% of the oldest old still claim to be in good health, in spite of activity limitations (Pol, May, and Hartranft, 1992). In addition to health concerns, the oldest old are also more likely to live alone and in poverty, more likely to be female, and less likely to be married than younger elderly.

Functional Age and Chronological Age

The pronounced differences in ability to function among the older population has created the need for a method to define the age of an individual in a more useful method than chronologically. Frequently, older adults are referred to according to their *functional age*. This age is determined by the individual's ability to carry out activities of daily living (ADLs) and to live independently. Consequently, an individual whose *chronological age* is 80 functionally may be younger than someone who is chronologically 65 if he or she requires less assistance with basic activities. Chapters 2 and 5 further discuss the importance of functional age in regard to the healthcare and health status of older adults.

Ethnic Differences

African Americans

Older African Americans comprise approximately 8% of the African-American population. The young outnumber the old among African Americans in a greater percentage than for the general population primarily because of the higher fertility of African-American women and higher mortality at midlife. In general, the life expectancy for African Americans is seven years less than it is for white Americans (Hooyman and Kiyak, 1991).

The toll of years of discrimination and racism is evident among older African Americans. Historically, the jobs available to older African Americans did not provide benefits such as pension plans. Furthermore, the low wages that were paid African Americans during their years of employment did not provide enough income for investments or savings. As a result, older African Americans are more likely than white Americans to rely on Social Security as a sole means of support (Ferrini and Ferrini, 1993).

Traditionally, the older black woman is viewed as the backbone of the family. Grandmothers frequently assume at least partial childcare responsibilities. Older black women are more likely than women of other ethnic groups to have children, grandchildren, and other relatives living in their homes (Yee, 1990).

Disabled older African Americans are more likely to be cared for at home as opposed to in an institution. Older African Americans are institutionalized at only 50% to 75% the rate of older white Americans. A number of factors have been suggested which may influence this trend including limited financial resources, lowered access to care, cultural values, and the tendency for extended families to live together in the African-American community (Belgrave, Wykle, and Choi, 1993).

Older African-American women's status in the family may be due to their history of independence (Yee, 1990). Since the time of slavery, black women have worked independently and not relied on the resources of men. Older black women today have long histories of employment which frequently began in childhood as field workers and domestic servants (Allen and Chin-Sang, 1990). Unfortunately, history of employment is not enough to help older black women stay out of poverty. An estimated 62% of black women over the age of 75 are poor. Allen and Chin-Sang (1990) described the status of older black women as that of "quadruple jeopardy." They are old, poor, female, and of minority status.

Native Americans

Older Native Americans represent 5% of their population (Hooyman and Kiyak, 1991). The small number of older Native Americans is due in part to a lower life expectancy. The life expectancy of Native Americans varies according to source, with an estimated range from 65 to 70 years (Ferrini and Ferrini, 1993; Hooyman and Kiyak, 1991). All estimates, however, are much lower than that of the general population.

Approximately 50% of older Native Americans live in the southwestern states. Many live in rural areas without much access to healthcare and social services. About 25% of older Native Americans live on reservations (Ferrini and Ferrini, 1993).

The older Native American has traditionally been viewed as a revered member of the extended family. Older adults provide spiritual guidance to younger family members and share cultural heritage. It is also common for older women to assume major childcare responsibilities (Yee, 1990).

The lack of resources and social support provided to this population is evident through widespread poverty and unemployment. Older Native Americans are more susceptible to a number of healthcare problems due to reduced access to healthcare. Alcoholism is a major health concern for many older Native Americans. Greater support through better healthcare, opportunities for education, and employment is needed to improve the quality of life for older Native Americans (Yee, 1990).

Asian Americans

The Asian and Pacific Island population in the United States is extremely diverse in terms of both cultural heritage and language. Some members of the population, such as Japanese Americans, have become highly westernized. Other members who have immigrated more recently still hold more traditional values.

Most Asian and Pacific Island cultures traditionally have placed a strong emphasis on prescribed gender roles. Older adults within these cultures were highly valued and respected for their wisdom and cultural knowledge. Interdependence between generations was strong. However, as younger Asian Americans have become accustomed to Western culture, they have begun to lose their reverence toward the elderly members of their population group, and the lines between gender roles have become less defined as well. Consequently, generational differences are strong.

Older adults represent 6% of the Asian-American population. The population is concentrated in California, Washington, and Hawaii (Ferrini and Ferrini, 1993). The largest concentration can be found in San Francisco. This is the only ethnic group in which the numbers of older men and women are almost equal. The difference is due primarily to immigration laws that have restricted the number of Asian immigrants allowed into the United States (Yee, 1990). The life expectancy of women is still greater in this population.

Hispanic Americans

In spite of sharing a common language, the older Hispanic-American population is culturally diverse. Mexican Americans represent the largest percentage of the Hispanic-American population. Many Mexican Americans are not first generation residents of the United States and have become acculturated to the *American way of life.* Intergenerational differences are evident in this population, as younger Mexican Americans are especially likely to reject traditional roles. Other Hispanic Americans, such as those originating from Puerto Rico and Cuba, are mostly first generation Americans and may be more accepting of traditional roles (Yee, 1990).

Traditional Hispanic culture is characterized by pronounced sex roles. The extended family also is an important element in Hispanic culture. Intergenerational exchange is common with older adults providing valuable cultural history and assistance with child rearing. Aging is accepted in the Hispanic culture and elders are viewed with respect (Yee, 1990).

Older Hispanic Americans represent less than 5% of the population (Hooyman and Kiyak, 1991) due to high fertility rates, immigration, and repatriation of some older and middle age adults (Yee, 1990). However, the number of older Hispanic Americans is expected to increase 400% by 2020. The majority of older Hispanic Americans live in urban areas. The population is especially concentrated in California, Texas, New York, and Florida (Ferrini and Ferrini, 1993).

Future Implications

The rate of growth of the older population has serious implications for healthcare and social policy planners. A greater number of older people will rely on Medicare,

Social Security, and other social programs without a substantial increase in the number of working taxpayers. Currently, the *dependency ratio,* the number of adults under age 65 to adults over age 65, is 8 to 1. This ratio will decrease to 6 to 1 or 5 to 1 by the year 2030 (AARP, 1995). As this ratio decreases, government will need to address issues associated with entitlement to social benefits and programs by older people. Specifically, decisions will need to be made regarding whether or not all older adults will continue to be entitled to the current level of support from Social Security, Medicare, and other social programs regardless of their ability to pay for services.

Greater demands will be placed on the healthcare system by older adults in the future. Chronic conditions requiring expensive, long-term care are projected to continue as the primary health concern of older adults. A growing debate already exists regarding the medical profession's obligation to preserve life and initiate treatment versus the right of a patient to refuse care and die peacefully without unwanted medical intervention when the quality of life becomes so low that the patient wishes to die. What obligations does society have to provide medical care to the dying elderly? Because the majority of medical expenses are incurred during the last month of life, should the healthcare system initiate and government pay for expensive treatments that will only prolong the inevitability of death for only a short time? Should these economic questions drive healthcare policy? These are tough questions that currently face society and the professionals who serve older adults.

The need for long-term care for the oldest old is a topic of growing interest as the size of that population segment expands. Traditionally, daughters, wives, and daughters-in-law have provided the majority of care to disabled older adults. Lower fertility rates, high rates of divorce, and increased female commitment to lifetime careers may reduce the number of women who are able to take on primary care responsibilities. In spite of this trend, family members and clients will probably continue to prefer home-based care as opposed to being institutionalized. The demand for home-based care services and increased levels of reimbursement from Medicare and private insurance companies are likely to grow.

The growing ethnic diversity among the older population can be expected to influence the delivery of services to older adults. Service providers will need to understand cultural differences to better serve a diverse older population. Traditional methods of reaching older adults to inform them of services will not be as effective for all members of this diverse population. New links between service providers and key members of ethnic communities (with access to this older population) must be established, and trust must be gained. The healthcare and social service systems need to be viewed not as symbols of majority bureaucracy, but as systems open to all members of the population.

Future implications for the healthcare system are not all negative. The current population of older adults is better educated, has greater access to healthcare services, and is more aware of living a healthy lifestyle than any previous generation of older adults. These are trends that will continue as the population ages. It is reasonable to expect that the majority of older adults will continue to remain independent until very old age. The percentage of young old requiring formal services may potentially decrease in the next few decades.

The growing healthy older population also will demand expanded service delivery. Adult education, community recreation, arts, exercise, and travel programs are examples of the types of services to which older adults may want increased access in their retirement. Older adults also may continue to seek opportunities to remain productive members of the community through volunteer work or part-time employment.

Summary

The older population has grown remarkably during this century and will continue to do so well into the next. This growth can be attributed to lifestyle and medical changes that have greatly increased the life expectancy of the average adult. The population of older adults is concentrated in those states with the largest populations. However, the states with the largest percentages of older adults are located in the rural south and midwest. Most older adults live with a spouse or other family member, although the number of older adults living alone has grown recently. The majority of older adults is not in poverty and can support themselves without financial assistance. Single women, some ethnic groups, and the oldest old are more likely to be living in poverty than other older adults. The majority of older adults are not employed. Their incomes typically come from Social Security, pension funds, income, and earnings from assets. The current population of older adults is more highly educated than any generation to come before them. Most have completed a high school education. Older adults generally are productive and independent individuals who do not utilize formal services or seek assistance with care until very late in life.

The older population can be characterized as diverse. Differences in functional ability are evident in the older population more than in any other age group. There are marked demographic differences between age groups within the older population. Gerontologists frequently refer to older adults as the young old, the old old, and the oldest old. However, there are still problems associated with these categories. Chronological age is not always a good indicator of functional ability. It may be more useful to refer to an individual's functional age rather than his or her chronological age. Diversity also is evident in terms of clear and distinct cultural differences between ethnic groups. It may be helpful for service providers to understand various cultures and, subsequently, to offer services with a sensitivity to cultural differences.

The older population will continue to grow well into the next century. Service providers will be faced with a variety of economic and ethical decisions regarding the types of services that can be offered to the disabled older population. The number of healthy older adults also will continue to grow in size, thus increasing the demand for leisure, travel, and other related services.

Comprehension Questions

1. Select three general characteristics of the older population and describe them in regard to recent trends.
2. Name two common misconceptions about older adults.
3. What does the feminization of poverty mean and describe the impact of this phenomena on older women.
4. What impact does cultural diversity have on the older adult population, now and into the future?
5. What does the future hold for older persons regarding health and social service programs?

References

Allen, K. R., & Chin-Sang, V. (1990). A lifetime of work: The context and meaning of leisure for aging black women. *The Gerontologist, 30*(6), 734-740.

American Association of Retired Persons & Administration on Aging (AARP). (1995). *A profile of older Americans.* Washington, DC: Author.

Aronson, J. (1992). Women's sense of responsibility for the care of old people: "But who else is going to do it?" *Gender and Society, 6*(1), 8-29.

Belgrave, L. L., Wykle, M. L., & Choi, J. M. (1993). Health, double jeopardy, and culture: The use of institutionalization by African Americans. *The Gerontologist, 33*(3), 379-385.

Crispell, D., & Frey, W. H. (1993, March). American maturity. *American Demographics,* 31-42.

Ferrini, A. F., & Ferrini, R. L. (1993). *Health in the later years* (2nd ed.). Madison, WI: Brown & Benchmark.

Hartman, A. (1990). Aging as a feminist issue. *Social Work, 35*(5), 387-388.

Hayslip, B. H., & Panek, P. E. (1993). *Adult development and aging.* New York, NY: HarperCollins College Publishers.

Hooyman, N. R., & Kiyak, H. A. (1991). *Social gerontology: A multidisciplinary perspective* (2nd ed.). Needham Heights, MA: Allyn & Bacon.

Kornhober, A., & Woodward, K. L. (1981). *Grandparents/grandchildren: The vital connection.* Garden City, NY: Anchor Press/Doubleday.

Neugarten, B. L., & Neugarten, D. A. (1991). Policy issues in an aging society. In M. Storandt & G. R. VandenBos (Eds.), *The adult years: Continuity and change* (pp. 147-167). Washington, DC: American Psychological Association.

Older Women's League. (1989). *Failing America's caregivers: A status report on women who care.* Washington, DC: Author.

Pol, L. G., May, M. G., & Hartranft, F. R. (1992, August). Eight stages of aging. *American Demographics,* 54-57.

Renzetti, C. M., & Curran, D. J. (1992). *Women, men and society.* Needham Heights, MA: Allyn & Bacon.

Schooler, K. K. (1975). Response of the elderly to environment: A stress-theoretic perspective. In P. G. Windley & G. Ernst (Eds.), *Theory development in environment and aging.* Washington, DC: Gerontological Society.

U.S. Bureau of the Census. (1989). *Population profile of the United States: 1987.* Series P-23, No. 159.

Yee, B. W. K. (1990). Gender and family issues in minority groups. *Generations, 15,* 39-42.

Key Terms

Acute Disease
Adult Daycare
Chronic Disease
Comorbidity
Continuing Care Retirement
    Community
Disability
Functional Competence
Functional Limitation
Health Promotion
Home-Bound

Impairment
In-Home Care
Life-Care Community
Morbidity
Nursing Facility
Nursing Home Care
Pathology
Prevention
Quality of Life
Rehabilitation

Learning Objectives

1. Describe functional status and heathcare needs as they pertain to older adults.
2. Define the concepts of pathology, impairment, functional limitation, and disability.
3. Describe the difference between chronic and acute disease.
4. Discuss how functional impairment and the need for healthcare are served in different settings.
5. Explain the difference between preventive intervention and rehabilitative intervention.
6. Discuss the importance of personal control and independence in the provision of intervention services to older persons.
7. Discuss current trends that are influencing healthcare and intervention services to older adults.

Chapter 2

Overview of Healthcare and the Elderly

Introduction

This chapter provides an overview of the need for healthcare services by older adults from the perspective of the process by which health conditions lead to impairment, functional limitation, and disability. Disability is described as an outcome that is not only related to level of impairment and functional limitation, but also as influenced by the social and physical environment in which the individual lives. Functional status of older persons is described as it relates to pathology, impairment, functional limitation, and disability. Each of these terms are defined and distinguished from one another.

Functional impairment and disability underlie the need for health-related services that are delivered on the basis of three levels of care (e.g., inpatient, outpatient, in-home) and across a variety of service settings. Services may be provided in institutions on an inpatient basis, or, for individuals who are not institutionalized, care may be provided in community-based or home-bound service settings by a range of service providers. Many service options exist on a continuum including adult day programs, in-home services, continuing care retirement centers, nursing homes, rehabilitation centers, and acute care hospitals. Each of these service settings is briefly described in this chapter.

Overviews of prevention and rehabilitation intervention services are provided in this chapter. Prevention strategies may be primary, secondary, or tertiary depending upon the functional status of the individual. Prevention services are aimed at preserving the optimal health and well-being of the individual. When functional limitations and disabilities are present, rehabilitative interventions often are directed toward restoring or preserving the individual's health and functional capabilities at the highest possible level. Prevention and rehabilitation form the basis for therapeutic activity intervention with elderly persons.

Health and Functional Status

At present, one-third of all healthcare services and products are consumed by the older adult population, and by the year 2030, it is projected that this proportion will increase to one-half (Pegels, 1988). While healthcare has steadily improved over the past two centuries, it remains a serious concern because of continually rising costs. The highest portion of healthcare expenditures among the elderly is for long-term care (e.g., placement in a nursing home). Only about 5% of the population over age 65, however, reside in nursing homes at any one time. In addition, the nursing home population continues to reflect an older, more frail and seriously impaired population. As a result, the percentage of the elderly population who reside in nursing facilities increases with each age group. For example, only 1% of the population between the ages of 65 and 74 live in nursing homes while 22% of adults over age 85 reside in these facilities (Pegels, 1988). The steady growth in the population groups who use a disproportionately higher share of health resources, of which the elderly is one, further exacerbates the healthcare problem.

The likelihood that older persons will need healthcare services and products increases with their age. In spite of positive gains in life expectancy, the quality of very old age is still problematic for a significant number of elderly persons. As a consequence, the prevalence of impairment and disability continue to rise among certain groups of older persons such as:

(a) those who have lower socioeconomic status,
(b) persons with less education,
(c) ethnic minorities, or
(d) very old females.

Another reason for the increase in disability and impairment among older adults is the increase in chronic diseases in the overall population. Chronic diseases are those that result from unhealthy lifestyles or behaviors that produce long-term impairment and disability. Two chronic conditions that are particularly problematic for older persons are heart disease and circulatory conditions (Pope and Tarlove, 1991). On the other hand, acute diseases, such as influenza, are largely managed through immunization, nutrition, improved public health practices, and sanitation. Acute diseases do not pose the same degree of pressure on the healthcare system and healthcare dollar as do chronic conditions. Because older persons experience functional limitations due to impairment from health problems, it is useful to examine the process by which pathological conditions result in impairment and disability.

Functional Status and Disability

It is not uncommon for adults, as they age, to experience the onset of chronic health conditions, many of which will result in impairment in normal functioning. Assessment can evaluate the overall impact of the condition on the individual's ability to perform daily tasks and activities, and make it possible to determine the degree of impairment in functioning. Not all health conditions, however, will result in disability. Disability is a status that places the individual's functional limitations within a social and physical environmental context that undermines independence. The degree of environmental demand and support determines whether the individual is seen as disabled or nondisabled. The functional competence or ability of the person to perform activities and tasks is related to the degree of impairment which may or may not result in disablement.

It is important to recognize that whether a person can and does:

> perform a socially expected activity depends not simply on the characteristics of the person but also on the larger context of social and physical environments. (Pope and Tarlove, 1991, p. 5–6)

A complex and interactive process involving both the functional capabilities of the individual and the social and physical environment influences the assessment of disabilities. Four basic concepts can be used to better understand the process by which a health condition impairs the individual and when the impairment becomes a disability. These concepts are: *pathology, impairment, functional limitation,* and *disability* (Pope and Tarlove, 1991).

Pathology is a direct result of changes in the tissues and cells of the human organism that are produced by injury, infection, disease, birth defects, or other agents (Pope and Tarlove, 1991). Pathological states in older persons involve either acute or chronic conditions. An acute condition is a bacterial or viral infection that results in immediate illness. Other distinguishing characteristics of acute illnesses are:

(a) abrupt onset,
(b) treatable with medication and sometimes surgery,
(c) short term in duration, and
(d) usually involve a low-cost cure (Ferrini and Ferrini, 1993).

Chronic illnesses, on the other hand, are characterized by:

(a) progressive onset,
(b) multiple causes usually associated with lifestyle behaviors and environmental carcinogens,
(c) a lifetime duration,
(d) irreversibility even with treatment,
(e) progressiveness, and
(f) management through medical care and rehabilitation (Ferrini and Ferrini, 1993).

Common acute illnesses among the elderly stem from respiratory infections (e.g., common cold, influenza, pneumonia) and gastrointestinal infections (e.g., indigestion, abdominal pain, heartburn, gas, diarrhea, constipation). Some of the common chronic conditions experienced by older persons include cardiovascular disease (e.g., high blood pressure, heart disease, stroke), cancer, respiratory disease (e.g., asthma, emphysema), sensory disorders (e.g., hearing loss, vision loss), skeletal disorders (e.g., arthritis, osteoporosis) and diabetes. These and other acute and chronic conditions are covered in greater detail in Chapters 5 and 6.

Impairment occurs when there is a loss in mental or physical function that results from the specific functioning of an organ or organ system. Impairment may be caused by more than one type of health problem, and all health conditions will result in some level of impairment. Depending upon the degree of impairment, individuals may experience limitations in their ability to function independently with normal activities and tasks in everyday life such as being able to get up and out of bed, or being able to move about their homes doing typical activities like bathing and dressing (Pope and Tarlove, 1991).

A *functional limitation* describes the effects that are present in the person's capacity to perform as a whole, as well as independently or with some assistance. For example, older persons have functional limitations when they are unable to open kitchen cabinets and remove items for use. Elderly persons respond to impairment on an individual basis. For example, the same pathological condition that is experienced by two individuals may manifest as different levels of impairment. One individual may experience limitations in overall functional capacity while another, based upon other factors that are influencing the capacity of the individual, may not. The manner in which all bodily systems work together to accomplish the demands of a specific activity has an impact upon the functional competence of the individual. For example, consider two individuals who have experienced the same degree of loss in visual acuity. If one individual has been an active athlete throughout his or her life while the second has been sedentary resulting in low overall physical fitness, it would then be expected that the first individual experienced less impairment in balance, spatial orientation, and mobility compared with the second person. As can be seen by this example, it is likely that impairments will result in functional limitations differently across elderly individuals. It is also true that "all functional limitations result from impairments" (Pope and Tarlove, 1991, p. 80).

Disability is an outcome that moves pathology, impairment, and functional limitation beyond the individual into the context of the social and physical environment. Disability is a limitation in the individual's ability to perform roles and tasks that are socially defined and expected:

> These roles and tasks are organized in spheres of life activities such as those of the family or other interpersonal relations; work, employment, and other economic pursuits; and education, recreation, and self-care. (Pope and Tarlove, 1991, pp. 81–82)

It is important to recognize that not all impairments or functional limitations result in disability. Disability is largely determined by sociocultural expectations and environmental demands. Other factors that also contribute to disablement include:

(a) the individual's definition of the situation and reactions, which at times compound the limitations;
(b) the definition of the situation by others, and their reactions and expectations— especially those who are significant in the lives of the person with the disabling condition (e.g., family members, friends and associates, employers and coworkers, and organizations and professions that provide services and benefits); and
(c) characteristics of the environment and the degree to which it is free from, or encumbered with, physical and sociocultural barriers (Pope and Tarlove, 1991, pp. 81–82).

A variety of determinants increase the risk of experiencing health-related conditions that can lead to impairment and disability. Primary sources of risk are:

(a) biological characteristics of the individual such as genetic predisposition to disease,
(b) features of the social and physical environment such as unsanitary or unsafe living conditions, and
(c) lifestyle habits or behaviors such as smoking or alcohol/drug abuse.

The risk for experiencing one or more chronic diseases increases with age and is related to socioeconomic status as well as level of education (Marge, 1988; Pope and Tarlove, 1991). Marge further identified the following disability-producing causes which are relevant for older persons: genetic disorders, accidents and injuries, nutritional disorders, lack of proper sanitation, stress, alcohol and drug abuse, poor environmental quality, lack of access to adequate healthcare, poor education, use of tobacco, lack of physical fitness, deleterious family or cultural beliefs, violence, and acute and chronic illness.

Generally, as age increases the risk of experiencing one or more chronic conditions also rises, therefore elevating the possibility of disablement. The rate for comorbidity (having more than one chronic condition at a time) rises dramatically with age. For example, the comorbidity rate for women who are between the age of 60 and 69 is 45% compared with 70% for women over age 80 (Guralnik, LaCroix, Everett, and Kovar, 1989). The need for assistance, which is directly related to the presence of functional limitation, increases with age and comorbidity. Poverty, lack of education, and social isolation also contribute to increased risk. Among the elderly who are over the age of 64, 37% have limitations with daily activities that would be identified as needing support and, therefore, are classified as a disability.

In summary, the profile of the older adult population in terms of the need for health-related services and products is complex. The continuing shift in the population age structure, coupled with the emergence of chronic disease as a leading cause of functional limitation and disability, have resulted in heightened national efforts to develop strategies for promoting health and functional independence across the life span. Health promotion and preventive health services have surfaced as popular approaches for impacting health and quality of life among older adults. As the number of choices for service settings and levels of care continue to improve in the service sector, new intervention strategies and activity programs will arise in an effort to meet the demands of the diverse and growing elderly population. It also is expected that healthcare technology and life expectancy will continue to improve and that the older adult segment of the population will be a growing service sector. These factors, as well as others, combine to make health-related services an important and challenging area—now and into the next century.

Service Settings and Scope of Care

Older persons who are in need of health-related services may seek different levels of care from a variety of service settings. Health-related therapeutic intervention may be provided on an inpatient, outpatient, or home-bound basis. Inpatient care is given in settings where the older individual is a resident. For individuals who remain in their own homes, in the homes of family members, or are living with others, community-based outpatient services provide an alternative to inpatient care. Finally, for individuals who are unable to leave their homes to obtain needed health services, in-home care may be the preferred option. These three broad levels of care (i.e., inpatient, outpatient, in-home) form a continuum that spans service settings ranging from residential institutions to noninstitutional programs and services. Figure 2.1 portrays this continuum of care with associated service settings.

Noninstitutional Care

Noninstitutional care is provided in various settings depending upon whether the older person is living at home on a fully independent basis or living in a retirement community (see Figure 2.1). One model of a highly successful community-based service setting is the *adult daycare center.* The adult daycare movement has been

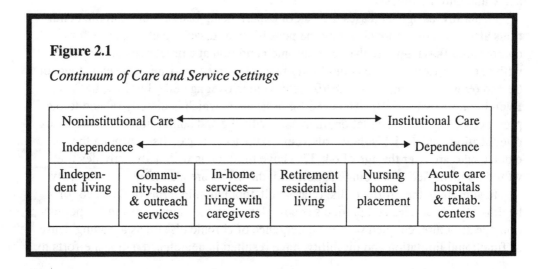

Figure 2.1

Continuum of Care and Service Settings

Noninstitutional Care ← → Institutional Care					
Independence ← → Dependence					
Independent living	Community-based & outreach services	In-home services—living with caregivers	Retirement residential living	Nursing home placement	Acute care hospitals & rehab. centers

beneficial for a growing number of elderly individuals, especially those who choose to remain in their own homes or with family members and who have needs that can be served by increasing the availability of a range of medical, social, health, and psychological support services in the community. Since the early 1970s when there were fewer than 25 programs nationwide, adult daycare has grown to more than 3,000 centers (Gunby, 1993; Mankoff, 1984; Pegels, 1988; Von Behren, 1986). There is a wide range in the character and scope of adult daycare programs. As a constellation of activities and services, adult daycare is designed to assist functionally impaired individuals, who would otherwise be at risk of institutionalization, to live at home while benefiting from community-based social, health, emotional, and medical care. Two general types of programs exist—adult day healthcare and adult day activity.

Adult day healthcare programs focus on providing health and rehabilitative services much like those that are available in hospitals and nursing homes. The individuals who attend adult day healthcare programs may either be experiencing increasing levels of disability as a result of a chronic health problem, or may have been recently discharged from a hospital or rehabilitation center. The primary purposes of adult day healthcare are to prevent further decline in health status and to provide rehabilitation services that restore the individual to his or her previous level of functioning.

Adult day activity programs, on the other hand, are more social in their focus. Activities are structured to provide maximum social, emotional, and physical stimulation, thus preventing loss and/or decline that is associated with a chronic and degenerative disease. Individuals in adult day activity programs typically do not need ongoing medical assistance or supervision. They usually need activity involvement and benefit from the social support that characterizes these programs. Their family members or caregivers also benefit by being able to work, enjoy some respite from caregiving, and have some time to take care of personal matters.

The costs of adult daycare vary based on the type of care (medical versus social) and the range of services provided (social and recreational activities to skilled nursing care). Basic adult daycare services include: client assessment and case management, meals (one to three plus snacks), personal care assistance (e.g., with eating, grooming, and going to the bathroom), ancillary services (e.g., occupational therapy, physical therapy, nutritional/dietary counseling, nursing, social work), therapeutic recreation and socialization, and education (Pegels, 1988).

Other community-based service models, in addition to adult daycare, include outreach services, multipurpose senior centers, area agencies on aging, and a plethora of voluntary organizations and agencies (e.g., religious, civic, and social groups). These community-based efforts provide a wide range of services including:

(a) volunteer opportunities such as the Retired Senior Volunteer Program (RSVP),
(b) friendly visitor services,
(c) handyman or homemaker assistance,
(d) health screening services,
(e) fitness programs,
(f) transportation assistance,

(g) recreational activities, and

(h) educational programs.

Often, the challenge confronted by elderly citizens and their caregivers is to find out what is available in their community and how to access these services and programs. Many community-based services and programs are essential for maintaining optimal health and functional competence in aging persons, especially as they reach very old age and the risks increase for disablement.

For many older adults, functional limitations coupled with other circumstances may mean that they are unable to use community-based services and yet, their overall need does not require residential care in a *long-term care facility* or nursing home. In some cases the individual may prefer to stay in his or her home or with family caregivers rather than be placed in a nursing home. In either or both cases, the degree of impairment has resulted in disablement such that ongoing care is needed and home healthcare may be an appropriate alternative.

There are many factors that support the choice for *in-home* or *home-bound* healthcare. The most prevalent reason given by older adults is to avoid institutionalization. Nursing home placement results in a loss in individual autonomy and independence that is not preferred by most adults. However, "[n]ational data shows that up to 60% of nursing home residents are placed for nonmedical reasons, i.e., lack of support in the community" (Central Indiana Council on Aging, 1988, p. 2). Other studies have shown that inappropriate placement in long-term care facilities occurs from 10% to 55% of the time (Holt, 1986-87; Kemper, Applebaum, and Harrigan, 1987). Receiving services on an in-home basis, if possible, is the preferred alternative by most older adults and their primary caregivers. Also, with continued growth in the size of the elderly population coupled with skyrocketing costs for healthcare, home-bound care is one possible means for containing service expenditures if, and only if, the individual's need is not as great as it would cost to provide services in a long-term care facility. Therefore, *in-home healthcare* is another alternative on the continuum of care settings.

In-home services are a priority area of the aging services network and refer to a range of services including:

> home health aid, family respite services, visiting and telephone reassurance and chore maintenance which enable older persons to remain in their homes for as long as possible. (Ficke, 1985, p. 104)

In-home services also can be grouped by categories such as:

(a) home health including "nursing care, medical social services, home health aide care, nutritional and dietary services, medical supplies and equipment, occupational therapy, speech therapy, and other specialized services;"

(b) social support including "housekeeping/chore services, personal care, transportation, pastoral services, telephone reassurance, friendly visiting, shopping, and laundry services;" and

(c) channeling or case management programs including "screening of clients, assessment of service needs, prescription of services, acquisition and coordination of services, monitoring of services, and reassessment." (Pegels, 1988, p. 95)

In summary, in-home healthcare is a constellation of services that includes assessment and diagnosis, rehabilitation and treatment, monitoring, and support services for maintaining noninstitutionalized living. "It is a wholistic concept of care that strives to restore, maintain, and enhance the quality of life" for both the elderly individual and his or her caregiver(s) despite:

> illness, infirmity, or even impending death. The term 'home care' is preferred within the industry because home care includes social and other human services, not health services alone. (Nassif, 1986, p. 6)

Retirement community living is a growing enterprise and many residential retirement complexes also include a variety of health and social support services (MacNeil and Teague, 1987). Within the planned retirement community, village, or complex, residents may be leading fully independent lifestyles or be receiving some level of assistance with health and social needs. While many retirement communities are established with the concept of providing housing units and social services for older adults who are primarily healthy, a growing number of organizations are developing the Continuing Care Retirement Community (CCRC) concept (Rivlin and Wiener, 1988). Some elderly persons find the concept of a CCRC or *life-care community* very appealing when making the decision to sell or move out of their home. The idea that they will be able to receive in-home assistance and social support, as well as be assured of short-term and long-term nursing care in a CCRC-based health pavilion, provides a sense of comfort and reassurance of stability throughout the remaining years of life. The CCRC may be thought of as a special case of community-based living with the same range of services one finds in a larger community such as in-home care, adult day assistance, and long-term care. While financing for CCRCs is costly, thus restricting enrollment to more wealthy individuals, current enrollment demand exceeds the available space. In 1987, about 680 CCRCs existed, each housing an average of 245 residents, and most were nonprofit organizations (Rivlin and Wiener, 1988). In a more recent study of CCRC oversight and regulation, 710 regulated CCRCs in 26 states were reported, thus indicating sustained and significant growth in this housing option (Netting and Wilson, 1994).

Institutional Care

Inpatient service settings typically represent institutional care and fall into the following types: nursing facilities, acute care hospitals, and residential rehabilitation centers (see Figure 2.1, page 24). Healthcare provided in hospitals or residential rehabilitation facilities is typically for a short period of time and ends in a transfer to some other level of care, either long term, community based, or home bound. In nursing facilities, a range of health and social services may be provided depending upon the needs of the individual and the type of nursing facility. The term *nursing facility* is a general term for facilities that provide long-term residential care for frail, infirm, and disabled individuals (MacNeil and Teague, 1987).

Some nursing homes are primarily concerned with providing a protective environment and assistance with basic daily living skills. These basic skills include being able to get out of bed, feed oneself, dress, bathe, and go to the bathroom. These facilities are known as Intermediate Care Facilities (ICFs) or, in some states, as Health Related Facilities (HRFs). Other nursing homes offer more intense medical care and usually individuals who are critically ill reside in these facilities. They are referred to as Skilled Nursing Facilities (SNFs) and are more like traditional hospital care. Elderly individuals typically reside in nursing homes for two main reasons: (a) their level of functional impairment is so disabling as to require ongoing care and possibly medical treatment; and (b) they do not possess the "psychological, social, and/or economic means for dealing with their condition outside an institution" (Pegels, 1988, p. 131). The nursing home industry is largely funded by public funds and, therefore, it is also closely regulated by laws in order to protect the clients' quality of care and safety.

The nursing home industry is a fast-growing enterprise. One reason for its growth is the general expansion in the over-age-65 population. Approximately 5.6% of the over-age-65 population reside in nursing facilities and one-third of this group are individuals over the age of 75 (Pegels, 1988). Older women who are poor and white are the dominant residents in long-term care facilities. The typical nursing home resident may suffer from heart disease, mental disorders, or from some type of physical impairment. Multiple conditions are common, and, thus the need for several kinds of assistance is not unusual. According to Pegels, the following percentages of the nursing home population will need assistance with basic activities of daily living: 55% with bathing, 47% with dressing, 11% with eating, and 33% with going to the bathroom. Because nursing home care is costly and the expenditure of public funds for acute as well as long-term care continues to grow, other alternatives to long-term care are being developed such as community-based and in-home care.

Acute care hospitals and rehabilitation facilities are the most expensive alternative and deliver the most extensive level of medical services of all healthcare settings. To be admitted to these facilities, the elderly person must be experiencing an acute health problem that is in need of the full range of diagnostic and treatment services. The level of care in this type of facility is the most costly alternative to the individual and society. New medical technology has further exacerbated the problem of rising healthcare costs associated with acute care. For example, advancements in medical technology have greatly impacted the number of older patients who are receiving kidney dialysis, cancer treatment, organ transplants, and open-heart surgery in acute care settings today (Evans, 1991). Because of the high costs associated with acute care, coupled with the rising incidence in chronic healthcare problems among the older adult population, the utilization of preventive healthcare is becoming an important trend in service delivery. The next section deals with the overall goals and purposes of intervention with the elderly in order to influence overall health status and quality of life.

Intervention through Prevention

The values and vision of today's society are exemplified by life that is abundant with good health and good fortune. The nation, however, is experiencing several trends that are placing strains on these values and vision. The growing size of the older adult population, the continuing rise in healthcare costs, the emergence of chronic disease as a major source of disability, and sustaining advancements in medical technology are collectively creating significant stress on the service delivery system. Consequently, professionals are looking for new ways to protect, as well as promote, the health and functional status of all older Americans. Health professionals, activity staff, caregivers, and citizens are focused on the rights of older persons to live with dignity and respect and to enjoy an acceptable quality of life. Activities, programs, and services are increasingly attending to the goals of improving, maintaining, and enhancing the health, functional status, and quality of life for all older citizens. Efforts have broadened beyond just the absence of disease to include optimal health through active lifestyles that emphasize physical fitness, intellectual stimulation, and social inclusion in the mainstream of community life.

Service delivery to promote health and well-being is guided by several levels of *prevention* that are designed to meet one or more purposes (Salamon, 1986). Three levels of prevention are *primary, secondary,* and *tertiary*. The purpose of primary prevention is to prevent illness, impairment, functional limitation, and disability. Typical approaches to primary prevention include educational programs and information distribution. The purposes of these activities are to prevent accidents, promote health, and inform elderly persons of risks that may result in injury, illness, or death. Classes, seminars, written materials, and audiovisual information all can be used productively in primary prevention. For example, videotaped adult fitness programs can be designed and marketed to help elders achieve optimal physical and mental functioning as well as to prevent acute and chronic diseases. Nutritional counseling, prescription education, and accident prevention programs are other examples of primary prevention strategies to enhance optimal health and well-being of older persons.

Primary prevention programs can be found in many places in the community. Primary prevention emphasizes more than just the prevention of illness; it also includes a focus on positive well-being and growth. Primary prevention through health promotion expands healthcare beyond the medical technologies of surgery, medications, and palliative care to include the *quality of life* dimension of the individual's health status.

For example, in 1985 the U.S. Department of Health and Human Services began a national effort to promote healthy lifestyles among the elderly. This primary prevention project was called Healthy Older People and it embraced six areas of concern: nutrition, safe use of medications, smoking cessation, exercise and fitness, injury control, and preventive and mental health (State of Indiana, n.d.). A variety of activities aimed at some or all of these targeted areas were carried out by state and local aging agencies under this program. All activities were intended to address the overall goal of preventing illness and disablement among older persons.

Secondary prevention targets the minimization of the illness's or disease's impact through screening, early detection, and treatment in order to contain or ameliorate the condition. Secondary prevention maintains the individual at a minimal level of health compromise, and/or restores the individual to a former level of health and functional capacity based on early detection. Some typical services in the secondary prevention area include high blood pressure screening, cholesterol screening, mammography, vision and hearing screening.

Tertiary prevention occurs after a pathological condition is present and has become serious (Salamon, 1986). This level of prevention is aimed at limiting the level of functional impairment and managing the process by which impairment becomes a disability. It is not unlike the restorative functions of rehabilitation. Tertiary prevention often focuses on reducing the risks of additional impairment based on the diffusion of the health condition to other areas of functioning. For example, a diagnosis of terminal cancer of the liver and lymphatic system will influence overall physical functioning and stamina. Added consequences of the disease may involve an emotional response by the individual to the diagnosis of a life-threatening disease. Therefore, tertiary prevention may involve mental health counseling to (a) assist the client with his or her adjustment to a terminal disease, (b) make plans for promoting a quality of life for the remaining time, and (c) help the person confront his or her disease with family members or friends. Tertiary prevention is useful in recognizing the holistic nature of the human organism and that illness in one area of functioning will usually influence the person in other areas of functioning.

Intervention through Rehabilitation

For elderly individuals who are living with functional limitations that are producing disablement, learning to live with dignity and control is a fundamental goal. The underlying philosophy of rehabilitation intervention services is best reflected in the question, "What can I help my patients do for themselves?" (Dominquez, 1988, p. 65). The purpose of rehabilitative intervention is to facilitate, cause, or maintain the individual's control over his or her physical, cognitive, emotional, and social capacities within the environment where he or she is living (Robinson, 1989). Activities that are applied in rehabilitation intervention are selected and implemented because they promote the maximum functioning and satisfaction within the individual. A sense of control through independence and autonomy are integral aspects of activity design and are used in meeting rehabilitation goals. Therefore, the individual's quality of life is dependent upon personal control over care and treatment in the process of promoting functional competence through activities of daily living, mobility, socialization, communication, and mental health.

Rehabilitation intervention often is achieved through a coordinated program of services that involves a team of professionals. Rehabilitative intervention involves an activity program where the emphasis is on the development or reacquisition of skills. Therapies, including activity therapy, are engaged to assist the individual in regaining functional capacity in one or more areas such as walking, getting out of bed, reaching, dressing, bathing, using community services, home care, and memory skills. For individuals whose skills are at the highest possible functional level, given the nature of their impairment and disability, a program of maintenance and prevention of further loss may be appropriately implemented. *Maintenance rehabilitation intervention* programs are integrated into the individual's everyday routines such as wheelchair exercises throughout each day for the purpose of preventing further losses in physical stamina due to excessive inactivity imposed by the necessary and constant use of a wheelchair. Maintenance rehabilitation programs are essential in order to prevent further declines when disability is permanent (Robinson, 1989).

Rehabilitation teams often include several professionals who represent a variety of areas of care including medicine, social work, psychology and psychiatry, pastoral/spiritual, legal, and various therapies. Rehabilitation intervention programs often involve several types of therapies including occupational therapy, physical therapy, mental health counseling, recreational activity therapy, and speech therapy. Understanding the whole individual is important in a successful rehabilitation program and, therefore, teamwork and communication among all professionals is important. Creating a match between optimal functioning, individual control, and professional service delivery lies at the heart of an effective rehabilitation program.

Summary

This chapter provides the reader with an overview of health status and the health-related needs of older adults as they are addressed through intervention services. The process by which an illness becomes a disability is instrumental in understanding healthcare needs. Older persons may seek a variety of services on either an inpatient, outpatient, or home-bound basis. Typical services and programs represent a continuum from noninstitutional to institutional care. Prevention and rehabilitation intervention are basic approaches to therapeutic care with older persons. Based on an understanding of the material presented in Chapters 1 and 2, the reader is now prepared to explore the process of normal aging, as well as common illnesses and diseases of the elderly, which are covered in greater detail in Unit II of the text.

Comprehension Questions

1. Describe health and functional status as they pertain to the older adult population.
2. By what process does impaired functioning become disablement?
3. What are three differences between a chronic condition and an acute illness?
4. Why is personal control important in the rehabilitation process?
5. Describe the continuum of care and service settings for the delivery of healthcare services to older persons.

References

Central Indiana Council on Aging. (1988, February). *A plan for home care in Indiana*. Indianapolis, IN: author.

Dominquez, S. E. (1988). Rehabilitation: A nurse's viewpoint. In R. D. Sine, S. E. Liss, R. E. Roush, J. D. Holcomb, & G. B. Wilson (Eds.), *Basic rehabilitation techniques: A self-instructional guide* (3rd ed.) (pp. 65-68). Rockville, MD: Aspen Publishers Inc.

Evans, R. W. (1991). Advanced medical technology and elderly people. In R. H. Binstock & S. G. Post (Eds.), *Too old for healthcare? Controversies in medicine, law, economics, and ethics* (pp. 44-74). Baltimore, MD: The Johns Hopkins University Press.

Ferrini, A. F., & Ferrini, R. L. (1993). *Health in the later years* (2nd ed.). Madison, WI: Brown & Benchmark.

Ficke, S. C. (Ed.). (1985). *An orientation to the Older Americans Act* (rev. ed.). Washington, DC: National Association of State Units on Aging.

Gunby, P. (1993). Adult day care centers vital, many more needed. *Journal of the American Medical Association, 269*(18), 2341–42.

Guralnik, J. M., LaCroix, A. Z., Everett, D. F., & Kovar, M. G. (1989). *Aging in the eighties: The prevalence of comorbidity and its association with disability* (Advance Data from Vital and Health Statistics, No. 170, DHHS Pub. No. 89-1250). Washington, DC: U.S. Public Health Service.

Holt, S. W. (1986-87, Winter). The role of home care in long-term care. *Generations, 11*(2), 9-12.

Kemper, P., Applebaum, R., & Harrigan, M. (1987). Community care demonstrations: What have we learned? *Home Care Financing Review, 8*(4), 87-100.

MacNeil, R. D., & Teague, M. L. (1987). *Aging and leisure: Vitality in later life*. Englewood Cliffs, NJ: Prentice Hall.

Mankoff, L. S. (1984, January). Adult daycare: A promoter of independent living. *American Healthcare Association Journal*, 19-21.

Marge, M. (1988). Health promotion for people with disabilities: Moving beyond rehabilitation. *American Journal of Health Promotion, 2*(4), 29-44.

Nassif, J. Z. (1986). There's no place like home. *Generations, 11*(2), 5-8.

Nassif, J. Z. (1985). *The home healthcare solution*. New York, NY: Harper & Row.

Netting, F. E., & Wilson, C. C. (1994). CCRC oversight: Implications for public regulation and private accreditation. *Journal of Applied Gerontology, 13*(3), 250-266.

Pegels, C. C. (1988). *Healthcare and the older citizen: Economic, demographic, and financial aspects*. Rockville, MD: Aspen Publishers Inc.

Pope, A. M., & Tarlove, A. R. (Eds.). (1991). *Disability in America: Toward a national agenda for prevention*. Washington, DC: National Academy Press.

Rivlin, A. M., & Wiener, J. M. (1988). *Caring for the disabled elderly: Who will pay?* Washington, DC: The Brookings Institution.

Robinson, K. M. (1989). Module 2.B: Rehabilitation services. In B. A. Hawkins, S. J. Eklund, & R. Gaetani (Eds.), *Aging and developmental disabilities: A training in-service package.* Bloomington, IN: Indiana University Institute for the Study of Developmental Disabilities.

Salamon, M. J. (1986). *A basic guide to working with elders.* New York, NY: Springer Publishing Co., Inc.

State of Indiana. (n.d.). *Healthy older people: Guidebook—A sourcebook for health promotion with older adults.* Indianapolis, IN: Indiana Department of Humans Services, Social Services Division.

Von Behren, R. (1986). *Adult daycare in America: Summary of a national survey.* Washington, DC: The National Council on the Aging, Inc.

Unit II

The Aging Process

The provision of care and activity programs to older adults requires a solid foundation of knowledge about the aging process and the diseases and illnesses that affect the elderly. Normal human aging can be explored from various perspectives including a theoretical view of the biology of aging and the systematic descriptions of changes that occur in humans as the bodily systems age. In addition to gaining an understanding of the physical processes of aging, caregivers and activity specialists will need background understanding of the social and psychological changes that take place in adults as they age. They can then distinguish pathological states from the normal process of aging. This distinction is particularly useful when activity intervention is intended to remedy, prevent, or rehabilitate in the case of an illness or diseased state.

Four chapters comprise Unit II of this text. Chapters 3 and 4 cover the normal aging process across the major domains of human functioning: physical, cognitive, and psychosocial. Following this background on normal aging, Chapters 5 and 6 introduce the reader to common physical diseases, illnesses, and disabilities (Chapter 5), and typical psychological illnesses and psychiatric disorders (Chapter 6) among older adults. Based upon the core information provided by the chapters in Units I and II, the reader will be prepared to approach the more practice-oriented information contained in the remaining chapters of the text.

Key Terms

Ageism
Cardiovascular System
Endocrine System
Gastrointestinal System
Genetic Theories of Aging
Geriatrics
Gerontology
Integumentary System
Intelligence
Learning
Life Expectancy
Lifestyle

Lymphatic System
Maximum Life Span
Memory
Musculoskeletal System
Nervous System
Reproductive System
Respiratory System
Sensory System
Social Gerontology
Stochastic Theories of Aging
Urinary System

Learning Objectives

1. Define gerontology, social gerontology, and geriatrics.
2. Identify three broad areas that are studied in gerontology.
3. Describe the aging process and factors that influence normal aging.
4. Describe biological theories of aging.
5. Describe how the process of normal aging influences physical functioning in humans.
6. Describe how normal aging affects psychological functioning in humans.
7. Discuss how lifestyle can influence the process of normal aging.

Chapter 3
Overview of Normal Aging

Introduction

In this chapter the reader is introduced to normal human aging. The concept of *ageism* is used to alert the reader to negative and inappropriate stereotypes about older persons. These negative views often result in lowered expectations of senior citizens by society. The systematic study of aging (i.e., gerontology and geriatrics) helps to dispel these myths and false ideas about the aging process and, thus, elderly persons.

The process of aging, including a cursory overview of biological theories of aging, is described. Following this section, the physical changes associated with human aging are described under key systems: sensory, integumentary, musculo-skeletal, cardiovascular and respiratory, gastrointestinal and urinary, lymphatic, nervous, endocrine, and reproductive. Cognitive changes in intelligence, learning, and memory are then presented. The chapter concludes with a section on lifestyle and how it influences the aging process.

Why Study Aging?

The significance of human life, whether one's own or that of a close friend, is something that everyone thinks about from time to time. On each occasion when one stops to reflect upon life, one usually notices how one has changed. This growth reflects one's human development as one moves through life: as one ages.

In the time that it takes to read this book, the reader will have aged. While perhaps only small, almost imperceptible changes will have occurred, it is through the passage of time that one grows and develops, and, thus, experiences *aging*. One of the most compelling reasons to study aging is to gain a personal perspective on one's own life so that one might anticipate what it will be like to grow older, what one can do to influence the aging process, and how one can be involved in shaping the best possible futures for oneself. Most people want to know about aging so that they can better understand themselves and their own destiny.

By building an understanding of the aging process, the reader will be better informed about one of the most significant changes taking place in the nation today—the graying of the population. Not only will the reader be empowered to manage his or her own life as he or she ages, but also he or she will have the knowledge needed to take care of aging family members and loved ones. Finally, if the reader happens to accept employment in a setting which provides ongoing care for older adults, it is essential that he or she has a solid understanding of the aging process. One of the most unfortunate situations that sometimes happens is when false stereotypes, myths, and inaccurate information form the basis on which professionals give care to and interact with older persons.

Negative stereotypes or false information about the aging process often lead to prejudice and discrimination toward older persons. Robert Butler, a well-known gerontologist, developed the term *ageism* to describe what happens when inaccurate views of the aging process influence the manner in which society, as well as individuals, treat the elderly. Ageism is a set of attitudes and behaviors that arise when society assigns certain characteristics (most of which are negative) to all older persons based solely on one shared attribute, chronological age (Hooyman and Kiyak, 1991).

Societal expectations of older persons, in general, are shaped by several factors of which chronological age is unfortunately the dominant force. As people grow older, society assigns certain expectations in terms of social roles, responsibilities, characteristics, and behaviors. For example, as individuals reach their 60s, society expects that they will retire from full-time work and, subsequently, that they will disengage from the social responsibilities typically associated with work. Likewise, when older persons reach very old age (i.e., 80s or 90s), the ageist stereotype implies that they will be frail, not very vigorous, and also helpless to some degree. Other inappropriate stereotypic views of older persons include rigid, senile, feeble, sexually inactive, and unattractive. Based on what is known about the aging process and older persons, however, these descriptors are both inaccurate and inappropriate (Neuhaus and Neuhaus, 1982).

An important reason for studying aging, then, is to dispel ageism from society, especially as increasing numbers of individuals are entering older adulthood. Distinguishing the normal changes that occur in the aging individual by learning about the aging process also will enhance society's understanding and service provision for the elderly. The concern for promoting an accurate understanding of the aging process has given rise to two broad fields of education and professionalism: *gerontology* and *geriatrics*.

Gerontology is a multidisciplinary field in which the biological, psychological, and social aspects of the aging process are studied. The field involves researchers, educators, and practitioners from many disciplines including biology, psychology, sociology and social work, economics, recreation and leisure studies, education, medicine, political science, and many others. The main concern of gerontologists from these disciplines is how to improve the quality of life for older adults, as well as to provide accurate information about the aging process from a biopsychosocial perspective. The biopsychosocial model of aging encompasses the total view of the aging process as it involves the following main areas of human functioning: biological aging which is concerned with the changes in physical functioning as the individual becomes older; psychological aging which includes mental, sensory, and perceptual functioning; and social aging which involves changing social roles and contexts with advancing age (Ferrini and Ferrini, 1993; Hooyman and Kiyak, 1991).

An area of particular interest to professionals who provide activity programs to older adults is *social gerontology.* Social gerontology can be distinguished as an:

> area of gerontology that is concerned with the impact of social and sociocultural conditions on the process of aging and with the social consequences of this process. (Hooyman and Kiyak, 1991, p. 4)

Of special interest to social gerontologists are the social and cultural factors that influence the aged and how an aging population impacts upon society. Some of the diverse issues that are studied today in the area of social gerontology are retirement, housing, income and poverty, health status and healthcare, leisure services, care for the elderly, ethnic diversity, and public policy.

Geriatrics, on the other hand, primarily refers to the medical care and management of disease in elderly persons. Geriatric medicine involves physicians, nurses, and other medical practitioners who are concerned with the changes that take place in older persons as a result of illnesses or diseases, and which are not primarily caused by growing older. The medical and health problems of older people form the central focus of geriatrics (Ferrini and Ferrini, 1993; Hooyman and Kiyak, 1991).

With sustained growth in the elderly population expected into the next century, gerontology and geriatrics will continue to be concerned with the issues and conditions of older adults. Accompanying this sustained growth in the senior segment of the population will be new cohorts of older persons who may be more politically active, have higher levels of education, and have greater financial resources with which to pursue the resolution of their concerns. Older persons can be expected to advocate for the development of appropriate health and social programs, as well as public policies that benefit the elderly population (e.g., the Americans with Disabilities Act). Thus, the knowledge that is gained from studying the aging process, thereby preparing professionals to work with the elderly, is vitally important for improving the quality of life and health status of all aging adults and their families.

The Aging Process

While early growth and development in humans is generally described in terms of increasing size and the development of complexity in structure and function, the same general description does not apply to the aging process when the individual reaches adulthood. The changes that occur after reaching maturity are differentiated from early development in several important ways. The rate of change slows and is not the same across all areas of human functioning (e.g., physical, cognitive, and social), nor does change occur the same across all individuals. There is a great diversity among individuals in how "aging-related change" is manifest and how each person adapts to the aging process. Also, it is extremely important to distinguish between normal aging change and the disease process. While the incidence of illness and disease increases among older persons compared to younger persons, not all older persons will automatically become ill or have a disease with advancing age. Aging and the normal changes associated with growing older, however, do happen to every human organism (Shock et al., 1984).

While there is no uniform course to aging for all individuals, six patterns can be used to characterize the overall process (Shock et al., 1984). First, relative stability across the adult years can be expected. The process of change is gradual. The human organism will adapt and adjust in order to provide for relative stability in performance overall. Second, declines due to illnesses that are associated with age can be expected, and third, in spite of good overall health, steady declines will occur for all individuals. A fourth pattern suggests that any changes that are precipitous (onset is rapid and acute) are associated with disease rather than aging-related change. A fifth pattern involves the human organism's tendency toward natural compensation for losses in order to maintain function. The sixth and final pattern relates to the influence that society and culture have on the aging process. The greater the understanding that a particular culture has about the aging process and the more progressive that culture is in promoting a conscious health milieu for elderly persons, the better the outcomes are for individuals as they move into their later years. For example, the promotion of physical fitness and activity in adulthood in order to preserve functional capacities is one way in which the rate of loss in physical performance due to aging may be slowed. In summary, the process of aging can be described as cumulative with all humans experiencing aging-related changes. The process continues from birth to death within each individual. The next section provides a general overview of biological theories of aging.

Biological Theories of Aging

One fact is evident in the research literature: no one theory adequately serves to explain the biology of aging (Arking, 1991). The changes associated with aging are complex and multileveled. Biological aging is a:

> sum total of many independent causes, some operating at the level of
> individual molecules, others at the level of individual cells, and still
> others at the level of tissues, organs, and whole organisms. (Schneider,
> 1992, p. 7)

Thus, several and different theoretical perspectives are required in order to gain a clearer understanding of the biology of aging. Biological theories of aging fall into two broad categories: programmed or genetic theories, and stochastic theories (Schneider, 1992).

Programmed or genetic theories describe the influence of human genes on the cell division and replacement process as it causes systemic change across the life span. The average human being expects to live about 75 years, and each individual's genetic endowment will contribute substantially to his or her chances of meeting this expectation. There are about 200 genes that specifically influence the aging process (Schneider, 1992). The cells of the human organism, however, do not continue to divide and replace themselves indefinitely; they are regulated by these 200 "aging" genes. Researchers have discovered that genes will direct the cells to divide and replace themselves about 40–60 times, thus limiting the maximum life span potential of the human organism (Ferrini and Ferrini, 1993; Schneider, 1992).

Genetically programmed aging can be readily recognized by several obvious changes in humans—the graying of the hair, the reproductive cycle of females from first menstruation to menopause, and the decline in immune system function after age 20 (Schneider, 1992). As cell division and replacement occurs, cell function declines due partly to loss in function and partly attributable to mutation. Often, the human organism dies before it reaches the maximum capacity for cell division as programmed genetically. Research findings about genetic endowment and the limits of genetically controlled cell division and replacement contribute greatly to our understanding of the biology of aging at both the cellular and the systemic level (Arking, 1991; Brookbank, 1990; Schneider, 1992).

Several stochastic theories of aging describe the influence of random or chance attacks on the body by accumulated external forces in the environment (e.g., toxins) and by internal factors (e.g., caloric restriction). One theory, the Metabolic Theory of Aging/Caloric Restriction, is based on the idea that the rate of metabolism is directly related to the length of life for the organism; that is, higher metabolism is related to shorter life and lower metabolism is related to longer life. Experiments with lowering caloric intake in animals have demonstrated this relationship. Similar experiments are needed with humans (Schneider, 1992).

The Free Radical Theory describes changes in cell function that are the result of damage caused by attacks from internal and/or external factors. Free radicals, or "parts of molecules that have either an extra or missing electron" (Ferrini and Ferrini, 1993, p. 37), attack cells. Free radicals are caused by normal cellular functions, as well as from environmental factors (toxins from cigarette smoke, poor drinking water, chemical additives in food, etc.). Free radicals have a short life but can damage the cell or genetic material (Ferrini and Ferrini, 1993; Schneider, 1992). Accumulated damage over time from free radicals is known to occur. What is not yet established is whether free radical damage causes aging per se.

Cross-Linkage Accumulation Theory of Aging suggests that as the human grows older, "an increasing number of cell molecules connect themselves with other molecules to form cross-linkages" (Ferrini and Ferrini, 1993, p. 38) as caused by free radicals. It has been proposed that the accumulation of these cross-linkages causes aging (Ferrini and Ferrini, 1993; Schneider, 1992). The ability of the cells to repair does not keep pace with the damage and, subsequently, the result is loss of cell function. Cross-linkage damage affects the connective tissues of the body causing them to be more rigid and less elastic. The outcomes of this kind of damage can be seen in skin damage (e.g., wrinkling) and losses in other bodily functions (e.g., lung movement in respiration, blood vessels, the lens of the eye).

Other biological theories of aging have been described in the literature but are beyond the scope of the present chapter. The preceding information serves to distinguish genetic theories from damage theories and thus, the reader is provided with a cursory orientation to biological theories of aging. For further or more detailed study of this topic, the reader is encouraged to consult the references at the end of the chapter.

The next two sections of this chapter provide brief overviews of the physical and cognitive changes that occur with normal aging. Social changes are covered elsewhere in the text (Chapter 4). Common illnesses or diseases of the body and mind are covered separately in Chapters 5 and 6.

Physical Changes

The physical body is a complex system of organs and structural components which are individually and interactively influenced by aging. As the human organism grows older, the body continues to change as a result of both cellular division and replacement and the accumulated effects of environmental factors. Taken together, these forces manifest uniquely in each individual. The following general information focuses on the physical changes that occur in each of the major bodily systems. It is important to be mindful of the fact that individuals vary greatly in their rate of change and the expression of age-associated physical change. Readers who are interested in knowing more detail are encouraged to consult the reference list at the end of the chapter. It is stressed that this chapter provides only a general introduction to normal aging. In each section an attempt is made to cover the composition, function, and aging-related changes that accompany the area under discussion.

The Sensory System

Changes in the senses are perhaps the most critical to the aging adult. It is through the senses that information is received and responses are made that govern our interactions with others and the environment. Decrements in vision, hearing, touch, pain, temperature sensation, taste, smell, and equilibrium influence the quality of these interactions. If the losses are great enough in one or more of these senses, everyday functioning becomes impaired. In general, however, sensory losses are gradual, and when they reach a level that impairs functioning, aids and environmental modifications may be implemented. The most common losses are experienced in visual and hearing acuity. Glasses and hearing aids can effectively offset decrements in these areas providing that the older adult is motivated to use them.

Vision

The changes in vision are primarily in the forms of acuity (seeing clearly at a distance), light perception, and accommodation (sharply focusing near images) (Ferrini and Ferrini, 1993; Neuhaus and Neuhaus, 1982). These changes are influenced by alterations in the structure of the eye and the loss of elasticity in the eye muscles. In general, the lens yellows, thickens, and clouds with age, thus impeding the amount of light that can pass through it and decreasing its elasticity. Also, the opening/closing of the pupil diminishes in speed, regularity, and size. When the eye can no longer adjust the lens and pupil quickly, the older adult has difficulty focusing near objects; this condition is called *presbyopia* (Ferrini and Ferrini, 1993).

The primary outcomes associated with vision changes include:

(a) the need for glasses to aid in focusing near objects with ease;
(b) the need for greater light in order to see;
(c) the need to be aware of a sensitivity to glare; and
(d) the need to accommodate difficulty in discriminating some colors, especially the blues, greens, and violets.

Other aging-related changes include the loss of facial muscle elasticity around the eye and the loss in fat around the eyeball. These changes can result in a drooping of the eyelid which affects facial appearance (Ferrini and Ferrini, 1993).

Hearing

Hearing loss is more common in the elderly than is the total loss of sight. Whereas vision usually begins to decline in the 40s, hearing losses begin in the 20s, gradually accumulating and becoming more pronounced by old age. Hearing losses are a result in changes in the ear structure and functioning (Neuhaus and Neuhaus, 1982).

The ear is constructed so that sound enters through the outer ear and is received in the middle ear as impulses which are processed by the auditory nerve to the brain and interpreted as sound. The ear also contains the structures that support the sense of equilibrium. Balance relies on special cells in the inner ear's semicircular canals that contain fluid. This vestibular system, working along with the visual system, helps the individual to maintain balance. As vision and hearing acuity decrease, problems with equilibrium may begin to occur, especially under certain circumstances such as nighttime when the eyes refocus more slowly or when the individual has a head cold.

In general, as the adult grows older, there is a stiffening of the inner ear structures such that the ear is less able to perceive and transmit sound. The resulting hearing loss most often manifests in an inability to perceive high-pitched tones. Older adults who experience age-associated hearing loss, or *presbycusis,* will have difficulty in discriminating between the following high-frequency sounds: *f, s, sh,* and *z* (Ferrini and Ferrini, 1993).

Another common hearing difficulty with age is the inability to sort out background noise from foreground conversation in crowded, noisy environments such as a party, conference, or large gathering of people with background music. This phenomenon is called the "cocktail party effect" and older adults may remark that they are unable to hear the person who is talking to them in a room filled with background noise. This kind of hearing loss creates discomfort for many older adults in social situations where there are many competing noise sources.

The natural aging of the human ear structure is not the only cause of hearing loss. For example, persistent high environmental noise (noise pollution) can hasten a decline in hearing acuity and can result in additional damage to inner ear structures such as the ear drum. Illnesses, diseases, and traumatic injuries also may impact hearing in later life. Some medications and dietary habits have known side effects on hearing such as causing ringing in the ears. Finally, some individuals "choose" not to hear as a result of psychological disturbances in their lives.

Unacknowledged and untreated hearing losses often result in lowered mental states and a lack of enjoyment of social activities. Paranoid ideas and behaviors, suspiciousness, withdrawal, disorientation with regard to reality, and depression may be observed when hearing loss becomes acute or prolonged without intervention. Providing hearing aid support and good, preventive healthcare to the ear (e.g., regular ear wax removal) can be effective in diminishing the impact of aging-related changes in hearing in everyday life.

Taste and Smell

The senses of taste and smell are governed by taste buds on the tongue and in the mouth and by smell receptor cells located high inside the nose. No clear evidence exists that shows distinct aging-related decreases in these senses. Most changes in taste and smell are experienced on a highly individual basis. Often lifestyle habits such as cigarette smoking are the cause for decreases in these senses.

Touch

Somatic receptors that are responsible for the sense of touch (e.g., pain, pressure, heat, cold, spatial relationship) are part of the skin, as well as the internal organ system of the body. As the body ages, a decrease in sensitivity to heat, cold, and pain has been documented (Ferrini and Ferrini, 1993). Environmental temperature management is important in supporting an appropriate and comfortable body temperature in older persons.

The Integumentary System

The integumentary system comprises the skin and related structures, the hair and nails. This system is by far the largest of the bodily systems and the most visible to us in terms of aging-related changes.

The skin is composed of the epidermis, dermis, and subcutaneous layer. The outermost layer, epidermis, protects the body from sunlight exposure by producing melanin. Dead skin cells are constantly being replaced by new cells produced by the epidermis. The inner layers, the dermis and subcutaneous layer, are composed of blood vessels, nerves, hair follicles, glands, connective tissue, and fat. The dermis and subcutaneous layers provide the primary functions of the integumentary system which are:

(a) protection from environmental elements, as well as from internal injury from bumps and falls;
(b) retention of vital bodily fluids;
(c) control of body temperature through sweating and shivering;
(d) elimination of body salts and waste products;
(e) sensation through touch or injury;
(f) production of vitamin D from exposure to sunlight;
(g) absorption of medication through patches;
(h) cushioning for other internal organs; and
(i) fat reserves for energy (Ferrini and Ferrini, 1993; MacNeil and Teague, 1987).

Heredity, hormones, and lifestyle habits are the primary influencing factors affecting changes to the integumentary system. For example, exposure to sunlight is one of the leading causes of wrinkles and drying of the skin. Cigarette smoking also is very damaging to the skin. The major changes to the skin with age are the appearance of wrinkles, folds, grooves, mottling, drying, thinning, and loss of elasticity. Hair becomes gray and less dense, as well as coarser on certain areas of the body such as ear lobes and eyebrows for men, and the upper lip and chin among women. It is not uncommon for men to bald with age, while balding is less common among women who will experience thinning hair (Ferrini and Ferrini, 1993; MacNeil and Teague, 1987).

Nails will grow slower, may become thinner with age, and may develop ridges. Some older adults have difficulty trimming their nails due to poor vision, arthritis, lack of flexibility or coordination, and obesity. Prevention of injury or disease associated with nail care is important to older adults, and a podiatrist may often be sought for assistance with toenail care.

When obvious changes in the integumentary system (e.g., wrinkles or gray hair) occur, many adults become aware for the first time that they are growing older. Fortunately good skin care through protection against excess sunlight and exposure, coupled with good nutrition and sleep, can do much to prevent premature aging of this system.

The Musculoskeletal System

The musculoskeletal system provides the support structure for the human body. Composed of bones, muscles, ligaments, cartilage, and tendons, it protects the other major bodily organs. The health and structural integrity of the musculoskeletal system also provides support for body shape, movement, stability, and posture (Ferrini and Ferrini, 1993; MacNeil and Teague, 1987).

The human skeleton consists of 206 bones that are held together by specialized connective tissues—ligaments, cartilage, and tendons (MacNeil and Teague, 1987). These connective tissues bind the musculoskeletal system together, bone to bone, muscle to bone, muscle to muscle. The elasticity of these connective tissues declines with age, which subsequently results in losses in joint function. As joints stiffen and range of motion becomes less, losses in flexibility and mobility result. The aging of joints begins before the skeletal system reaches full maturity; thus, the cumulative effects of joint degeneration are associated with old age (Ferrini and Ferrini, 1993; MacNeil and Teague, 1987).

Bones are built as calcium and minerals are stored (Ferrini and Ferrini, 1993). Regular exercise will promote bone growth along with sufficient amounts of nutritional intake of calcium and essential minerals. Losses in bone strength and mass are hastened by poor diet and/or the lack of adequate exercise (MacNeil and Teague, 1987).

Bone demineralization with age results in bones that are more porous; consequently, bones are weaker and prone to being easily broken. Women experience greater bone loss than do men, with as much as 20–30% bone density loss over the average life span among women compared with only 10–15% in men (Ferrini and Ferrini, 1993). Bone loss, over time, results in functional decline, increased susceptibility to disease, and elevated risks for injury. Changes in gait, stance, posture, height, and overall neuromotor performance occur with progressive losses in bone density, mass, and strength in old age.

There are over 700 muscles in the body that are grouped into three types: skeletal or striated, cardiac, and smooth. The skeletal muscles help to support the skeletal frame and provide the mechanisms for controlled movement. The cardiac muscle, or the heart, maintains the heart-pumping actions in support of the cardiovascular system. Smooth muscles, which are muscles that are not consciously controlled, maintain internal functions such as the digestive system, the bladder, and the lungs. Smooth muscles function on a rhythmic, wave-like, sustained movement basis (Ferrini and Ferrini, 1993; MacNeil and Teague, 1987).

The muscles of the body atrophy at a fairly rapid rate when not regularly used. The decline in muscle mass and strength with age, therefore, may be greater or lesser depending upon exercise and diet. The rate of loss in musculature is small until late in life (the 70s and 80s). Leg strength loss is greater than that of arm strength; however, all losses can be greatly influenced by whether the individual has a sedentary or active lifestyle. Overall, decreases in strength and endurance will vary greatly among individuals based on activity patterns.

The long-term impact of aging-related decreases in bone and musculature will occur in several areas of human performance:

(a) lowered strength,
(b) restricted/reduced range of motion,
(c) increased stiffness and pain,
(d) gait changes,
(e) diminished height,
(f) postural change,
(g) reduced movement (slower),
(h) cramping,

(i) declined motor performance,

(j) increased susceptibility to injury and disease, and

(k) restricted lifestyle (Ferrini and Ferrini, 1993; MacNeil and Teague, 1987).

One of the most important thoughts to keep in mind about aging and declines in the musculoskeletal system is the important influence that diet, exercise, and other lifestyle habits (cigarette smoking and alcohol use) have on the rate of decline.

The Cardiovascular and Respiratory Systems

The cardiovascular and respiratory systems are closely related systems that together provide major support for the transport of nutrients and oxygen to the body. The respiratory system's major function is to provide oxygen from the air to the bloodstream and to remove carbon dioxide from the blood transporting it back into the environment. The cardiovascular system is instrumental in transporting oxygen-rich blood throughout the body and returning carbon dioxide laden blood to the lungs for the exchange with fresh oxygen.

The major structures of the respiratory system are the nose, oral cavity, pharynx, larynx (voice box), trachea (wind pipe), bronchi (bronchial tubes and bronchiole), and lungs. Air passes through these structures to tiny air sacs in the lungs called alveoli. In the lungs are close to a billion alveoli which are covered with capillaries where the exchange of oxygen and carbon dioxide takes place. With each inspiration and expiration of air, the lungs expand and constrict thereby taking in oxygen-rich air and transporting out carbon dioxide. Breathing rate and depth are controlled by the brain according to oxygen and carbon dioxide levels in the blood (Brookbank, 1990).

Aging-related changes in the respiratory system are primarily in the loss of elasticity and thus, the hardening or stiffening of support tissues, airways, and diaphragmatic function. The bronchi degenerate with age also. These changes result in a reduction in overall vital capacity (amount of air moved in and out of the lungs) so that the uptake and diffusion of oxygen is reduced. The chest wall and skeleton become more rigid, influencing breathing functions. Reserve capacity of the lungs declines with age. These changes are somewhat inevitable; however, aerobic exercise can be helpful in minimizing the functional effects. It is appropriate to recognize that environmental pollution is as much a hazard to respiratory decline and wellness as is any other single factor including advancing age and exercise:

> In general, elders have decreased capacity to cope with environmental
> pollutants and are more susceptible to pulmonary distress or death
> during periods of high pollution. (Ferrini and Ferrini, 1993, p. 78)

The heart and blood, along with a vast network of veins, arteries, and capillaries, comprise the cardiovascular system. This system, while transporting oxygen to cells and carrying away carbon dioxide for removal through the lungs, also delivers other nutrients to body cells. Nutrients from the digestive track, antibodies from the immune system, and hormones from the endocrine system are provided to the body's cells via the circulatory system. Body wastes also are transported to the kidneys and lungs by this complex network. Finally, body temperature is regulated by the circulatory system (Brookbank, 1990).

The major pump for the circulatory system, the heart, is composed of four main chambers: two atria (upper chambers) and two ventricles (lower chambers). In the process of pumping about 170 gallons of blood each hour, the right chambers of the heart receive and distribute deoxygenated blood to the lungs while the left chambers receive the oxygen-rich blood from the lungs and distributes it to the rest of the body. Arteries transport the blood to the capillaries which supply body cells; there are specialized arteries (coronary arteries) which supply the heart muscle cells. Veins carry the blood back to the heart for distribution to the lungs for oxygenation.

As the body ages, some structural changes occur to the cardiovascular system. Aging-related declines in maximal function and efficiency can be expected. The heart muscles become less elastic with some calcification and degeneration of the internal valves is to be expected. The walls of the heart thicken. This influences contractibility and oxygen consumption by the heart muscle cells. With gradual thickening the weight of the heart increases, and the pumping force may increase as compensation. Increased pumping force contributes to an elevated blood pressure which can, if high enough, damage other bodily organs. It is well-known, however, that cardiovascular function is greatly influenced by physical activity. Thus, highly active older adults tend to have much higher cardiovascular function than do inactive elders (Ferrini and Ferrini, 1993).

Throughout the body the arteries progressively become less elastic and harden due to a process called arteriosclerosis (Ferrini and Ferrini, 1993; MacNeil and Teague, 1987). Arteriosclerosis is a stiffening of the connective tissue and calcification in the arterial walls. This process will occur regardless of the level of activity the elder may exhibit. Lifestyle will not slow or alleviate arteriosclerosis. Along with this change to the body's arteries, blood flow to internal organs will decline with age. The general impact of cardiovascular changes on functioning can be summarized as follows:

(a) diminished cardiac reserve;
(b) reduced exercise capacity;
(c) decreased blood flow to the coronary arteries;
(d) decreased ability of the heart to use and distribute oxygen;
(e) increased blood pressure;
(f) lowered ability of the heart to recover, especially following exercise; and
(g) lowered blood flow to other organs thus impacting upon their functioning (Brookbank, 1990; Ferrini and Ferrini, 1993; MacNeil and Teague, 1987).

The Gastrointestinal and Urinary Systems

The digestive (gastrointestinal) system consists of the mouth and salivary glands, pharynx, esophagus, stomach, liver, pancreas, gallbladder, small intestine, large intestine, rectum, and anus. This modified muscular tube is responsible for receiving and processing food for the usable nutrients that maintain the human body. As food passes through this system, it is broken down and moved along by rhythmic, wave-like motions to that portion of the intestine where nutrients are absorbed, and waste products are passed on for elimination via the bowels. It is the least likely system to be overly affected by aging-related change. Because the cells of the digestive system are replaced often and there is a large capacity in reserve, serious decrements need to accrue before functional losses are noticed (Ferrini and Ferrini, 1993).

Aging-related changes in the stomach and small intestine are manifest as decreases in the enzyme content necessary for food digestion. In addition, the production of saliva may decrease along with a generalized slowing in the swallowing reflex. These changes, coupled with muscle fiber changes in the digestive tract, result in a slowing of digestive capacity and the absorption of nutrients. Liver weight and functions decline between age 60 and 90 which results in a lessened capacity for the metabolism of hormones and drugs. It is known that some drugs take much longer to be absorbed and utilized in elderly persons which has serious implications for the medical management of diseases and illnesses (Brookbank, 1990; Ferrini and Ferrini, 1993; MacNeil and Teague, 1987).

If older persons are healthy, then the changes that do occur to the digestive system will be minimally noticed with age. Other disturbances that are of concern to the elderly tend to be induced by poor diet or dental hygiene. Although teeth will wear down with age, normal diets and good care of the teeth will minimize the effects. Receding gums and tooth loss are not normal consequences of aging.

The urinary tract consists of the kidneys, ureters, bladder, and urethra. The primary function of the urinary system is to cleanse the blood of waste products produced by body cell use of nutrients. The blood transports waste and other toxic substances to the kidneys where it is removed from the blood. Along with this cleansing, the urinary system controls body fluid composition and amount. Kidneys filter the waste and toxins from the blood. This waste becomes urine which is then transported out of the body through the ureters, bladder, and urethra. The bladder is an expandable muscular sac which contains sensory receptors that signal the brain when the sac is about half-full (Ferrini and Ferrini, 1993).

Changes with age in the urinary tract system consist of decreases in weight and volume of the kidneys, thus influencing filtration. The decreases in filtration rate accelerate after age 40, constituting a decrease of 1% per year (Brookbank, 1990). A weakening in the bladder wall and lowered capacity with age influences the ability to completely empty the bladder. The result of aging-related changes in bladder structure and functioning are more frequent filling of the bladder, more frequent need to urinate, and increased incidence of incontinence. The combined changes in the kidneys and bladder produce the need to get up in the night to void, a common occurrence among the elderly.

The Lymphatic System

The lymphatic or immune system consists of the thymus and bone marrow as principal organs with the spleen and lymph nodes as secondary organs. The thymus is located in the upper chest and the spleen in the upper left part of the abdomen. Lymph nodes are located in the following areas: the underarm, neck, inside the chest, abdomen, groin, and around joints. Bone marrow, of course, is located inside the bones. When the body is invaded by a virus, bacteria, fungi, or other foreign substance, the immune system goes into action. The first mechanism to mobilize is the immune system's ability to identify "self" from "nonself." When the invader is detected as nonself, the immune system goes into action protecting the body from the invader. Thus, two important functions are performed by the immune system: (a) it is the body's military system against infections that would mean death if not destroyed; and (b) the immune system is responsible for the collection of excess fluids from around the body's cells (Arking, 1991).

Aging-related changes in the immune system stem from the deterioration of the thymus beginning at sexual maturity and subsequent decrease in the levels of thymic hormones. There is evidence that supports a functional decline in the immune system with age although the underlying causes are not completely known at this time (Arking, 1991).

The Nervous System

The nervous system consists of the brain, spinal cord and peripheral components. All knowledge and information that we have about ourselves and the automatic regulation of bodily functions are controlled by the brain and nervous system. The brain receives sensory input from nerves connecting the senses (e.g., eyes, nose, ears) to it, and messages from the other bodily systems through the spinal cord. The brain receives, organizes, processes, and sends messages that govern all aspects of bodily function, as well as our personality and identity (Arking, 1991; Brookbank, 1990; Ferrini and Ferrini, 1993).

A detailed discussion of the different regions of the brain, including the structure and functioning of each, is beyond the scope of the present chapter. The most predominant structural change to the brain is a gradual reduction in weight and size with age. The rate of loss is accelerated after age 60 (Arking, 1991; Brookbank, 1990).

The brain is made up of billions of neurons, or nerve cells, which conduct and store information. Nerve cells transmit information to other nerve cells by impulses which are chemically and electrically induced. With age there is a gradual reduction of the number of neuron cells which results in some loss in function. A noticeable consequence of losses in neurons and neuron functioning is in reduced reaction time. Nerve conduction velocity slows, and it takes longer for an impulse to cross the synapse. Additionally, the number of synaptic interconnections declines (Arking, 1991; Brookbank, 1990; Ferrini and Ferrini, 1993).

While it may take older people longer to learn new material or to react to a stimuli, the loss in reaction speed has not been shown to influence memory function or intelligence. Also, many other factors may influence nervous system functioning and, subsequently have an impact on memory functioning. Changes in hormone levels, blood transmission of nutrients to the brain, as well as the influence of medications on brain functioning are as common as are the effects of structural changes. The brain and nervous system, while experiencing changes with age, function well into very old age in the absence of illness or a pathological condition such as dementia. Cognition and functional changes in cognition with age are covered under a separate section later in this chapter. Diseases of the brain and nervous system are covered in Chapter 6.

Endocrine System

The endocrine system consists of a group of glands located in the brain and through-out the body that are responsible for the production and secretion of chemical messengers. These chemicals or hormones regulate a broad range of bodily functions. The pituitary gland which is attached to the front of the brain produces a wide range of hormones that govern the other glands in the endocrine system. The thyroid is located in the central part of the neck in front of the trachea, regulates metabolism, and lowers calcium levels in the bloodstream. The parathyroid, located on the back of the thyroid, increases blood calcium levels as needed. The adrenal glands, which are located above the kidneys regulate the body in response to stress, maintain potassium and sodium balance, and supplement sex hormone production. The pancreas, located behind the stomach, provides glycogen which stimulates the liver to break down sugar and produces insulin which promotes the utilization of glucose. The thymus gland, which atrophies after puberty, is located in the lower neck and produces certain white blood cells. The ovaries (in women) are located in the pelvic area and the testes (in men) within the scrotum behind the penis. These glands secrete hormones that govern the development and maintenance of sex characteristics and reproduction (Arking, 1991; Brookbank, 1990; Ferrini and Ferrini, 1993).

Aging-related changes in the production of hormones are complicated by changes in the nervous and circulatory systems. More is known about the aging-related changes in the pancreas and changes associated with insulin in the break-down and utilization of sugars than is known about other aging-related changes in other hormones. Hormones are released by the pancreas and then are used when they link with target cells. The response of target cells in the utilization of insulin may be slowed significantly with age and, in some cases, may result in noninsulin-dependent diabetes, which is discussed in Chapter 5.

With the exception of the female reproductive hormones (e.g., estrogen), de-creases in the amount of other hormones produced by the endocrine system are not consistent with advancing age. There may be a lowered sensitivity, however, in the stimuli that cause the glands to respond; thus, hormone deficiencies can occur with age. In the case of females, reproduction ceases with menopause when estrogen declines. However, other sex hormones (i.e., testosterone) continue to be produced after menopause, and sexual interest is maintained. While testosterone levels in males decrease gradually, sexual activity is maintained well past age 70 (Brookbank, 1990; Ferrini and Ferrini, 1993).

Reproductive System

As can be seen by the information presented in each previous section, some aging-related changes do occur in the functioning of each bodily system. However, no system will shut down completely with age in the absence of illness or disease. The one exception to this general statement is in the female reproductive system which ceases to function typically sometime between age 45 and 55. It is wise, however, to separate reproduction from sexual activity which does not cease with age.

The reproductive system is governed by hormones (from the hypothalamus, testes or ovaries, and pituitary gland) and the reproductive organs (in females: ovaries, uterus, vagina, and external reproductive organs; in males: testes, penis, seminal vesicles, and prostate gland). Hormones control arousal and sexual activity, egg and sperm production, and the development of characteristics associated with gender (e.g., facial hair in men, and hip and buttock fat in women). Hormones also govern the bearing and nursing of children by women. In later life, hormones generally maintain sexual activity and sex characteristics (Ferrini and Ferrini, 1993).

The major aging-related change in the reproductive system occurs in women at menopause (the cessation of reproduction). As women experience a reduction in the production of estrogen, other secondary sex characteristics may change somewhat. Hair pattern, skin texture, and a loss in breast mass may occur.

Men also experience a decline in fertility around the same time that women do, 40s–50s. The main difference between men and women is that men are capable of fertilizing an egg well into late life whereas women cease reproduction at menopause. Men do experience an enlargement of the prostate gland that may begin in their 40s and be fairly common among men in their 80s. Sexual activity will be unaffected by this enlargement, but other bodily functions may be affected (e.g., urination frequency and urgency, urinary retention). Dysfunction in sexual activity or performance in older men is more often due to psychological reasons. For example, men who are aging may experience anxiety over performance, negative effects of medications, or declines in health. Any of these factors may influence male sexual activity in late life (Neuhaus and Neuhaus, 1982). The point is well-made that there is no physiological reason for a decrease in sexual activity for men and women in old age.

Cognitive Changes

Cognitive functioning consists of intelligence, learning, and memory, which taken together, support normal psychological and social functioning in everyday life. Without normal cognitive functioning, many of life's tasks (e.g., family responsibilities, work roles, and leisure activities) are more challenging and this may present added stress for the individual. Much of the research on cognitive functioning throughout the life course, including in older people, suggests that abilities in this area do not decline with age (Hooyman and Kiyak, 1991).

Intelligence, for example, is difficult to define, measure, and verify across the life span. Intelligence is, theoretically, the ability to deal with information, new situations, symbols, abstractions, and ideas. Intelligence can only be estimated rather than definitely known, and this estimate is easily influenced by environmental factors rather than actual abilities. IQ (intelligence quotient) is the measure used to estimate intelligence by evaluating performance in a number of areas such as those listed above and then comparing performance with that of other people of the same age (Hooyman and Kiyak, 1991).

Intelligence is composed of different dimensions and abilities in those dimensions. A theoretical model that is commonly used to understand intelligence and aging-related change in older adults describes two broad categories of ability: fluid intelligence and crystallized intelligence (Cattell, 1963; Horn, 1972, 1988; Horn and Cattell, 1966). Fluid intelligence is represented by skills that are biologically determined—abilities or skills that are not learned through experience. Crystallized intelligence, however, represents accumulated knowledge or abilities that are learned (e.g., words, concepts). While research has been controversial regarding whether older people experience a decline in intelligence compared to younger persons, it is believed that fluid abilities do decline with age but crystallized abilities continue to show improvement throughout the life course.

The *Classic Aging Pattern*, used for describing cognitive performance in old age, has emerged from the results of much research in this area. The Classic Aging Pattern purports that verbal scores (measures of crystallized intelligence) will remain stable while performance scores (measures of fluid intelligence) will decline with age. Because performance-related intelligence tasks require the use of other noncognitive functions (psychomotor skills, perceptual abilities, and sensory abilities), aging-related declines in fluid intelligence may be a finding that is influenced by many factors that are difficult to separate. Other research in this area suggests that the speed of cognitive processing declines with age which will then result in slower performance in other cognitive performance measures (Hooyman and Kiyak, 1991). Verbal skills, however, remain stable across the life span. When and if declines are exhibited in the ability to recall verbal information, they are usually in persons who are very, very old.

Other factors also affect performance on intelligence-related tasks. Health status, sensory loss, hypertension, education, and occupation have been shown to influence performance on intelligence tests. Therefore, given that intelligence is a difficult concept to define and measure, a more definitive understanding of cognitive performance with age remains a topic of continuing research.

Learning and memory are cognitive processes that also must be considered when understanding aging and cognitive functioning. Learning involves the processing and storing of new information, while memory is the process of retrieving the learned information. Memory contains all the information that has been learned across the life course. Three types of memory have been identified: short-term memory, long-term memory, and sensory memory (Hooyman and Kiyak, 1991).

When new information is received by the senses (sensory memory), it is passed along to either short-term or long-term memory. There are two primary types of sensory memory: visual (iconic) and auditory (echoic). Stimuli that we see and hear are received by our sensory memory and passed along for processing and storing.

Short-term (primary) memory is where information is organized and temporarily held. While information is received by sensory memory and temporarily held in short-term memory, true learning occurs when material is stored in long-term (secondary) memory. Rehearsal, memorization, or repeated use of information is necessary for the storage of information in long-term memory. Because short-term memory has a limited capacity and may be affected by declines in reaction time, long-term memory is unlimited in its capacity.

Learning, therefore, takes place when information is received (sensory memory), encoded (short-term memory), and stored (long-term memory). Research on recognition and recall (or memory utilization) does not support aging-related declines in the capacity of these aspects of memory. However, older people may be less efficient in accessing long-term memory and in retrieving information that was stored long ago (Hooyman and Kiyak, 1991).

Learning and memory in older persons can be maintained or even enhanced through providing stimulating activities and environmental supports. Cognitive performance in memory and learning can be as good as when the person was younger, with more time given for task performance; large lettering; adequate lighting; relevant tasks to do; visual, auditory, and gestural cues; nonthreatening environments; and greater opportunity for repetition. Most of the current research evidence supports small, if any, aging-related declines in intelligence, learning, and memory. By maintaining mentally active lifestyles, most older people can enjoy good mental functioning throughout their later years.

Lifestyle and Aging

In spite of gradual and eventual declines in the body's physiological systems with age, the rate of decline can be slowed in many areas of functioning based on lifestyle. Regular exercise, a good diet, and the absence of hazardous health habits (e.g., cigarette smoking) can modify aging-related changes in physical and mental functioning. Older people who are active often have quicker reaction time and movement speed compared with sedentary adults. It is widely accepted that lifestyle influences health and functional status in elderly persons. More important, however, motivating older adults to engage in healthy lifestyles is a contemporary problem, at least in the United States (Ferrini and Ferrini, 1993; MacNeil and Teague, 1987).

Lifestyle factors (exercise, eating, and other health habits) have a significant impact not only on the rate of aging decline but also on the quality and longevity of life. A longer life expectancy has not necessarily meant longer healthier lives for many older persons. It is important to differentiate between human life span, life expectancy, and a healthy life in old age.

Life expectancy is the projected number of years that an individual is expected to live based on environmental conditions and the genetic heritage of the individual. Individuals will have different life expectancies at different points throughout their lives depending upon conditions within that time period and also the functional status of other members of their families at the same age. Disease, sanitation, health service availability and quality, familial genetic dispositions, and other factors combine to influence the statistically projected life expectancy (Ferrini and Ferrini, 1993; MacNeil and Teague, 1987).

Life span, on the other hand, is a fixed maximum age for the human species. The human life span is generally thought to be between 113 and 114 years (Brookbank, 1990). That is to say that few, if any, members of the species will survive past this age if no disease, genetic disposition, or environmental conditions were to affect the life of the individual.

While life expectancy has continued to dramatically improve throughout the twentieth century, few people survive much past 100 years of age. Many older people in their 70s, 80s, and 90s experience aging-related declines that impose serious impairment to independent functioning and health. Advances in medicine, sanitation, nutrition, and other facets of lifestyle have dramatically affected life expectancy, but life span has not been altered as of yet. Lifestyle factors, especially, are important in not only slowing aging-related declines but also in improving the quality of life and independent functioning of older adults. The accumulated effects of the physiological aging process coupled with sedentary living, poor diets, and lifelong participation in hazardous health habits have resulted in a significant portion of the elderly population experiencing impairment, disablement, morbidity, and early mortality. Three major areas of lifestyle that are primary targets of health promotion and prevention in older adults are diet, exercise, and hazardous habits (Public Health Service, 1990).

Far too many adults in the U.S. are overweight. Obesity is a national concern and specific health threat to the elderly. Diet and proper nutrition are current targets of the U.S. Department of Health and Human Service's national health promotion and disease prevention plan (Public Health Service, 1990). The reduction of body weight and sodium intake are instrumental in controlling the risk of disease as well as in promoting independent functioning in late life. Obesity increases the risk for:

> hypertension, heart stress, adult on-set diabetes, increased serum fats, respiratory difficulties, and pain from overstressed joints. (Brookbank, 1990, p. 187)

The control of fat, sugar, and overall caloric intake also are dietary concerns of the elderly. Diets not exceeding 1,800 kcal for women and 2,400 kcal for men are recommended for older adults.

A second major lifestyle concern of the elderly is the lack of regular physical activity. A significant amount of research supports the impact that exercise has on health, rate of functional declines, and life quality in general for older adults (Arking, 1991; Brookbank, 1990). For example, regular physical activity promotes the following benefits:

(a) increased blood volume;
(b) decreased blood pressure;
(c) increased maximal stroke volume and cardiac output;
(d) improved respiration during exercise;
(e) increased bone, ligament, and tendon strength; and
(f) increased musculature.

Unfortunately, a very low percentage (10%) of the adult population exercises at the minimal amount (e.g., 20 minutes on three or more days per week) needed to promote health, improve overall functioning and to slow the rate of aging decline. The problem of inactivity or a sedentary lifestyle is much higher among elderly persons. It is generally observed that more physically active older people are healthier than sedentary persons.

Hazardous health habits are a national concern and a problem of the elderly. The long-term negative consequences of cigarette smoking and tobacco chewing are widely known. Nicotine is an alkaloid substance that causes heart rate to significantly increase (tachycardia) and vascular contractions that may result in elevated blood pressure (Brookbank, 1990). Tobacco tars are known to cause cancer of the mouth and lungs. Finally, cigarette smoke causes damage to lung function and reduces the uptake of oxygen into the bloodstream. While recent national efforts aimed at reducing cigarette smoking in the U.S. population probably have decreased the overall numbers of smokers, tobacco use continues to present a significant health threat among the elderly.

Alcohol abuse (i.e., the consumption of alcohol in harmful amounts) is problematic in the older adult segment of the population much the same as it is in the rest of the population. Barnes (1982) reported that 14% of males and 7% of females over age 60 are classifiable as heavy drinkers. It has been estimated that between 2% and 10% of the elderly have alcohol problems so severe as to be identified as alcoholics (Brookbank, 1990). In addition to these percentages, periodic overconsumption is not uncommon among older adults. The long-range effects of alcoholic consumption are greater for older adults than they are for younger people due to changes in metabolic and liver function with age. The accumulated effects of alcoholism on cognitive function include losses in visual-spatial ability, sensory-motor functioning, and verbal ability. The aging process has a profound effect on the older person, reducing his or her ability to regain cognitive function that was damaged from alcoholism (Brookbank, 1990).

It is clear from the research that lifestyle factors have a great influence on how individuals are affected by the aging process. The increased risk for health problems and functional declines to the severity that the individual experiences impairment is a direct outcome of lifestyle habits such as poor diet, overconsumption of alcohol, cigarette smoking, and lack of regular exercise. On the other hand, a slowing in aging-related decrements in some areas of functioning and an overall increased quality of life and perceived well-being are often experienced by older individuals who engage in positive lifestyles. While it is true and inevitable that all humans age and eventually die, much can be gained by cultivating a health-promoting lifestyle. It is on this positive note that this chapter on the aging process ends.

Summary

It is important to know about the human aging process for personal as well as professional reasons. Negative myths and stereotypes abound in reference to growing older and being an older adult. By studying aging, caregivers and activity specialists can learn more about how aging will affect their own lives and how to provide appropriate activities and programs to older persons whom they serve.

The aging process follows certain patterns of change but is highly influenced by individual genetic makeup and personal lifestyle habits. While many of the body's systems will decline in efficiency, memory and learning abilities hold up quite well through later life. As life expectancy continues to improve for each new birth cohort, the manner in which the society promotes healthy lifestyles will have a great impact on the quality of health and well-being of tomorrow's elderly. In this chapter the process of aging is connected with the habits of lifestyle in order to help the reader appreciate the role of activities in the overall quality of life of older adults.

Comprehension Questions

1. Discuss the difference between gerontology and geriatrics.
2. Describe six patterns that characterize the aging process.
3. Compare and contrast programmed or genetic theories of aging with stochastic theories of aging.
4. Select three physical systems of the human body and briefly describe the aging-related changes that occur in each system.
5. Describe how aging affects intelligence, learning, and memory.
6. Discuss the influence that lifestyle has on the aging process and quality of life for older persons.

References

Arking, R. (1991). *Biology of aging: Observations and principles.* Englewood Cliffs, NJ: Prentice Hall.

Barnes, G. M. (1982). Patterns of alcohol use and abuse among older persons in a household population. In W. G. Wood & M. F. Elias (Eds.), *Alcoholism and aging.* Boca Raton, FL: CRC Press Inc.

Brookbank, J. W. (1990). *The biology of aging.* New York, NY: Harper & Row.

Cattell, R. B. (1963). Theory for fluid and crystallized intelligence: A critical experiment. *Journal of Educational Psychology, 54,* 1-22.

Ferrini, A. F., & Ferrini, R. L. (1993). *Health in the later years* (2nd ed.). Madison, WI: Brown & Benchmark.

Hooyman, N. R., & Kiyak, H. A. (1991). *Social gerontology: A multidisciplinary perspective* (2nd ed.). Needham Heights, MA: Allyn & Bacon.

Horn, J. L. (1988). Cognitive diversity: A framework for learning. In P. L. Ackerman, R. J. Sternberg, & R. Glazer (Eds.), *Learning and individual differences.* New York, NY: W. H. Freeman and Co.

Horn, J. L. (1972). State, trait and change dimensions of intelligence. *British Journal of Educational Psychology, 42,* 159-185.

Horn, J. L., & Cattell, R. B. (1966). Refinement and test of the fluid and crystallized intelligence. *Journal of Educational Psychology, 57,* 253-279.

MacNeil, R. D., & Teague, M. L. (1987). *Aging and leisure: Vitality in later life.* Englewood Cliffs, NJ: Prentice Hall.

Neuhaus, R., & Neuhaus, R. (1982). *Successful aging.* New York, NY: John Wiley & Sons, Inc.

Public Health Service, U.S. Department of Health and Human Services. (1990). *Healthy people 200: National health promotion and disease prevention objectives* (conference edition). Washington, DC: U.S. Government Printing Office.

Schneider, E. L. (1992). Biological theories of aging. *GENERATIONS—Journal of the American Society on Aging, 16*(4), 7-14.

Shock, N. W., Greulich, R. C., Andres, R., Arenberg, D., Costa, P. T., Lakatta, E. G., & Tobin, J. D. (1984). *Normal human aging: The Baltimore longitudinal study of aging,* NIH Publication No. 84-2450. Washington, DC: U.S. Government Printing Office.

Key Terms

Activity Theory

Age Stratification Theory

Apportioned Grandparent

Caregiving

Cohort Effect

Continuity Theory

Deep Friendship

Disengagement Theory

Ego Integrity

Empty Nest Syndrome

Erikson's Psychosocial Model

Ethnocentric

Exchange Theory

Individualized Grandparent

Interest-Related Friendship

Modernization Theory

Remote Grandparent

Social Breakdown

Stage Theories of Personality

Subculture Theory

Symbolic Grandparent

Symbolic Interactionism

Learning Objectives

1. Define and compare the various social theories of aging.
2. Discuss stage theories of adult personality.
3. Discuss the impact of marriage in later life.
4. Describe the nature of intergenerational relationships and their value in later life.
5. Explain the impact of widowhood and divorce in later life.
6. Explain the importance of friendship in later life.
7. Explain the impact of retirement on older adults.

Chapter 4

Psychosocial Aspects of Aging

Introduction

The period of older adulthood is a time of many changes in the life of an individual. Changes in family and work status may adversely affect the older adult; being a retiree and grandparent may be perceived as quite positive. Social networks are utilized by older adults to support transitions and life changes. This chapter will focus on common psychosocial aspects of the aging process including personality development, marriage, widowhood, intergenerational exchange, friendship, and retirement.

Social Theories of Aging

Social theories of aging have been developed to describe what successful aging means in our society. A number of theories have been developed which range from very simplistic to highly involved. The following section briefly highlights some of the major social theories of aging discussed in the gerontological literature.

Disengagement Theory

Disengagement Theory was developed in the early 1960s by researchers working with data from a cross-sectional study of older adults (Cumming and Henry, 1961). The primary tenet of the theory was that a mutual withdrawal of the elderly and society from each other would result in higher life satisfaction among the elderly (Hendricks and Leedham, 1991). As they aged, individuals would be released from responsibilities which subsequently would be passed on to younger generations. Personal satisfaction among the elderly was present when acceptance of withdrawal occurred.

This theory drew immediate criticism from social gerontologists. Efforts to disprove the theory led to research that was critical in the development of other social theories of aging. Additional research was unable to duplicate the original findings, and eventually the authors modified their opinions. Today disengagement theory is rarely referred to as a viable theory.

Activity Theory

Activity Theory is a widely accepted theory of aging that is particularly significant for activity specialists. The popularity of the theory may be partially due to the manner in which it intuitively seems rational (Hooyman and Kiyak, 1993). Activity Theory is based on the premise that high levels of activity are associated with perceptions of high life satisfaction in old age (Havighurst and Albrecht, 1953).

Although there has been empirical support for Activity Theory, it has been criticized as being too simplistic to fully explain life satisfaction in old age. One limitation is that personal differences in activity level across the life span are not taken into account (Hooyman and Kiyak, 1993). For example, an individual who lived a sedentary lifestyle in middle age may be satisfied with that lifestyle in old age. Additional research has indicated that activity which is personally meaningful correlates with life satisfaction, while highly structured activity does not (Hendricks and Leedham, 1991; Hooyman and Kiyak, 1993).

Continuity Theory

Continuity Theory suggests that personality remains stable over the life span (Hooyman and Kiyak, 1993). Relationships and orientations present in midlife are continued into old age (Hendricks and Leedham, 1991). The older adult will develop new roles to replace lost ones. Based on individual personality characteristics, the older adult develops his or her own expectations for successful aging.

Continuity Theory certainly addresses the shortcomings of Activity Theory. Recent empirical evidence indicates that personality remains stable over the life course (Costa and McCrae, 1989). However, this theory has its own limitations. The continuation of roles in old age may be difficult for people with functional impairments. In such situations the inability to change patterns of behavior may be detrimental (Hooyman and Kiyak, 1993).

Subculture Theory

The premise of Subculture Theory is that older adults interact primarily with each other, consequently forming their own subculture (Rose, 1965). It is from this subculture that older people develop their social identities (Hooyman and Kiyak,

1993). Demographic trends that support Subculture Theory include the voluntary segregation of older people into retirement communities and the concentration of older people in urban centers vacated by younger residents (Hendricks and Leedham, 1991). The elderly certainly constitute a subculture in the political arena. Social Security and Medicare are examples of government programs administered on the basis of age. In recent years, older people have joined forces to increase their political clout with the government.

Subculture Theory must be criticized for not taking individual differences into account. Individuals do not become more alike as they age. In fact, the opposite is true (Hendricks and Leedham, 1991). Socioeconomic and race differences are discounted by Subculture Theory, as well.

Modernization Theory

According to Modernization Theory, the status of older people declines as a society increases modernization (Hendricks and Leedham, 1991). In preindustrial societies older men owned the land and held the power that accompanied such ownership. As societies industrialized, land became less of a source of power and older men lost their status.

Modernization Theory also is open to a number of criticisms. The primary criticism is that it is *ethnocentric.* The power in all preindustrial cultures is not based on the ownership of land. Furthermore, lower socioeconomic classes and minority groups who are not allowed to own land are excluded from this model.

Comparison of modern societies to preindustrial societies is difficult because of the great differences which exist between them. In most preindustrial societies, few people lived to an age that is considered old by modern standards. The idea that older people were honored and revered universally in old age is a misconception. Historical evidence indicates older people in many preindustrial societies were victims of harsh treatment (Hendricks and Leedham, 1991).

Age Stratification Theory

At the core of Age Stratification Theory is the concept that people are stratified by society into categories based on age (Riley and Foner, 1972). Roles, responsibilities, and resources are assigned according to these categories. *Cohort effects* make the aging process for each generation unique. Cohort effects reflect the impact that history has upon a specific age group that distinguish that group from people who grew up during another time period.

Age Stratification Theory addresses important considerations for gerontological research. Primarily it provides evidence that cross-sectional research which compares members of different cohorts is not sufficient to explain aging-related changes in the older population. Differences between generations may be due to the historical experiences of a cohort rather than chronological age. Other criticisms of the Age Stratification Theory include the fact that it does not sufficiently take into account individual class, race, and gender differences (Hendricks and Leedham, 1991).

Social Breakdown Theory

Social Breakdown Theory refers to the spiral that occurs when criticism and negative feedback of older people leads to lowered self-esteem and decline in performance which then leads to more criticism. Loss of self-confidence due to social breakdown may cause older people to reach out for assurance which may be interpreted as another sign of decline (Hendricks and Leedham, 1991). The negative spiral of social breakdown can be interrupted when older adults are provided the opportunity to demonstrate their abilities (Hendricks and Leedham, 1991). Social Breakdown Theory is particularly useful as a model to guide the planning of therapeutic activity interventions with older people.

Exchange Theory

Exchange Theory is based on the premise that the status of older people is largely based on the balance between contributions made by older people to society and the cost of supporting them (Hooyman and Kiyak, 1993). According to Exchange Theory, individuals and groups in society will act to maximize gains and minimize costs. Relationships are maintained only as long as benefits outweigh costs. Because older adults are often perceived as not being productive, they have a lowered social status. The major problem with Exchange Theory is the basic assumption that the primary motivation for human behavior is personal gain (Hendricks and Leedham, 1991).

Symbolic Interactionism

Symbolic interactionism perspectives of aging view the interaction of the environment, the individual, and situations as key to the aging process. Older people who believe they are capable of dealing with the demands placed on them by the environment are more satisfied than those whose environment is too challenging or not challenging enough. Individual outcomes can be improved by altering the environment to fit the functional ability of the older person. This theory is particularly useful for service providers with control over the level of stimulation in the older person's environment. Unfortunately, circumstances do not always allow for environmental modifications. The person-environment fit model will be further addressed in Chapter 10.

Leisure and Life Satisfaction

Some of the various social theories of aging discussed in the previous section are based, at least in part, on the relationship between involvement in activities and satisfaction with life in older adulthood. Life satisfaction has been found to be positively related to leisure participation in a number of studies (Haley, Levine, Brown, and Bartolucci, 1987; Kelly, Steinkamp, and Kelly, 1986; Riddick, 1985). In fact, the positive relationship between activity and life satisfaction served as the basis for Activity Theory.

Recent research, however, suggested that the relationship between activity and life satisfaction may not be as straightforward as believed. In a study of 92 retired older adults, Mannell (1993) found that older adults who had a greater investment in their daily activities tended to have higher life satisfaction than did individuals with a lower level of investment. Consequently, older adults who primarily invested their leisure time in watching television or other passive activities experienced pleasure while engaged in the activity, but over a period of time these activities contributed little to perceived life satisfaction.

Mannell's research is important for therapists to understand. Often these activity specialists work with older adults who are resistant to putting forth the energy to invest in potentially highly satisfying activities. Specialists are challenged to provide programs that do more than amuse. They are encouraged to utilize motivational techniques to ensure participation in high investment activities.

Theories of Adult Personality

Prior to the 1930s, psychologists tended to believe that the psychological development of humans was completed by about age 30, and that little, if any, change in personality was evident after this time (Costa and McCrae, 1989). In 1933, C. G. Jung presented a bold alternative view in his seminal work, *Modern Man in Search of a Soul.* According to Jung, a number of changes in personality occurred throughout the life span. In the decades that followed, a number of psychologists developed theories of adult development and personality. This section will focus on five of the most important theoretical works: Erikson's psychosocial crises, Levinson's life structure approach, Gilligan's work on women's development, Neugarten's cluster of personality types, and Costa and McCrae's work on personality change/stability.

Erikson's Psychosocial Model

Stage theories of personality define personality development as a step process. According to stage theories, people pass through a series of developmental stages throughout the life course. At each step they are required to complete a developmental task. Failure to complete the task will prevent successful passage to the next step. Erik Erikson's (1959) Psychosocial Model is perhaps the most frequently cited stage theory of human development throughout the social sciences. According to Erikson's model, the individual moves through eight stages of development throughout the life course. The final four stages in his model are completed in adulthood. Stage five, ego identity versus role diffusion, begins in adolescence and involves efforts to define clearly one's identity and social roles. Stage six, intimacy versus isolation, typically begins in the early to middle 20s and continues into the middle 30s. This stage is characterized by the establishment of long-term intimate relationships. Marriage is more common during this stage. Stage seven, generativity versus stagnation, generally begins in the middle 30s and continues into the early 50s. Generativity may be defined as the need to build something that lasts or the need to provide for future generations by looking toward the future. Parenting is an excellent example of generativity. The final stage, ego integrity versus despair, is completed in late life. During this stage, the older person strives to establish a sense of meaning and purpose in life. Resolution of conflicts in earlier stages of life and integration of past experiences into the present are elements of ego integrity. Successful completion of this final stage should result in higher life satisfaction and acceptance of the inevitableness of death.

Levinson's Life Structure Approach

Levinson (1978) also developed a stage theory of adult personality. His work was based on the concept of life structure, the basic patterns of an individual's life during a given period. Life structure encompasses three factors:

(a) the individual's participation in the sociocultural world through work, family, and other social groups;

(b) the extent to which aspects of the self are expressed or inhibited, including wishes, conflicts, and anxieties; and

(c) the manner in which the individual participates in the external world.

According to Levinson (1978), the following 10 stages characterize life structure in adulthood:

1. Early Adult Transition (17–22 years)—This stage is characterized by severing or altering significant relationships of childhood. During this stage, the individual experiments with relationships, careers, and other aspects of adult life.

2. Entering the Adult World (22–28 years)—This stage is characterized by making important decisions about occupation, lifestyle, and relationships which will determine the life course of the individual. Independence is established during this period.

3. Age-Thirty Transition (28–33 years)—This stage is characterized by adjustments made by the individual to tentative decisions made during the previous stage. During this stage, family and occupational choices tend to be more permanent.

4. Settling Down (33–40 years)—Individuals in this stage have made a strong commitment to family, occupation, and a secure future. Career advancement is important during this stage.

5. Midlife Transition (40–45 years)—This stage is characterized by a change in life orientation. In the past, achievement was the primary life orientation. During this stage, the individual becomes more reflective and evaluative of what has been accomplished in life. The individual may modify his or her life path or form a new one.

6. Entering Middle Adulthood (45–50 years)—In this stage, the individual makes choices regarding the life structure of middle age. Changes in feelings towards work and family/marriage may occur during this stage. Divorce, illness, and loss of loved ones may be a theme.

7. Age-Fifty Transition (50–55 years)—This stage does not significantly differ from the previous one. According to Levinson, all adults must experience some type of a midlife crisis. This may occur during this stage.

8. Culmination of Middle Adulthood (55–60 years)—This stage is characterized by stability and a solidified life structure.

9. Late-Adult Transition (60–65 years)—Middle adulthood is terminated during this stage. Adults prepare a life structure for late adulthood. Levinson did not actually interview men of this age, so his ideas regarding this stage are mostly speculative.

10. Late-Adulthood (65+ years)—Levinson did not interview men in this stage. Consequently, this life structure is not well-developed.

What about Women's Development?

A criticism of Levinson's and Erikson's work is that both theories are based on research conducted with male samples. Although some research has indicated that the lives of women can be imposed into these stages (Harris, Elliott, and Holmes, 1986; Reinke, Holmes, and Harris, 1985), other research has indicated that women's development is different than men's. According to Gilligan (1982), the emphasis Levinson places on achievement is not appropriate for women.

Gilligan (1982) has theorized that women's moral development is based on their involvement in relationships, whereas men's moral development revolves around achievement. In other words, women judge the success of their lives by their ability to maintain relationships with those around them. Men, on the other hand, judge their lives in terms of personal achievement.

Gilligan (1982) identified a common characteristic of women as the *ethic of care*. This concept described the tendency of women to put the needs of others before their own and to make sacrifices in order to provide care for others. Research has indicated that caregiving is a central theme throughout the lives of many women because they often assume primary caregiving responsibilities for children, aging parents, and finally, their spouse.

Aging and Personality

The Kansas City Studies

The Kansas City studies are a classic set of studies of personality conducted by well-known gerontologist and psychologist, Bernice Neugarten (Neugarten and Hagestad, 1976). Data for these studies were collected during the 1960s from 100 adults in the Kansas City area. A cross-sectional comparison of 700 adults ranging in age from 40 to 70 and a six-year longitudinal study of 300 individuals ranging in age from 50 to 90 were conducted at this time.

The results of the Kansas City studies indicated that there were four clusters of personality types which encompassed most of the adults in the studies. The personality types were:

1. *Integrated* people have high life satisfaction, high cognitive skills, and have successfully adjusted to aging. People with integrated personalities may have high, moderate, or low levels of participation in activities. What is important is whether or not their level of involvement is voluntary or involuntary.

2. *Armored* or defensive people have not adjusted to the idea of aging and are actively combating the effects of aging. Some individuals may be struggling to maintain high levels of involvement in past activities. Others may withdraw from relationships in order to isolate themselves from the losses associated with aging. Armored or defensive people have moderate life satisfaction and high cognitive skills.

3. *Passive/dependent* people have a lower life satisfaction than the previous groups. Individuals in this group rely on others to meet their physical and emotional needs. Members of this group have moderate to low involvement in activities.

4. *Unintegrated* people have considerable physical and cognitive decline. They have low life satisfaction and involvement in activities. In spite of dysfunction, they are able to remain in the community.

Costa and McCrae: Stability or Change?

Early studies of personality indicated some personality changes in later life. These included a tendency for adults to disengage and become more self-oriented in later life. Research also indicated that men and women became more alike in later life. Women took on more masculine traits and became more assertive, while men became more nurturing.

More recent research indicated that age is only weakly related to personality (Costa and McCrae, 1989). Adults of all ages show considerable variation in personality. These individual differences tend to remain stable throughout the adult years, even when individuals perceive change has occurred.

Adjusting to Change in Older Adulthood

Later adulthood is a period of life that is often accompanied by many role changes and stressful life events. Retirement, potential loss of health, and the death of one's spouse, friends, and siblings are common. The ways that older adults adapt to these events vary greatly between individuals. Some older adults may adjust to significant life changes without much stress, while others may need professional support and guidance.

Whitbourne (1987) developed the concept of identity style to explain adaptation to aging and related events. According to Whitbourne, older adults generally fall into one of three types of identity style. The first identity style is *assimilative.* An individual with this style attempts to integrate new experiences into his or her existing identity. This identity style may lead to denial of the aging process. While older adults with this style generally have a perception of good health, they also may project problems to others instead of themselves (Hayslip and Panek, 1993). Adults with an *accommodative* identity style take the opposite approach. Accommodators change identity to fit the environment. While accommodation is generally more successful, it may be problematic on occasion. For example, loss of some functional abilities in old age may lead the individual to believe that he or she is *falling apart.*

Whitbourne (1987) suggested the *balanced* identity style as the most stable. Individuals with this identity style are able to assimilate or accommodate when necessary. They also tend to have a more realistic view of the aging process. As a consequence, they are likely to take preventive steps to combat the effects of aging, but will seek therapeutic services when necessary (Hayslip and Panek, 1993).

Self-Concept and Self-Esteem in Older Adulthood

The remainder of this chapter will discuss common role changes and adjustments in later life. In order to understand these changes, it is necessary to be familiar with self-concept and self-esteem. Self-concept refers to the individual's self-identity or self-image. Hooyman and Kiyak (1993) refer to self-concept as the "cognitive definition of one's identity" (p. 198). Poor self-concept may be a concern for older adults who base feelings about their identity on a role—worker or parent—which may be lost in later life.

Self-esteem can be defined as the emotional assessment of self (Hooyman and Kiyak, 1993). Since self-esteem is related to emotions, it is more likely to be affected by changes in social roles than self-concept. In older adulthood, if the changes in social roles involve loss, the loss very well may have a negative impact on self-esteem. The following factors suggested by Morgan (1979) are important for maintaining self-esteem:

1. Older adults need to define self free from previous roles. It is more beneficial to focus on internal and individual qualities. For example, "I am a caring person" rather than "I am a good nurse."
2. Older adults need to accept the realities of the aging process. An individual is less likely to suffer loss of self-esteem if he or she is aware of what physical and social losses are inevitable, and what losses can be negotiated.
3. Older adults need to be able to reevaluate goals throughout the life cycle. Life circumstances sometimes change unexpectedly, and, as a consequence, life goals need to be readjusted to reflect the new circumstances.
4. Older adults need to be able to reevaluate their lives objectively in terms of failures and successes. According to Hooyman and Kiyak (1993), an older adult who can do this will be better able to utilize successful past coping responses in current situations.

Social Networks in Older Adulthood

Social support networks in later life are crucial to the maintenance of high life satisfaction. The social needs of older adults can be met by both family and friends. The following sections discuss common changes in the social networks of older adults.

Marriage

The majority of older adults are or have been married at some point in their lives. Research indicates that marriages generally remain stable (given that they were stable in middle age) into retirement and old age (Vinick and Ekerdt, 1989). The majority of older couples report satisfaction with their marriage. Comparisons of three generations of spouses have indicated that older couples report higher levels of life satisfaction than do middle-aged couples, but lower than newlyweds (Gilford and Bengston, 1979; Markides and Hoppe, 1985).

Although the quality of marriages appears to remain stable in old age, some changes can be expected to occur. A benefit that many older adults report is an increase in opportunities to spend time with children and grandchildren. In a study of retired veterans and spouses, about one-half of the respondents reported an increase in companionship activities or activities with the company of others in retirement. Generally, women maintained responsibilities for daily household tasks in old age. Men tended to increase participation in home maintenance tasks, often "projects" they had been saving for retirement (Vinick and Ekerdt, 1989). The *empty nest syndrome* is commonly perceived to be a crisis for older adults, especially women. Research indicates, however, that children not leaving home at the appropriate time may create more stress for both the parent and the child (Neugarten and Neugarten, 1987).

Some conflicts can be expected in later life marriages, as in marriages of all ages. Most late life marriages do not produce serious problems, however. Women who were used to being at home alone have reported feelings of impingement on their time from their husbands (Vinick and Ekerdt, 1989). Conflict also may arise when one partner is still working and the other retires (Siegel, 1990). Working women may feel exploited if their retired husband does not assume responsibility for more household responsibilities (Vinick and Ekerdt, 1989). The problem that potentially has the greatest negative impact on a marriage usually arises when the illness or disability of one spouse forces the other into assuming primary care responsibilities (Shamoian and Thurston, 1986; Vinick and Ekerdt, 1989).

Divorce

Divorce is rare among older adults. Today's older adult couples grew up during a time in history when divorce was viewed as a personal failure (Grambs, 1989). However, future cohorts will have more members who have divorced and perhaps will exhibit greater rates of divorce in old age. The number of never-divorced individuals declines with each 10-year cohort (Cherlin, 1981). When older people do make the decision to divorce, the recovery process may be much more difficult than for younger adults (Grambs, 1989; Shamoian and Thurston, 1986). It also is very difficult for older divorcees, particularly women, to find new partners.

Widowhood

Widowhood is a situation that the majority of older women will face. Widows exceed widowers in the U.S. by a margin of five to one. This trend is largely due to:

(a) a longer life expectancy among women,
(b) the common practice of men marrying younger women, and
(c) the decreased incidence of remarriage by widowed women.

Regardless of gender, older adults consider the death of a spouse to be the most stressful life event. Porcino (1983) lists the following situations that are most likely to create high levels of stress for older persons:

- when husbands die unexpectedly;
- when the widow (or widower) was very dependent on the spouse or the spouse was heavily dependent on her (or him) for social and emotional support;
- when the widow (or widower) did not have a career;
- when the widow (or widower) has attempted to be totally independent of relatives and friends or if her (or his) life has only revolved around the family;
- when teenage children are at home; and
- when the widow's (or widower's) income drops significantly as a result of the death.

The continuation of long-term relationships with other family and friends provides crucial support to widows and widowers (Heinemann, 1983). Often these relationships are renegotiated, and new roles are defined during the bereavement period. In addition to family support, bereavement groups and programs, such as a Widow-to-Widow Program, may be helpful to the grieving spouse. Regardless of type of support, bereaved individuals need permission and encouragement to express their feelings.

Health declines often occur during the first year of widowhood. The lack of human companionship which results from the death of a spouse contributes to increased incidents of physical and emotional illness (Porcino, 1983). Increased rates of chronic illness, mortality, and suicide also are found. A wide range of emotions (e.g., sadness, longing, loneliness, sorrow, guilt, and anger) are commonly expressed during the grieving process (DeSpelder and Strickland, 1992). These emotions may be evident particularly during holidays, anniversaries, birthdays, or other special days in the couple's life.

Intergenerational Relationships

Relationships with Adult Children

In spite of the modern day myths that elderly individuals are forgotten by their busy children, most older adults maintain satisfying relationships with children and other family members. The extended family of the past was, in fact, never the prominent family arrangement. The nuclear family dominated even in early America when grandparents rarely lived to see their grandchildren (Hareven, 1992). As life expectancy has lengthened in recent decades, modern families find themselves providing increased amounts of intergenerational care.

The relationship between older adults and their adult children is typically interdependent and mutually satisfying. The relationship between parent and adult child is likely to remain stable until the parent experiences significant losses in functional ability. As health status declines, the adult child may have to assume some caregiving responsibilities.

Caregiving can be defined as provision of emotional support and physical services (Allatt, Keil, Bryman, and Bytheway, 1987). Tasks involved in caregiving may range from daily telephone calls to personal assistance with feeding, bathing, and toileting. Often the caregiver assumes responsibilities for infrequent or irregular assistance while moving into a more time-consuming role as functional status of the older adult continues to decline.

Grandparenting

The grandparenting role is one that many older adults look forward to assuming in old age. Ninety-four percent of older adults with children have grandchildren (Hooyman and Kiyak, 1993). Nearly 50% of this group see their grandchildren almost every day (Smyer and Hofland, 1982). Grandparents who do not live close by are likely to maintain close ties with their grandchildren if they have a close relationship with their children (Kornhober and Woodward, 1981).

A strong relationship between grandparent and grandchild can benefit both. Grandparents can offer children unconditional love and prevent them from developing negative stereotypes of older people (Hooyman and Kiyak, 1993; Kornhober and Woodward, 1981). Grandchildren can provide support and reinforce feelings in the grandparents that the family line will be continued (Robertson, 1977).

Variables that influence the style of grandparenting include education, lifestyle, marital status, and age. Wood and Robertson (1976) classified grandparents into four groups:

1. *Apportioned type*—This grandparent views social norms and personal needs as important in achieving satisfaction in the grandparenting role.
2. *Symbolic type*—This grandparent views social norms as important, but has low personal need. The symbolic grandparent finds the status of grandparent to be most rewarding.
3. *Individualized type*—This grandparent views the personal benefits of grandparenting as most rewarding and is less concerned with social norms.
4. *Remote type*—This grandparent does not draw any satisfaction from personal interactions or the social role.

Generally the relationship between grandparents and grandchildren is warm and indulgent. Most grandparents do not interfere with the parent/child relationship under normal circumstances. A family crisis such as divorce often changes this norm. Grandparents with children who are divorcing often provide financial support and also may provide grandchildren with a place to live during or following the divorce.

Friendships

Friendships provide an important network of social support for older adults. Intimacy, a sense of belonging, and interdependency are important needs related to the life satisfaction that friendships can help to foster. Relationships with friends differ from those with family members because of their voluntary nature and emphasis on mutual gain.

Defining friendship is difficult because of its subjective nature. One definition of friendship relates the importance of mutuality (Stevens-Long, 1984). Specifically, friendship involves mutual self-disclosure, mutual commitment, and mutual expectations. Most friendships can be placed into one of two broad categories: interest-related friendships and deep friendships (Hayslip and Panek, 1993). Interest-related friendships are developed on the basis of common lifestyles and interests between two individuals (Bensman and Lilienfield, 1979). Deep friendships are more intimate and focus less on mutual interests. These friendships tend to last throughout life and the individuals involved are less concerned with equity (Roberts and Scott, 1986).

Not surprisingly, older adults living alone have higher levels of contact with peers than those who live with a spouse or other family member (Wister, 1990). Healthy older adults also have greater levels of contact with friends. Functional impairment can put older people at risk of losing friends when the impairment prevents the individual from fulfilling obligations and meeting the other person's expectations. Friends provide some informal support for disabled older adults while support from family members is preferred by most older people (Adams, 1986). Typically, friends provide support when it is convenient, or the need for help is unpredictable.

Retirement

Retirement is a social institution largely unique to the twentieth century. Prior to that time, few individuals lived to what could be considered retirement age. In addition to the longevity that is associated with higher standards of living, industrialization and surplus labor were major factors in the development of widespread retirement (Hooyman and Kiyak, 1993). The passage of Social Security legislation in 1935 insured the right to financial security in old age. Today, the vast majority of adults can look forward to spending several years in retirement.

The median age for retirement in the United States is 62.3 years for men and 62.0 years for women (Gendell and Siegel, 1992). Employers commonly encourage retirement prior to age 65 in order to reduce expenses. Currently, an estimated nine out of 10 pension plans offer incentives for early retirement (Hooyman and Kiyak, 1993). While the majority of older adults do retire from the work force during their early 60s, it also is not uncommon for individuals to retire during their 50s or to continue working on a part-time basis into their 70s (Neugarten and Neugarten, 1987).

The majority of American workers find the prospect of retirement desirable (Hooyman and Kiyak, 1993). Factors that typically influence the decision to retire are: adequate income, health status, family preference, informal norms of the workplace, and long-range plans (Hooyman and Kiyak, 1993).

Satisfaction in retirement depends on a number of variables. Health status is correlated with retirement satisfaction. The nature of retirement also may be a significant variable. Individuals who retire on a voluntary basis tend to regard retirement more favorably than those who are forced to retire. An income that sustains the preretirement standard of living appears to be important. Family members often impact retirement satisfaction. Retirement may be more satisfying if the family supports the individual's decision to retire. The nature of family relationships also is significant. Individuals who are involved in mutually satisfying relationships tend to rate higher on measures of retirement satisfaction than those who are involved in relationships that involve primary care responsibilities. Other factors related to retirement satisfaction include work values, job history, and the perception that daily activities are useful (Hooyman and Kiyak, 1993).

In the past, retirement was often viewed as a time of declining vigor, social disengagement, and isolation (Neugarten and Neugarten, 1987). In contrast, contemporary older adults often view retirement as a time of continued activity. The emphasis today embraces a *retirement to something* (e.g., involvement in a retirement lifestyle) rather than a *retirement from something* (e.g., the job) (McCluskey, 1989).

Summary

Social gerontologists utilize a number of social theories of aging to describe successful aging in our culture. Although many of the theories have limitations, some are useful in understanding aspects of the aging process and guiding interventions. Theories also have been developed to describe personality changes in old age. Erikson's Psychosocial Model defines eight stages of personality development throughout life. Recent research has indicated that personality remains relatively stable throughout life.

Social relationships frequently undergo significant changes in later life. The young old are likely still to be married and have mutually satisfying relationships with their children. This situation is likely to change, however, as the individual gets older and begins to show signs of functional decline. The assumption of primary caregiving responsibilities often has negative consequences for the spouse or child who is doing the caregiving. Widowhood is common for older women. Family and social support networks are important to the bereaved spouse as a mechanism through which to resolve grief. Grandparenting is often viewed as a positive social role. Generally, grandparents take an indulgent role of noninterference with grandchildren. The exception occurs when there is a family crisis.

Prior to the twentieth century, retirement was nonexistent. Although retirement has previously been viewed as a time of disengagement and inactivity, many older adults now view retirement as a time of retiring to a new, active lifestyle. Retirement is usually viewed as a positive experience.

Comprehension Questions

1. Select two social theories of aging and comparatively discuss them in terms of how well they describe successful aging.
2. Describe how adult personality changes over the adult life stages. Include in your discussion how personality remains stable.
3. How does retirement affect older persons?
4. Discuss factors that influence older persons' social networks and why social networks are very important to the elderly.
5. Describe four types of grandparents.

References

Adams, R. G. (1986). A look at friendship and aging. *Generations, 10*(4), 40-43.

Allatt, P., Keil, T., Bryman, A., & Bytheway, B. (Eds.). (1987). *Women and the life cycle.* New York, NY: St. Martin's Press, Inc.

Bensman, J., & Lilienfield, R. (1979, October). Friendships and alienation. *Psychology Today, 55-66.*

Cherlin, A. J. (1981). *Marriage, divorce, remarriage: Changing patterns in the post-war United States.* Cambridge, MA: Harvard University Press.

Costa, P. T., & McCrae, R. R. (1989). Personality continuity and the changes of adult life. In M. Storandt & G. R. VandenBos (Eds.), *The adult years: Continuity and change* (pp. 41-77). Washington, DC: American Psychological Association.

Cumming, E., & Henry, W. E. (1961). *Growing old: The process of disengagement.* New York, NY: Basic Books.

DeSpelder, L. A., & Strickland, A. L. (1992). *The last dance: Encountering death and dying.* Palo Alto, CA: Mayfield Publishing Co.

Erikson, E. H. (1959). Identity and the life cycle. *Psychological Issues, 1.*

Gendell, M., & Siegel, J. S. (1992). Trends in retirement age by sex, 1950–2005. *Monthly Labor Review, 175,* 22-29

Gilford, R., & Bengston, V. (1979). Measuring marital satisfaction in three generations: Positive and negative dimensions. *Journal of Marriage and the Family, 41*(22), 387-98.

Gilligan, C. (1982). *In a different voice: Psychological theory and women's development.* Cambridge, MA: Harvard University Press.

Grambs, J. D. (1989). *Women over 40: Visions and realities.* New York, NY: Springer Publishing Co., Inc.

Haley, W. E., Levine, E. G., Brown, S. L., & Bartolucci, A. A. (1987). Stress, appraisal, coping, and social support as predictors of adaptational outcome among dementia caregivers. *Psychology and Aging, 2*(4), 323-330.

Hareven, T. K. (1992). Family and generational relations in the later years: A historical perspective. *Generations, 17*(3), 17-22.

Harris, R. L., Elliott, A. M., & Holmes, D. S. (1986). The timing of psychosocial transitions and changes in women's lives: An examination of women aged 45 to 60. *Journal of Personality and Social Psychology, 51,* 409-416.

Havighurst, R. J., & Albrecht, R. (1953). *Older people.* New York, NY: Longmans, Green.

Hayslip, B. H., & Panek, P. E. (1993). *Adult development and aging.* New York, NY: HarperCollins College Publishers.

Heinemann, G. D. (1983). Family involvement and support for widowed persons. In T. H. Brubaker (Ed.), *Family relationships in later life* (pp. 127-148). Newbury Park, CA: Sage Publications, Inc.

Hendricks, J., & Leedham, C. A. (1991). Theories of aging: Implications for human services. In P. K. H. Kim (Ed.), *Serving the elderly: Skills for practice* (pp. 1-25). New York, NY: Hawthorne Aldine de Gruyter.

Hooyman, N. R., & Kiyak, H. A. (1993). *Social gerontology: A multidisciplinary perspective* (3rd ed.). Needham Heights, MA: Allyn & Bacon.

Jung, C. G. (1933). *Modern man in search of a soul.* New York, NY: Harcourt, Brace, and Company.

Kelly, J. R., Steinkamp, M. W., & Kelly, J. R. (1986). Later life leisure: How they play in Peoria. *The Gerontologist, 26*(5), 531-537.

Kornhober, A., & Woodward, K. L. (1981). *Grandparents/grandchildren: The vital connection.* Garden City, NY: Anchor Press/Doubleday.

Levinson, D. J. (1978). *The seasons of a man's life.* New York, NY: Alfred A. Knopf, Inc.

Mannell, R. C. (1993). High-investment activity and life satisfaction among older adults: Committed, serious leisure, and flow activities. In J. R. Kelly (Ed.), *Activity and Aging: Staying Involved.* Newbury Park, CA: Sage Publications, Inc.

Markides, K., & Hoppe, S. (1985). Marital satisfaction in three generations of Mexican Americans. *Social Science Quarterly, 66,* (March), 147-154.

McCluskey, N. G. (1989). Retirement and the contemporary family. *Journal of Psychotherapy and the Family, 5*(1-2), 211-224.

Morgan, J. C. (1979). *Becoming old.* New York, NY: Springer Publishing Co., Inc.

Neugarten, B. L., & Hagestad, G. (1976). Aging the life course. In R. H. Binstock & E. Shanas (Eds.), *Handbook of aging and the social sciences* (pp. 35-37). New York, NY: Van Nostrand Reinhold.

Neugarten, B. L., & Neugarten, D. A. (1987, May). The changing meanings of age. *Psychology Today, 21*(5), 29-33.

Porcino, J. (1983). *Growing older getting better: A handbook for women in the second half of life.* Reading, MA: Addison-Wesley Publishing, Co.

Reinke, B. J., Holmes, D. S., & Harris, S. L. (1985). The timing of psychosocial changes in women's lives: The years 25 to 45. *Journal of Personality and Social Psychology, 48,* 1353-1364.

Riddick, C. (1985). Life satisfaction determinants of older males and females. *Leisure Sciences, 1*(1), 47-63.

Riley, M. W., & Foner, A. (1972). *Aging and society.* New York, NY: Russell Sage Foundation.

Roberts, K. A., & Scott, J. P. (1986). Friendships of older men and women: Exchange patterns and satisfaction. *Psychology and Aging, 1,* 103-109.

Robertson, J. F. (1977). Grandmotherhood: A study of role conceptions. *Journal of Marriage and the Family, 39,* 165-174.

Rose, A. M. (1965). A current theoretical issue is social gerontology. In A. M. Rose & W. A. Peterson (Eds.), *Older people and their social worlds.* Philadelphia, PA: F. A. Davis Co.

Shamoian, C. A., & Thurston, F. D. (1986). Marital discord and divorce among the elderly. *Medical Aspects of Human Sexuality, 20*(8), 25-34.

Siegel, R. J. (1990). Love and work after 60: An integration of personal and professional growth within a long-term marriage. *Journal of Women and Aging, 2*(2), 69-79.

Smyer, M., & Hofland, B. F. (1982). Divorce and family support in later life. *Journal of Family Issues, 3,* 61-77.

Stevens-Long, J. (1984). *Adult life: Developmental processes* (2nd ed.). Palo Alto, CA: Mayfield Publishing Co.

Vinick, B. H., & Ekerdt, D. J. (1989). Retirement and the family. *Generations, 13*(2), 53-56.

Whitbourne, S. K. (1987). Personality development in adulthood and old age: Relationships among identity style, health, and well-being. In K. W. Schaie & C. Eisdorfer (Eds.), *Annual review of gerontology and geriatrics* (pp. 189-216). New York, NY: Springer Publishing Co., Inc.

Wister, A. (1990). Living arrangements and informal social support among the elderly. *Journal of Housing for the Elderly, 6*(1-2), 33-43.

Wood, V., & Robertson, J. F. (1976). The significance of grandparenthood. In J. F. Gubrium (Ed.), *Time, roles, and self in old age* (pp. 278-304). New York, NY: Human Sciences Press.

Key Terms

Accident
Activities of Daily Living (ADLs)
Acute Disease
Arthritis
Cancer
Cardiovascular Disease
Chronic Disease
Chronic Obstructive Pulmonary
    Diseases (COPD)
Diabetes
Functional Independence

Health Status
Heart Disease
Impairment
Influenza
Instrumental Activities of Daily
    Living (IADLs)
Metabolic Disease
Oral Disease
Osteoporosis
Pneumonia
Thyroid Disease

Learning Objectives

1. Explain differences between normal aging versus disease processes in older adults.
2. Describe the health status of older Americans.
3. Distinguish between acute and chronic health problems.
4. Describe the common chronic physical health problems of older adults.
5. Define the concepts of activities of daily living (ADLs), instrumental activities of daily living (IADLs), and functional independence.
6. Describe the prevalence of functional limitations among elderly populations.

Chapter 5

Common Physical Diseases, Illnesses and Disabilities

Introduction

Good health in later life is of great importance to most adults. Declines in body functions that are associated with growing older do not necessarily mean that all adults will automatically suffer from illness or disablement when they are elderly. Health status, good or bad, is highly individual in the older adult population. There is a great deal of variability in how acute and chronic conditions are experienced from one older person to the next.

In this chapter health-related conditions are distinguished from the normal aging process. Health status is discussed, especially as it influences functional limitations and independence. An overview of chronic and acute conditions that are common among older adults is given. The chapter concludes with a discussion of functional independence and the management of health status in old age.

Health and Normal Aging

In spite of the inevitable declines in physical functioning that are expected with age, poor health is not necessarily a consequence of growing older. Health status, in large measure, is determined by several factors both within the individual, as well as the environment in which he or she lives. A lowered resistance and/or genetic predisposition in older persons may increase the risk for disease or illness in later life from environmental carcinogens and infections. Also, losses in other bodily functions (e.g., bone demineralization) may place an elderly person at greater risk for accidents or injuries from falls. Selected sociodemographic factors (poverty, education, race, gender) also are related to increased incidence of illness or disease. Stress may influence the older person's ability to fight infections or cope with long-term disease. Therefore, health maintenance and promotion are vital concerns of the elderly. Older adults are very aware of the consequences of poor health. For example, the loss of financial security, personal autonomy, and social network in the wake of one or more chronic diseases can be overwhelming and threatening to long-term survival. Health status, therefore, is a significant concern of the older population.

Traditionally, the health status of the nation has been measured on the basis of key vital statistics such as life expectancy, mortality rates, morbidity statistics, and the control of infectious disease (Thompson, 1981). This view, however, leaves certain gaps in our understanding of the health status of older people. The World Health Organization (WHO) (1947) envisioned health as more than the absence of disease, illness, or disability. According to the WHO, health is the combination and interaction of physical, mental, and social well-being. Good health is a sense of well-being that is experienced when the body, mind, spirit, and social aspects of life are in harmony.

While growing older may increase the risk of experiencing *chronic* (long-term) disease, most older people perceive their health positively and do not feel that their health is limiting their daily activities. Those older adults who are happier and more satisfied with their lives also tend to be healthier. The fact that the elderly have a higher risk for chronic disease, as well as a lower resistance to *acute* (short-term) illnesses, does not mean that growing old guarantees a poorer health status. Most chronic diseases are the product of long-term engagement in hazardous habits and a lower resistance to disease may be combated by maintaining a vigorous lifestyle.

Chronic Disease versus Acute Disease

Chronic diseases are distinguished from acute diseases in several ways. Chronic diseases are usually the most troubling in old age because they are difficult to diagnose and manage. As adults experience changes associated with normal aging, distinguishing the symptoms associated with chronic disease is often complicated. Aches and pains, fatigue, transient changes in appetite, vision disturbances, occasional feelings of depression or confusion may be experienced as part of growing old, as well as associated with a chronic disease (Ferrini and Ferrini, 1993).

Chronic diseases are ongoing, have progressive deteriorative effects, and usually are irreversible or incurable. Chronic diseases often start much earlier in life (e.g., heart disease) but become manifest in later life when treatment and management is more difficult or impossible. It is not uncommon for older persons to experience long-term financial, social, and psychological adversity in the presence of a newly diagnosed chronic disease. Seven of the 10 leading causes of death among persons age 65 and older are the following chronic conditions: heart disease, cancers, cerebrovascular disease, chronic obstructive pulmonary disease, diabetes mellitus, atherosclerosis, and chronic nephritis or nephrosis (National Center for Health

Statistics, 1990). Among the elderly, four of every five persons suffer from at least one chronic disease (Ferrini and Ferrini, 1993).

The older the person becomes, the greater the risk of experiencing one or more chronic disease. Among people who are over age 80, 70% of the women and 53% of the men have more than one chronic disease (Guralnick, LaCroix, Everett, and Kovar, 1989). While some individuals and some chronic diseases do not seriously impair daily functioning, other conditions are devastating. The incidence of chronic disease is much higher among the elderly than any other age group in the U.S. population.

Acute diseases, on the other hand, are episodic and short-term in duration. They are caused by viral, bacterial, or fungal infections. These illnesses come on rapidly and are usually curable through medical treatment. The cost of healthcare for acute diseases is typically much lower than for chronic diseases due to the short-term, curable nature of the condition. Older people have about the same risk for infectious or acute diseases as do younger people. The complications that may result from an acute illness episode, however, can be deadly for older persons whose immune system resistance is lower. The occurrence of pneumonia and influenza is especially high in the elderly, and these infections combined account for the fifth leading cause of death among persons over age 65.

The presence of one or more chronic diseases increases the risk for secondary, acute infections. Also, poor management of environmental quality (e.g., clean, temperature controlled air) may increase the incidence and severity of acute diseases among elderly persons. Some viruses and bacteria remain in the body in a latent state to reoccur in older adulthood (e.g., herpes zoster or shingles, and tuberculosis). The diagnosis of acute diseases, like that of chronic diseases, is more difficult in older persons. Symptoms (e.g., loss of interest or appetite, depression, fatigue) may be confused with existing chronic diseases, aging-related declines, or medication interactions. Thus, acute diseases present special challenges in the diagnosis and treatment as well as in the management of health status in the elderly.

In summary, older people suffer from more chronic and acute diseases than do younger persons. The risk for multiple chronic and acute diseases increases with age. These conditions may go unrecognized, and thus untreated, because of the extra attention needed to identify symptoms and to render a proper diagnosis. The elderly have increased susceptibility to secondary infections and adverse drug interactions. The psychological impact of chronic and acute diseases often goes unreported and undetected, thus complicating treatment and health management. Finally, the care and management of health in elderly persons may be challenged by a shrinking social support system (especially among the very old), as well as a healthcare system that discriminates against the very old (Kemp, 1993).

Chronic Diseases Common among Older Adults

Heart disease is the leading cause of death among older persons, followed by cancer and cerebrovascular diseases. These three chronic conditions account for more than 75% of all deaths in people over age 65. Cardiovascular disease increases dramatically with age in both men and women. Other common chronic conditions of the elderly include arthritis, osteoporosis, chronic obstructive pulmonary diseases, diabetes, urinary system diseases, and intestinal diseases (Ferrini and Ferrini, 1993).

Cardiovascular Disease

Heart disease accounts for nearly 50% of all deaths among the elderly. Atherosclerosis, coronary artery disease, high blood pressure (hypertension), and congestive heart failure are the most common diseases of the cardiovascular system (Ferrini and Ferrini, 1993).

Atherosclerosis is a narrowing of the blood vessels that occurs over time with the deposition of fat on the lining of the vessel wall. This condition begins in childhood and progresses throughout life as a result of a diet that is high in cholesterol or fat-saturated foods. Atherosclerosis is a form of arteriosclerosis, which includes a number of pathological conditions in which there are thickening, hardening, and a progressive loss of elasticity in the blood vessels. Atherosclerosis is a disease condition that results primarily from a diet that is high in animal-based fat. Other factors that increase the risk of atherosclerosis are high blood pressure, stress, diabetes mellitus, obesity, sedentary lifestyle, cigarette smoking, and familial predisposition to heart attacks (Ferrini and Ferrini, 1993; MacNeil and Teague, 1987).

As atherosclerosis progresses slowly cutting off blood supply due to thickened vessel walls and fatty deposits, the risk of injury to the affected organ increases. Clogged arteries can occur anywhere throughout the body but the most life-threatening areas that can be affected are the coronary (heart) arteries as well as the vessels leading to the brain. The reduced blood flow to the heart results in coronary artery disease (heart disease). If the blood supply is compromised or blocked too long, the heart muscle is damaged and a heart attack may ensue. Symptoms of a heart attack are pain in the neck, arm and/or chest; shortness of breath; weakness; dizziness; confusion; and/or numbness.

Atherosclerosis in the legs can cause cramping and pain in the legs. Coldness or numbness also may be experienced. Modifications in diet, increased exercise, and the cessation of other hazardous health habits have been shown to slow the development of atherosclerosis.

Hypertension, or high blood pressure, also increases the risk for heart disease and stroke. Blood pressure that is higher than 140 hg systolic and 90 hg diastolic represents an increased risk for organ damage and heart attack. Arteriosclerosis will normally elevate blood pressure with age but not to the extent necessary to present a risk factor for a heart attack or stroke. A variety of factors are suspected of causing hypertension including age, gender, stress, genetics, race, diet (especially high intake of salt), and obesity (Ferrini and Ferrini, 1993). In most cases of high blood pressure, however, the cause is not known. Untreated hypertension results in damage to the heart and other organs of the body. Hypertension may be treated with drug therapy, reduced salt intake, exercise, reduced fat intake, the elimination of cigarette smoking, and reduced alcohol consumption.

Congestive heart failure results when the heart muscle can no longer pump adequately to meet the demands of the body. When the heart is unable to pump sufficiently, damage to other organs results because an insufficient blood supply is delivered to them. Symptoms associated with congestive heart failure are shortness of breath and swelling from the accumulation of blood and fluid in the body (edema). Hypertension is the leading cause of congestive heart failure followed by heart attacks, diabetes, and diseased heart valves. Congestive heart failure can be managed with medications, rest, and dietary modifications (Ferrini and Ferrini, 1993; Hooyman and Kiyak, 1991; MacNeil and Teague, 1987).

Cerebrovascular Disease

Atherosclerosis and arteriosclerosis also can affect the blood vessels to the brain, thus increasing the risk for stroke or cerebrovascular injury. Stroke is the disruption of the blood supply to the brain or an area within the brain which causes brain injury, malfunction, or death of brain cells. Stroke or cerebrovascular disease is the third leading cause of death among persons age 65 years and older. The risk of stroke increases in persons who have heart disease (Ferrini and Ferrini, 1993; Hooyman and Kiyak, 1991; MacNeil and Teague, 1987).

Strokes can be caused by either a blood clot (cerebral thrombosis) that cuts off or reduces blood to the brain, or when a weak area of a blood vessel in the brain bursts causing a brain hemorrhage. Hemorrhage occurs primarily among persons with high blood pressure, and strokes caused by clots are more common among the elderly in general. Strokes are a major cause of disability among the elderly. Depending on what part of and how much of the brain is damaged, the stroke victim will experience damaged functioning to some area of the body. Paralysis to one side of the body or damage to the speech center are sometimes permanent. Some areas of functioning, however, can be regained through rehabilitation that makes use of unaffected areas of the brain (Ferrini and Ferrini, 1993; Hooyman and Kiyak, 1991; MacNeil and Teague, 1987).

One of the warning signs of a pending stroke is called a transient ischemic attack (TIA) or mini-stroke. TIAs are small disruptions that often only last for a short time (e.g., a few minutes to a few hours). The symptoms associated with TIAs include weakness, dizziness or blackout, disturbances in speech, and changes in personality or affect. Strokes are preventable by reducing the risk factors (i.e., high blood pressure), medical management of diabetes, and drug therapy to thin the blood (Ferrini and Ferrini, 1993).

Cancer

Cancer, or malignant neoplasm, is the second leading cause of death among the elderly. There are different types of cancers, the most common of which are: lung, colon and rectal, stomach, pancreatic, prostate, and breast (Ferrini and Ferrini, 1993; Hooyman and Kiyak, 1991; MacNeil and Teague, 1987). Lung cancer is the leading cancer-related cause of death in older persons followed by colon and rectal (colorectal) cancer.

The incidence of lung cancer is much higher in men than in women; however, more women die from lung cancer compared with breast cancer. The leading cause of lung cancer is cigarette smoking, which is responsible for more than 90% of all lung cancer. Other causes of lung cancer include environmental toxins such as air pollution and secondhand cigarette smoke. Smokers are more likely to get mouth cancers and if the smoker also consumes alcohol, the risk of developing oral cancer increases (Ferrini and Ferrini, 1993; MacNeil and Teague, 1987).

Colon and rectal cancers constitute the second leading source of death among elderly Americans, with colon cancer the more common of the two forms. If colon cancer is diagnosed when localized, survival rates are higher; however, if it is not identified until after spreading, the probability of survival is seriously diminished. Colorectal cancer's contributing factors are:

(a) family history of cancer;
(b) persistent colon inflammation;
(c) polyps in the colon;
(d) high fat, low fiber diet; and
(e) sedentary lifestyle.

The most common symptom associated with colorectal cancer is rectal bleeding which is easily detected through regular health screening. Most colon cancer is treated with surgery followed by chemotherapy and radiation to help prevent recurrence. The recurrence rate for colorectal cancer is quite high at 50% (Ferrini and Ferrini, 1993).

Breast cancer is the second most common cancer which causes death in older women. Approximately 75% of all breast cancer is diagnosed in older women with the causes still not definitely known. Suspected risk factors include higher levels of estrogen, high-fat diet, sedentary lifestyle, obesity, inadequate exposure to sunlight which results in an inadequate production of vitamin D, and family history. Early detection through regular screening and early treatment are effective in reducing the morbidity and mortality rates associated with breast cancer (American Cancer Society, 1991). The appearance of a suspicious lump is the most common symptom of breast cancer. Treatment can range from radiation and lumpectomy to the removal of the breast (mastectomy) or, in some cases, a radical mastectomy to remove the breast, lymph nodes, and surrounding tissue. Radical mastectomy is typically only pursued when the cancer has spread beyond the localized lump to the lymph nodes. Treatment success for breast cancer is quite high, especially with early detection through self-examination and mammography. Older women, however, engage in self-examination and routine mammography screening at a significantly lower rate than do younger women. When breast cancer is identified in older women, aggressive treatment is sometimes not pursued with parallel vigor to that for younger women. Thus, improvement in the rate of self-examination and more aggressive treatment of breast cancer among older women is a needed service area (American Cancer Society, 1991).

Men experience prostate cancer at a rate that makes it the second leading cancer-related cause of death with 80% of all cases found in elderly men. Prostate cancer is a slow-growing cancer which makes it amenable to early detection and treatment. Risk factors for prostate cancer include age, race (more black men experience prostate cancer than white men), and testosterone levels. Detection is through either an annual internal examination for nodules on the prostate and/or a specific blood test. Cancer that is just in the prostate can be surgically removed. If the cancer has spread (metastasized), surgical removal of the testes or hormone therapy are used to manage the disease (American Cancer Society, 1991).

Skin cancer is the last cancer that will be discussed in this chapter. Death from skin cancer is generally not common; however, the risk of skin cancer with age makes it a concern of the elderly. There are several types of skin cancers, of which only one is deadly—melanoma. The primary cause of skin cancers is excess exposure to sunlight, and people with a history of sunburning are at greater risk for skin cancer. With ozone depletion and the sociocultural value attached to suntanned skin, the rate of skin cancers is increasing in recent years. In fact, 90% of all melanoma cases have occurred in the past 10 years (Glass and Hoover, 1989). Symptoms of skin cancer include abnormal mole-like growths that continue to grow, change in color, and easily bleed with injury. Early detection of basal cell, squamous, and melanoma cancers are treatable through surgical removal of the cancer cells. If melanoma has spread to other parts of the body, chemotherapy is used to treat the cancer (American Cancer Society, 1991).

Often the symptoms associated with cancers are not easy to detect in the early stages because they are confused with normal aging-related changes. Weakness and fatigue, depression, weight loss, and changes in appetite are some of the symptoms difficult to differentiate. The warning signals of potential cancer are:

(a) changes in bowel or bladder functions,
(b) nagging cough or hoarseness,
(c) rectal discharge or bleeding,
(d) a lump or thickening in the breast or elsewhere on the body,
(e) an unhealed sore,
(f) difficulty swallowing or intestinal disturbance, and
(g) changes in a wart or mole (Ferrini and Ferrini, 1993).

Cancer is treated using radiation, chemotherapy, and/or surgery. The course of treatment is determined by the overall health status of the individual, the type of cancer, and the growth rate of the cancer. The high incidence of cancer in the elderly may be related to the length of time it takes for most cancers to develop and be detected, in addition to immune system declines with age. Diet, lifestyle, and environmental carcinogens also have been implicated in the increasing incidence of cancer.

Chronic Obstructive Pulmonary Diseases

The occurrence of chronic respiratory conditions increases with age due primarily to declines in pulmonary functioning, genetic disposition, and long-term exposure to environmental carcinogens of which cigarette smoking is the leading cause. Decrements in the immune system also may contribute to increased episodes of acute respiratory infections which eventually lead to chronic obstructive pulmonary disease (COPD). COPD is characterized by seriously damaged lung tissues, resulting from several conditions including chronic bronchitis, emphysema, fibrosis, and asthma. Each of these COPDs develop slowly, are progressive, may result in frequent hospitalization, produce major changes in lifestyle, and often end in death.

Chronic bronchitis, the most common COPD, is characterized by the production of abundant sputum and a chronic cough. Breathing becomes more difficult as the condition progresses (Boss and Seegmiller, 1981).

Emphysema is the destruction of the lung air sacs which reduces oxygen intake and the excretion of carbon dioxide. Emphysema is common among longtime smokers and is irreversible. Modifications in lifestyle and pain-reducing exercises can be used to manage the effects of this disease (Ferrini and Ferrini, 1993).

The treatment of COPD includes respiratory therapy, drug therapy, breathing exercises, environmental management to reduce exposure to air pollution, and lifestyle modifications (e.g., smoking cessation). As individuals age, the debilitating aspects of COPD sometimes dominate their attention, thus reducing the ability to attend to other activities. It is not uncommon to find a COPD patient totally preoccupied with his or her disease (Ferrini and Ferrini, 1993).

Diabetes Mellitus

There are two types of diabetes mellitus: Type I or insulin-dependent diabetes which usually is first diagnosed in youth, and Type II or noninsulin-dependent diabetes which generally presents in middle through later adulthood. The prevalence of diabetes, primarily Type II, in older adults is approximately 20% of all people over age 65. This percentage increases among African-American, Hispanic, and Native-American populations (Ferrini and Ferrini, 1993).

Diabetes is caused by the lack of production or utilization of insulin in the metabolism of glucose (sugar) by the body's cells. In older adults, Type II diabetes is characterized by elevated levels of glucose in the blood and urine. Insulin, even if produced, is inadequately used by the body's cells in the metabolism of glucose. The result is an over-releasing of glucose in the blood by the liver, as well as an elevated production of insulin by the pancreas (Ferrini and Ferrini, 1993).

Symptoms associated with Type II diabetes are increased appetite, increased urination, weight loss, fatigue and weakness, excessive thirst, and slowed healing of wounds. These symptoms may be confused with other aging-related changes in elderly persons. The detection of diabetes in older persons is often discovered through routine eye examination, medical testing, and hospitalization for other conditions. Predisposing factors that increase the risk for diabetes in old age include obesity and persistent overeating behavior (Ferrini and Ferrini, 1993; Hooyman and Kiyak, 1991).

The treatment of Type II diabetes includes:

(a) weight loss through specified diets that are low in sugar and saturated fats while high in complex carbohydrates and fiber;
(b) regular exercise; and
(c) medications, in some but not all cases.

Diabetes can have long-term, deleterious effects on other body systems including eye infections, vision loss, kidney failure and infections, and peripheral nerve damage (Ferrini and Ferrini, 1993). Therefore, it is very important that older adults strictly manage their diets and exercise regimens in order to minimize subsequent damage to other organs. Increased risk of cardiovascular and cerebrovascular disease is common among older adults who have Type II diabetes. Once Type II diabetes is diagnosed, medical management of the disease is required in order to prevent additional complications (Ferrini and Ferrini, 1993; Hooyman and Kiyak, 1991).

Skeletal Conditions

Osteoporosis and arthritis are the most common chronic skeletal conditions affecting the elderly. These conditions often result in functional activity limitations among older adults with the number of activity limitations increasing with age. Not all older persons, however, experience functional limitations, but most suffer from the excruciating pain associated with these skeletal disorders. These disorders are progressive, often beginning in middle adulthood. Arthritis is the leading cause of loss in functioning among all age groups in the U.S. (Ferrini and Ferrini, 1993; Hooyman and Kiyak, 1991).

Arthritis

Arthritis includes over 100 inflammatory, degenerative conditions of the skeletal system's joints and bones. Osteoarthritis, the most common type of arthritis, is a degenerative joint disease that occurs through a wearing away of the protective cartilage of the joint. Aggravating causes of osteoarthritis include aging-related deterioration of the joint, overuse wear and tear, injury, genetic disposition, and obesity. Pain, decreases in function (e.g., range of motion), and joint crackling are commonly experienced symptoms of the disease. Treatment for osteoarthritis includes weight loss, low-impact exercise (e.g., walking), heat, and painkillers (e.g., aspirin) (Ferrini and Ferrini, 1993; Hooyman and Kiyak, 1991).

Rheumatoid arthritis is caused by persistent inflammation of the joint membranes. The small bones of the feet and hands are more commonly affected but other joints can be involved also. Rheumatoid arthritis is a degenerative, deteriorative disease of the joints. Left untreated, the disease will result in loss of function. Rheumatoid arthritis is episodic; that is, it typically begins by middle adulthood and recurs as acute attacks interspersed with inactive periods. As the disease progresses throughout middle and older adulthood, severe symptoms may be experienced during acute attacks (fatigue, weight loss, fever, pain, redness and swelling, stiffness in many joints, and malaise) (Hooyman and Kiyak, 1991). Treatment involves initial rest, exercise, painkillers, as well as other anti-inflammatory medications, and corticosteroids. Joint repair through surgery is used to correct severe degeneration and deformity. Medical management and treatment of rheumatoid arthritis can prevent crippling effects of the disease (Ferrini and Ferrini, 1993; Hooyman and Kiyak, 1991).

Osteoporosis

Osteoporosis is the aging-related loss of bone mass at an accelerated rate which causes serious structural weakness and vulnerability to fractures. As bone mass is lost, the accumulated effects in later life include weak bones, height loss, slumped posture, dowager's hump, and backache (Ferrini and Ferrini, 1993; Hooyman and Kiyak, 1991).

Bone density and bone loss are conditions associated with normal aging. The building of bone density peaks somewhere between age 20 and 35 after which progressive, gradual declines in bone mass occur under normal aging conditions. Osteoporosis is the abnormally accelerated loss in bone density which is why it is considered a disease condition. Fractures of the hip are the most common and problematic consequence of osteoporotic bones. Among the very old (over age 80), hip fractures often portend a poor recovery and an increased risk for mortality (Ferrini and Ferrini, 1993; Hooyman and Kiyak, 1991).

The risk factors associated with osteoporosis include family history and genetic disposition, estrogen and calcium losses during menopause, sedentary lifestyle, cigarette smoking, excessive alcohol consumption, race (Caucasian), gender (females), and high caffeine consumption (Hooyman and Kiyak, 1991). Since prevention is the preferred treatment approach, changes in diet and lifestyle should begin long before old age. Increasing dietary intake of calcium, vitamin D, and fluoride are recommended, as is modified weight-bearing exercise (e.g., stair climbing, walking). Therapeutic doses of estrogen also are increasingly being recommended for women, especially those in menopause.

Genitourinary Conditions

As adults age, the incidence of genital and urinary problems increase. Chronic conditions are a result of gradual deterioration in the excretory system. As kidney function declines, the probability of disease increases. Incomplete emptying of the bladder in women may bring about inflammation or cystitis. Older men frequently experience a gradual enlargement of the prostate which interferes with urination. Noncancerous enlargement is called benign prostatic hyperplasia and is caused by changes in testosterone production. This condition is experienced by as many as 70% of men between the ages of 60 and 70, and 90% of men age 90 and older (Ferrini and Ferrini, 1993).

Enlargement of the prostate affects urinary functioning because of the anatomical proximity of the prostate to the urethra. Typical symptoms include hesitancy when beginning urination, reduced force, increased frequency of urination, dribbling, and the lack of ability to completely empty the bladder (Ferrini and Ferrini, 1993). Currently, if proper urinary function is disrupted by an enlarged prostate, balloon dilation is used to widen the urethra. Drug-induced prostate shrinkage is being studied as an alternative course of treatment (Loughlin, 1991).

Chronic urinary incontinence is a fairly common problem among the elderly which increases in prevalence with age. The rate of incidence varies for noninstitutionalized older persons compared with those people who are in hospitals or nursing homes. Herzog, Diokno, Brown, Normolle and Brock (1990) estimated that as many as 19% of men and 38% of women who were noninstitutionalized experienced urinary incontinence. This disorder is caused by a number of factors including nervous system problems, infection, muscle weakening, and medication interactions

(Ferrini and Ferrini, 1993). Medical management of incontinence ranges from drug therapy to special exercises, biofeedback, surgical repair, urination flow devices, and other supportive measures.

Four types of urinary incontinence are experienced by the elderly. When uncontrolled leakage of urine coincides with sneezing, coughing, laughing, lifting, or exercise it is called stress incontinence. This form of incontinence is a result of muscle weakness around the bladder and urethra. It is common among women and is related to childbirth, surgery, and estrogen deficiency (Ferrini and Ferrini, 1993).

Enlargement of the prostate often influences the ability to sense when the bladder is full, thus resulting in overflow incontinence when a full bladder leaks out a small amount of urine. Urge incontinence, on the other hand, is the inability to hold urine when experiencing the urge to urinate. Urge incontinence is frequently associated with neurological disorders (e.g., stroke, dementia) or infection.

The fourth type of incontinence is a result of an unwillingness or inability to urinate normally. It is called functional incontinence and may be cause by any number of reasons including medications, psychiatric disturbances, the presence of other diseases, or impaired mobility (Ferrini and Ferrini, 1993; Hooyman and Kiyak, 1991).

Urinary incontinence presents both a chronic health problem and a social problem. It is socially unacceptable in public while also representing a highly personal health behavior. Incontinence is often a deciding factor in nursing home placement. For these reasons and others, the management of this disorder is of great interest and importance to elders, their caregivers, and the healthcare system.

Other Chronic Conditions

Elders also can experience a variety of other chronic health conditions including skin irritations, thyroid dysfunction, oral diseases, and intestinal disorders. While these conditions may be less problematic in terms of long-term survival, they are still bothersome and may create additional difficulties when combined with more serious chronic diseases (e.g., cancer).

Skin Conditions

Older adults suffer from skin disorders primarily due to gradual changes in the integumentary system, long-term exposure to sunlight, the effects of environmental pollutants, and familial history. Psoriasis, or scaly skin, tends to run in families and can be quite bothersome to the older adult (Hooyman and Kiyak, 1991).

Chronic itching, or senile pruritus, is very common among older adults. This disorder can be very distressing if it is severe. It may be caused by any number of factors including underlying disease (diabetes, cancer, etc.); drug reaction; lice, flea, or mite infestation; or stress, tension, and emotional upset (Hooyman and Kiyak, 1991).

Finally, older diabetic adults may experience stasis dermatitis on the legs due to diminished circulation. The skin will appear scaly, reddened, shiny, and will have reduced growth of hair. The treatment of most skin conditions primarily consists of controlling irritation with creams, relieving symptoms by warm water bathing, light therapy, and prescription drugs to avoid additional infection (Hooyman and Kiyak, 1991).

Thyroid Dysfunction

Older adults, particularly women, may experience thyroid dysfunction either as an excess of thyroid hormone (hyperthyroid) or as a deficiency (hypothyroid). Hypothyroidism is the more common of the two conditions and can cause death if not treated. Typical symptoms include constipation, weight gain, cold intolerance, depression, psychic disturbances (e.g., hallucinations), slowed mental processes, and the inability to respond to stress. Treatment is by thyroid hormone replacement and is usually effective in reversing the symptoms of this dysfunction (Ferrini and Ferrini, 1993).

The less common hyperthyroidism has the opposite symptomatology (e.g., irritability, tremors, diarrhea, weight loss, heat sensitivity, sweating, and increased heart rate). Hyperthyroidism is also treatable.

Intestinal Disorders

Intestinal disorders in the elderly are primarily caused by poor or unbalanced diet. Diverticulitis, or inflamed intestinal sacs, results from inadequate intake of dietary fiber. Symptoms include disrupted bowel function, bleeding, abdominal discomfort, and nausea. Treatment involving dietary changes and antibiotics are effective in alleviating this condition (Hooyman and Kiyak, 1991).

Older adults also frequently complain about constipation. Most constipation is caused by inadequate exercise, stress, other diseases of the gastrointestinal system, poor diet, and overuse of catheters and laxatives. Probably too much attention by elders is given to the regularity of their bowel movements which, in turn, may result in the inappropriate utilization of laxatives. The overuse of laxatives will eventually damage normal functioning of the intestinal tract.

Oral Diseases

Older adults primarily suffer from the loss of teeth, gum disease, and dental caries of the root of the tooth. As preventive dental care has steadily improved, the incidence of these problems may decline among older persons.

Acute Diseases of the Elderly

The two leading causes of acute health problems in elderly persons are influenza/pneumonia and accidents. Influenza and pneumonia are the fifth leading cause of death among older adults while accidents are the seventh leading cause. Because these acute conditions result in high medical care expenditures, they are important considerations in understanding the health status of older people (Ferrini and Ferrini, 1993; MacNeil and Teague, 1987).

Influenza/Pneumonia and Other Infections

Older adults frequently suffer from infections for a variety of reasons. Normal aging changes in the immune system which result in a lowered resistance to infection coupled with the presence of one or more chronic conditions, will often leave the elder more vulnerable to infections. Other bodily changes in the respiratory system may increase the risk of pneumonia due to a lowered ability to adequately clear the lungs. Two acute infections that pose significant risks for the elderly are influenza and pneumonia. Other infections that may be secondary outcomes associated with chronic disease also are threatening to the health and survival of the elderly. Finally, latent infections (e.g., tuberculosis, herpes zoster or shingles) can suddenly reoccur in late life, producing acute illness episodes (Ferrini and Ferrini, 1993; MacNeil and Teague, 1987).

Respiratory infections, particularly the common cold, flu, and pneumonia, are significant acute illnesses that often increase the risk of mortality among older persons. Increased risk is primarily due to lowered resistance, complications, secondary infection, and a lowered ability to clear the lungs and airways of infectious material. The older the person is, the higher the risk of complications and mortality from acute respiratory infections (Ferrini and Ferrini, 1993; MacNeil and Teague, 1987).

Diagnosis and treatment of respiratory infection can be complicated when in the presence of a chronic condition. Medications taken for chronic conditions may mask the typical symptoms used to diagnose acute infections (e.g., fever, elevated white blood cell count). Other symptoms (e.g., confusion, fatigue, appetite loss) can be misinterpreted as an aging-related change rather than associated with an illness.

Because pneumonia and influenza are particularly threatening to elders, immunizations are highly recommended. Type A influenza, the most deadly of three types (A, B, and C), can be avoided through yearly vaccination. Pneumonia, on the other hand, is a serious threat to older people, especially those who are inactive and/or institutionalized in hospitals or nursing homes. Treatment of bacterial pneumonia, which generally is the more dominant type in older persons, is with antibiotics. Vaccines have been developed to protect against pneumonia, but their usefulness among the very old and frail is questionable (Gable et al., 1990).

Other infections that are troubling for elders include appendicitis which is caused by bacterial infection, infected diverticula in the intestine, diarrhea, urinary tract infections, genital infections (vaginitis), bedsores or pressure sores (decubitus ulcers), shingles (latent herpes zoster from childhood chicken pox), tuberculosis, and AIDS. In elders, AIDS is typically contracted either from blood transfusion or homosexual intercourse. The identification of AIDS in older people is confounded by normal aging-related changes and the presence of other chronic conditions. Treatment, therefore, is complicated by lowered immune system functioning and other bodily changes associated with growing older.

Accidents and Injury

Death by accident or injury constitutes the seventh leading cause of death in older persons. The most common types are falls, pedestrian accidents, and motor vehicle accidents. Other causes of injury include medical complications, fires, choking, drowning, and poisoning. Falls and motor vehicle accidents are the leading type of accidental death among older people (Ferrini and Ferrini, 1993).

Elders are more susceptible to accidents and experience more severe injury based on several factors. The most common risk factor is functional loss due to normal aging-related declines. Declines in the nervous and sensory systems result in a slower reaction time and to a decreased awareness of a hazardous situation. Lowered perception of temperature extremes, pain, vision, and hearing contribute to an increased risk for accidents to occur.

Changes in the musculoskeletal system may influence motor abilities (i.e., balance, strength, endurance). Poor nutrition, emotional stress, and medication side effects all may produce lowered capabilities and slower reactions to pending hazardous situations. The existence of other chronic or acute illnesses further impair the elder's functional capabilities which increases the risk for injury and accidents. For example, impaired cognition due to diseases of the central nervous system may influence memory and judgment.

Environmental design factors also significantly contribute to the rate of injury and accidents among the elderly. Personal functional capabilities coupled with poor environmental designs that are not user-friendly to older people produce increased risks for accidents in this segment of the population. Older people are much more vulnerable to extremes in temperature, slick walking surfaces, stairs without handrails, cluttered environments, and traffic lights that change too quickly, just to name some of the aspects of the environment that pose risks to the health of older people.

In the case of accidents in older people, prevention can be very effective in controlling risk and reducing the incidence of death by accident. The placement and kind of furniture, walking surfaces, handrails, room layout, placement of cupboards and shelves, exterior supports and walkways, lighting, and temperature control are special considerations to which professionals who serve the elderly pay close attention. Injury and accidents can be reduced to some degree through environmental design and management as well as by an increased awareness among elders of their vulnerabilities.

Impact of Chronic and Acute Illness on Functional Independence

The older person's ability to maintain his or her independent functioning is an important indicator of his or her overall quality of life and subsequently, his or her health status. As the incidence of chronic and acute illness increases, the individual will potentially experience limitations in his or her daily activities. Limitations in daily activities increase with age and in the presence of illness. Approximately 39% of all people over age 70 experience activity limitations (LaPlante, Rice, and Krauss, 1991). The main cause of activity limitation is impairment due to chronic conditions.

In this section, how functional limitations are impacted by health status and what functional independence means to older persons is explored. According to the National Center for Health Statistics (1984), older people experience three times the number of days of restricted activity compared with younger people. This restricted activity is primarily influenced by health problems. The most prevalent conditions that affect activity limitation are arthritis, high blood pressure, impaired hearing, and heart disease. As age increases, the presence of activity limitation increases, as does the need for assistance.

Functional limitations can be described in two broad categories of activities: activities of daily living (ADLs) and instrumental activities of daily living (IADLs). Typical ADLs are bathing, dressing, getting out of bed, going to the bathroom, and other essential tasks associated with basic daily functioning. IADLs are activities that are concerned with the more instrumental tasks of everyday life, such as meal preparation, managing one's finances, shopping, using community services, etc. Activity limitations begin to occur when an older person needs partial or full assistance with one or more of these ADLs or IADLs. Help with one activity does not necessarily mean dependence with others. However, when older adults need help with three or more ADLs, they are considered unable to perform major activities associated with functional independence (Dawson, Hendershot, and Fulton, 1987; LaPlante, Rice, and Krauss, 1991). In other words, elders who need assistance with IADLs may still demonstrate functional independence within their residence; however, when impairment affects ADLs to the extent that partial or full assistance with three or more ADLs occurs, the elderly may be considered functionally dependent.

The leading personal care or ADL activity with which adults over age 65 experience difficulty is walking (19%). Walking is followed by each of these successive activities: bathing (10%), getting outside (10%), getting in and out of bed (8%), and dressing (6%). The proportion of the elderly who need assistance increases as the over-age-65 group is further subdivided into age strata. For example, 40% of persons over age 85 were reported to have difficulty with walking, 31% with getting around outside, 28% with bathing. Older women tend to report having more difficulty than do older men (Dawson, Hendershot, and Fulton, 1987).

In regard to home management activities or IADLs, almost one fourth of all adults over age 65 report having some problems. Again, the percentages increase with age so that 55% of all persons over age 85 report having some difficulty with IADLs (Dawson, Hendershot, and Fulton, 1987).

According to one study, approximately 23% or 6 million noninstitutionalized adults over age 65 are functionally limited (Dawson, Hendershot, and Fulton, 1987). These difficulties range from personal care activities (ADLs) to instrumental activities (IADLs) such as home management. While functional impairment does not necessarily mean a loss of overall quality of life, the interactive effects of functional losses coupled with the presence of chronic and acute illness does place stress on the older person's lifestyle. Good health in older adulthood means more than the absence of disease. Health status, particularly if it is good, impacts functional independence and therefore, ultimately increases the quality of life in later life. Assisting the elderly in managing, maintaining, and promoting their health will help them to lead active and functionally independent lifestyles in old age.

Summary

In this chapter the differences between normal aging-related change and the illnesses and diseases common among older people are presented. An overview of common chronic and acute conditions that are experienced by elderly persons helps to clarify this difference. It is clear that health status and healthy lifestyle habits influence the functional independence of older adults. Readers who would like to know more about common illnesses and diseases of the elderly are encouraged to consult the references that accompany this chapter.

Comprehension Questions

1. Discuss health status in older adults.
2. Discuss three factors that influence health status in the elderly.
3. Distinguish acute illness from chronic disease.
4. Describe three chronic conditions that are common among older persons.
5. Discuss the most common forms of cancer among elderly men and women.
6. Describe the most common skeletal condition of older women.
7. Why is incontinence a problem among older persons?
8. What is COPD and what treatment approaches can be used with COPD?
9. Describe the two leading causes of acute illness among older persons.
10. Discuss how the ability to perform ADLs and IADLs, or loss thereof, affects the functional independence of older persons.

References

American Cancer Society. (1991). *Cancer facts and figures: 1991.* Atlanta, GA: Author.

Boss, G., & Seegmiller, J. E. (1981). Age-related physiological changes and their clinical significance. *Western Journal of Medicine, 135,* 13-19.

Dawson, D., Hendershot, G., & Fulton, J. (1987). Aging in the eighties: Functional limitations of individuals age 65 years and older (Advance Data from Vital and Health Statistics, no. 133). Washington, DC: U.S. Public Health Service.

Ferrini, A. F., & Ferrini, R. L. (1993). *Health in the later years* (2nd ed.). Madison, WI: Brown & Benchmark.

Gable, C. B., Holder, S. S., Engelhart, L., et al., (1990). Pneumococcal vaccine: Efficacy and associated cost savings. *Journal of the American Medical Association, 264,* 2910-2915.

Glass, A. G., & Hoover, R. N. (1989). The emerging epidemic of melanoma and squamous cell skin cancer. *Journal of the American Medical Association, 262*(15), 2097-2100.

Guralnick, J. M., LaCroix, A. Z., Everett, D. F., & Kovar, M. G. (1989). Aging in the eighties: The prevalence of comorbidity and its association with disability (Advance Data from Vital and Health Statistics, No. 170, DHHS Pub. No. 89-1250). Washington, DC: U.S. Public Health Service.

Herzog, A. R., Diokno, A. C., Brown, M. B., Normolle, D. P., & Brock, B. M. (1990). Two-year incidence, remission and change patterns of urinary incontinence in non-institutionalized older adults. *Journal of Gerontology, 45*(2), M67-74.

Hooyman, N. R., & Kiyak, H. A. (1991). *Social gerontology: A multidisciplinary perspective* (2nd ed.). Needham Heights, MA: Allyn & Bacon.

Kemp, B. (1993, Winter). Critical aspects of geriatric rehabilitation: How older people are different. *Aging and Vision News, 5*(1), 4-5.

LaPlante, M. P., Rice, D. P., & Krauss, L. E. (1991). *Disability Statistics Abstract: People with activity limitations in the U.S.* San Francisco, CA: University of California School of Nursing.

Loughlin, K. R. (1991). Medical and nonmedical therapies for benign prostatic hypertrophy. *Geriatrics, 46*(6), 26-34.

MacNeil, R. D., & Teague, M. L. (1987). *Aging and leisure: Vitality in later life.* Englewood Cliffs, NJ: Prentice Hall.

National Center for Health Statistics. (1990). Advance report on final mortality statistics: 1988. *NCHS Monthly Vital Statistics Report, 39*(7), Supplement No. 21.

National Center for Health Statistics. (1984). Changes in mortality among the elderly, United States, 1940-78 supplement to 1980. *Vital and health statistics,* Series 3. DHHS Publication No. (PHS) 82-1406a.

Thompson, F. J. (1981). *Health policy and the bureaucracy: Politics and imple-mentation.* Cambridge, MA: The MIT Press.

World Health Organization. (1947). Constitution of the World Health Organization. *Chronicle of the World Health Organization,* 29-43.

Key Terms

Alcoholism
Alzheimer's Disease
Anosognosia
Antidepressant Drugs
Anxiety Disorders
Bereavement
Bipolar Disorders
Counseling
Delirium
Delusions
Dementia
Depression
Drug Abuse
Electroconvulsive Therapy
Excess Disability
Family Therapy
Functional Mental Disorders

Group Therapy
Hallucinations
Iatrogenic Disorders
Multi-Infarct Dementia
Organic Cognitive Disorders
Paraphrenia
Paranoia
Perseveration
Polypharmacy
Pseudodementia
Psychosis
Psychotherapy
Schizophrenia
Sundowning
Tardive Dyskinesia
Wandering Behavior

Learning Objectives

1. Identify conditions and diseases that cause cognitive dysfunction in elderly persons.
2. Describe the types, origins, causes, and symptoms of organic cognitive disorders in elderly populations.
3. Describe the types, origins, causes, and symptoms of functional mental disorders in elderly populations.

Chapter 6
Psychological Illnesses and Psychiatric Disorders

Introduction

Psychological and psychiatric disorders/diseases of the elderly are often neglected or are thought to be of little importance. Therefore they may receive minimal attention. Depression and organic brain syndrome are the most common disorders exhibited by the elderly. While depression is the most common mental health problem of the elderly, organic brain syndrome is the most feared and the least understood (Edinberg, 1985; Jenike, 1989).

The organization of this chapter proceeds with an overview of the diseases that cause cognitive dysfunction. Organic cognitive disorders are discussed with an emphasis on dementia and its various types including Alzheimer's disease, multi-infarct dementia, Pick's disease, and other dementia-related syndromes. An introduction to the factors that characterize delirium and other reversible causes of mental impairment is included.

Functional mental disorders also are described with an emphasis on depression, anxiety disorders, psychotic illness, alcoholism, and other drug abuse. It is difficult to determine whether the symptoms of functional disorders and organic mental syndromes accurately depict true disorders of aging, reactions to stressful life events and circumstances, or the overt expression of enduring disorders.

Diseases that Cause Cognitive Dysfunction

Diseases and disorders of the elderly that cause cognitive dysfunction may be divided into two general categories: organic and functional. Organic mental syndrome is not a diagnosis; instead, it refers to psychological and behavioral symptoms such as loss of orientation to person, place, and time without reference to a specific cause for the symptoms. *Organic cognitive disorder* is the designation for a particular variety of organic mental syndromes for which the cause has been identified. The most well-known organic mental disorders are delirium and dementia, especially dementia of the Alzheimer's type (Edinberg, 1985; Jenike, 1989).

Organic brain syndromes are recognized by various symptoms including: (a) changes in judgment such as in the capacities for decision making, evaluation, and comprehension; and (b) changes in affect such as either a flat affect or an excessive display of emotions. Other symptoms common to organic brain syndromes are memory impairment; loss of cognition such as in mathematical or learning abilities; and loss of orientation to time (day, date, month, year), place (current location), and person (identity of self and others) (Edinberg, 1985).

Multiple psychological and social factors are involved in both organic and functional mental disorders. Estimates of those older persons who suffer from mental illness range from 15% to 25% of the elderly population. Depression is considered the most prevalent mental disorder among the elderly, affecting nearly 20% of those persons over 65 years of age. However, many other conditions such as anxiety, alcoholism, drug abuse, and schizophrenia also are common among the elderly. Additionally, psychiatric symptoms often occur in older persons suffering from Alzheimer's disease and other chronic medical conditions (Butler, Lewis, and Sunderland, 1991).

Organic Cognitive Disorders

Approximately 25% of elderly individuals suffer from serious diseases of the brain at some point in their lives (Jenike, 1989; Katzman, 1985). The primary organic cognitive disorders are termed dementias. *Dementia* is widely used in reference to many cognitive disorders of the elderly. There are about 50 known types of dementia (Stuart-Hamilton, 1991). Dementia is defined as a loss of intellectual abilities to the degree that it interferes with social or occupational functioning; memory impairment; and at least one of the following: impairment in abstract thinking, judgment, higher cortical function, or personality change (American Psychiatric Association, 1987).

The onset and course of dementia depend upon the underlying cause. Most dementias are considered to be irreversible. Some dementias, however, may be irreversible and progressive; some may be stable; or some may even be reversible to an extent depending upon the cause and the course of treatment (Butler, Lewis, and Sunderland, 1991).

Dementia is characterized by a complex set of symptoms that may be caused by a variety of disorders and these must be considered before diagnosis is complete (Katzman, 1985). The vast majority of dementias are caused by specific brain diseases, lack of adequate blood supply to the brain, or a combination of the two. A careful medical evaluation is required in order to exclude other causes which may be reversible (Butler, Lewis, and Sunderland, 1991; Edinberg, 1985). Common symptoms that are associated with dementia are summarized in Table 6.1 (page 106).

Perseveration, the tendency to emit the same verbal or motor response continually and *anosognosia,* "the apparent unawareness of or failure to recognize one's own functional defect" (Butler, Lewis, and Sunderland, 1991, p. 159), also are consistent with a diagnosis of dementia. Jenike (1989) reported, however, that many patients with progressive dementia are clearly aware of their impairments.

Alzheimer's Disease

One type of dementia is *Alzheimer's disease.* This disease may be referred to as primary degenerative dementia, primary degenerative dementia of the Alzheimer's type, Alzheimer's disease, and senile dementia. It is the most common form of dementia in the U.S. Alzheimer's disease has been diagnosed in 5% to 7% of older persons over the age of 65 and in 20% of those over the age of 80. The likelihood of developing dementia of the Alzheimer's type increases dramatically with age (Blazer, 1990; Jenike, 1989) and it occurs more frequently in women than in men, apparently due to their longer life expectancy (Butler, Lewis, and Sunderland, 1991).

Although a specific cause for Alzheimer's disease has not been found, several types of brain abnormalities that are related to Alzheimer's disease have been discovered. Low levels of acetylcholine, which appear to be related to loss of memory functions, have been found in older persons with dementia. Senile plaques which exist in small amounts in all older adults' brains correlate positively with loss of orientation (Edinberg, 1985). Neurofibrillary tangles in the brain may be related to problems in protein metabolism. They also represent degeneration, interfere with nerve transmission, and lead to the death of brain cells (Butler, Lewis, and Sunderland, 1991; Edinberg, 1985).

Alzheimer's disease is a devastating brain disorder. The predominance of behavioral symptomatology in Alzheimer's disease distinguishes it from many other brain disorders (Cohen, 1989). Memory loss is progressive and severe and is marked by few complaints or concerns about the loss. Memory loss for recent events is greater than for events from the distant past (Edinberg, 1985). Impairment in intelligence and cognition are common with difficulties in abstract thinking, simple calculations, understanding directions and questions (perceptual problems), and communication. Attention, and orientation to time, place, and person also become impaired (Blazer, 1990; Edinberg, 1985). Difficulties in judgment include the inability to plan or make decisions. Judgmental problems may be increased by a lack of interest in the activities of living. Lapses in self-care often become evident and can present management problems (Edinberg, 1985).

Wandering is a demanding problem for caretakers of persons with Alzheimer's disease. Those who do wander are potentially at risk for harm. There are many possible causes for wandering including physical discomfort, disorientation, restlessness, and agitation. Wandering in some individuals becomes greater at night (Leng, 1990).

Table 6.1

Symptoms Associated with Dementia

Area of Loss	Symptoms	Onset
Cognition	Loss of memory	Early onset; gradual and
	Disorientation—confusion	progressive decline
	concerning time, place,	
	people, eventually	
	forgetting own name	
	Poor judgment	Onset in middle stages
	Decreased abilities in	
	calculation	
	Impairment in abstract	
	thinking	
	Anosognosia	Onset in later stages
Affect	Excessive, inappropriate	
	or lack of emotional	Onset in later stages
	response	
Behavior	Irritability	Onset at any stage
	Withdrawal	Onset in middle stages
	Agitation	Onset in later stages
	Apathy	
	Occasional violence	
Psychological	Depression	Onset at any stage
	Denial	
	Anxiety	
	Paranoia	Onset in later stages
	Hallucinations	
	Delusions	
	Personality change	
Language	Speech disorders, including	Onset at any stage;
	perseveration	progressive decline
Physical	Visual impairments	Early onset
	Impaired motor function,	Onset in later stages
	including perseveration	
	Incontinence	
	Sleep disorders	
	Weight loss	
	Sexual disorders	
	Seizures	

Note: Developed from information contained in Butler, Lewis, & Sunderland, 1991; McKhann, Drachman, & Folstein, 1984; and Reisberg, Ferris, DeLeon, & Crook, 1982.

Early in the disease, moderate to severe depression is a common symptom. As the disease progresses, victims can become agitated, restless, and uncooperative. Suspiciousness, paranoia, delusions, and hallucinations may occur and are often accompanied by angry outbursts and verbal abuse. Incontinence, speech difficulties, disturbed sleep patterns, and eating problems also can emerge in the final stages of the disease (Blazer, 1990; Leng, 1990).

According to Katzman (1988), the clinical diagnosis of Alzheimer's disease has improved markedly and currently approaches 90% accuracy. If the patient's dementia has had a deceptive onset, a generally progressive and deteriorating course, and the patient meets the other criteria for dementia, a clinical diagnosis of Alzheimer's disease may be made. All other specific causes of dementia must be excluded by history, physical examination, and laboratory tests. The importance of evaluating demented patients in order to document the course of illness should be emphasized, thereby further increasing the accuracy of diagnosis in patients suspected of having the disease. The onset of Alzheimer's disease is between ages 40 and 90, most often after the age of 65, and the diagnosis of probable Alzheimer's disease is supported by a family history of similar disorders (Jenike, 1989).

Multi-Infarct Dementia

The second most common form of dementia is *multi-infarct dementia.* In this disorder, the dementia results as a consequence of multiple small strokes throughout the brain. Although the symptoms are similar to those described for Alzheimer's disease, the course of multi-infarct dementia is not gradual. It occurs rather unevenly, and the deficits tend to be differentiated (e.g., agitation and depression can be severe, but memory loss may only be minimal) (Blazer, 1990). Multi-infarct dementia is a chronic disorder and can occur simultaneously with Alzheimer's disease in the same patient. Onset is generally between the ages of 50 and 70 and is usually associated with hypertension (Butler, Lewis, and Sunderland, 1991).

Infarcts occur randomly in multi-infarct dementia; therefore, the course of illness is difficult to predict and symptoms vary greatly between patients (Stuart-Hamilton, 1991). Many multi-infarct patients die but those who survive may experience a remission of symptoms with varying amounts of intellectual impairment (Butler, Lewis, and Sunderland, 1991). Table 6.2 (page 108) summarizes the differences between depression, Alzheimer's disease, and multi-infarct dementia.

Pick's Disease

Pick's disease is clinically very similar to Alzheimer's disease, and differentiation may be impossible until autopsy. The age of onset is usually between 40 and 60 years. Behavioral symptoms can include a lack of initiative, social misconduct, personality change, and variable memory impairment (Butler, Lewis, and Sunderland, 1991; Jenike, 1989).

The cause of Pick's disease is unknown, but genetic factors appear to be relevant. The prognosis is always fatal with survival ranging from two to 15 years. The course of illness is steadily progressive and the treatment of symptoms is all that can presently be done (Butler, Lewis, and Sunderland, 1991). Clients with Pick's

Table 6.2

Comparative Differences between Depression, Alzheimer's Disease and Multi-Infarct Dementia

	Depression	Alzheimer's Disease	Multi-Infarct Dementia
Onset	Relatively rapid changes in mood and behavior	Deceptive; poorly defined	Abrupt, step-wise
Mood and Behavior	Stable, depressed, or agitated	Unstable and/or depressed	Variable with periods of recovery
Mental Competence	Unaffected except for attention, concentration, and interests	Increasingly defective	Defective with recovery; step-wise losses
Complaints	Memory; concentration; self-image; overly concerned with symptoms; loss of interest	Others' complaints about him or her; denial of symptoms	Memory and behavioral losses appropriate to area of infarct
Somatic Symptoms	Anxiety, sleep, eating, fatigue	Sleep disorders, anxiety	Anxiety, neurological disorders
Prognosis	Generally self-limited; 20–30% of cases are chronic	Chronic and progressive	Progressive unless treatable
Past History	Episodes of depression	None specifically related	Hypertension
Brain Scan	Normal	Generalized atrophy	Localized evidence of stroke
EEG	Normal	Generalized slowing	Localized abnormalities

Note: Developed from information contained in Belsky, 1990; Jenike, 1989; and Zung, 1980.

disease are often more difficult to manage than clients with Alzheimer's disease. Nursing home placement is often indicated at earlier stages of the illness (Butler, Lewis, and Sunderland, 1991; Jenike, 1989).

Other Dementia-Related Syndromes

Parkinson's disease and Huntington's disease are often accompanied by dementia. In Parkinson's disease, the clinical symptoms may include forgetfulness, slowing of thought processes, altered personality, and other impaired intellectual functioning. The characteristic features are involuntary movement, rigidity of muscles, slowness of movement, and tremor (Butler, Lewis, and Sunderland, 1991; Jenike, 1989; Leng, 1990). The overt motor functioning of Parkinson's patients can differentiate them from those suffering from the other dementias (Butler, Lewis, and Sunderland, 1991; Leng, 1990).

Huntington's disease is hereditary and usually begins in middle age. The early symptoms of the illness are involuntary movements (Leng, 1990; Stuart-Hamilton, 1991). Subsequently, Huntington's disease patients develop symptoms of dementia. Huntington's disease is progressive and life expectancy is usually about 15 years. It is also characterized by cognitive impairments such as loss of memory and decreased skills in organizing and sequencing (Butler, Lewis, and Sunderland, 1991; Stuart-Hamilton, 1991).

Treatment is disease-specific. Currently there is no therapeutic agent available that has proven effective in the treatment of Huntington's disease. Treatment is directed at controlling the symptoms. Patients with Parkinson's disease receive drug therapy. However, accurate diagnosis and treatment are essential (Butler, Lewis, and Sunderland, 1991; Jenike, 1989).

Prolonged use of alcohol also may cause dementia. In order to make the diagnosis of dementia associated with alcoholism, all other causes of dementia should be excluded and three weeks must have elapsed since the prolonged heavy ingestion of alcohol (Jenike, 1989).

Delirium

Delirium is an organic psychiatric syndrome characterized by acute onset and impairment in cognition, perception, and behavior (Beresin, 1988). Delirium also is termed transient cognitive disorder (McPherson, 1991) and acute confusional state, which refers to confusion with a relatively sudden onset that is potentially of limited duration (Leng, 1990; Stuart-Hamilton, 1991).

Delirium is characterized by acute episodes of confusion, fluctuating levels of awareness, and impairment in attention. Hallucinations and delusions may be present. A predominant feature of delirium is disturbance in the sleep-wake cycle and impairments are usually most severe at night. The term *sundowning* is used to describe the agitated and confused behaviors that often occur in the evening and night. Disorganized thinking also is indicated by rambling, irrelevant, or incoherent speech (Blazer, 1990; Butler, Lewis, and Sunderland, 1991; Jenike, 1989). There are many possible causes of delirium. Overmedication, medication interactions, and improper use of medication by older clients are among the most common sources of delirium in the elderly (Edinberg, 1985).

Delirium is a critical symptom in the elderly. As many as 15% to 40% of delirious patients progress to stupor, coma, and death (Butler, Lewis, and Sunderland, 1991; Liston, 1982). Delirium is frequently undiagnosed; however, when diagnosed and treated early, delirium is often completely reversible (McCartney and Palmateer, 1985).

Treatment of delirium must include attending to any organic or disease-related factors (Jenike, 1989). The immediate environment of the delirious patient is extremely important. The environment must be consistent, familiar, and simplified in order to moderate sensory input, personal contact, activities, and physical aspects of the environment. Supportive reassurances may be provided to diminish anxiety, provide comfort, and promote an affirmation of reality (Butler, Lewis, and Sunderland, 1991; Jenike, 1989).

Reversible Causes of Mental Impairment

The dementia that is associated with depression in the elderly is perhaps the most important of all the reversible dementias. Antidepressant medications are available for this condition, yet a large percentage of depressed patients are consistently misdiagnosed as suffering from dementia (Butler, Lewis, and Sunderland, 1991). Complaints of poor memory may accompany depression and disappear when the depression is treated (Jenike, 1989).

The term *pseudodementia* is often used to describe reversible depression-related cognitive disorders (Jenike, 1989). A lack of progressive symptomatology is a typical characteristic of pseudodementia. Patients who are pseudodemented are usually oriented to time and place, whereas demented patients are not. Pseudo-demented patients often perform better in the afternoon than in the morning. Also, patients who are pseudodemented are usually aware of their poor performance while true dementia victims may not be reconciled with their deficiencies. The intellectual performance of pseudodemented patients often improves as the depression is treated (Jenike, 1986; Kermis, 1986; Sahakian, 1991; Stuart-Hamilton, 1991).

Cognitive impairment in depression is distinct from that of the dementias. However, more than 50% of elderly depressed patients subsequently develop true dementia (Reding, et al., 1986; Sahakian, 1991; Stuart-Hamilton, 1991). The impact of depression compounded with dementia increases cognitive impairment to a degree greater than either disorder alone—a state referred to as *excess disability*. When excess disability is treated, an increase in overall functional capacity of patients with dementia may occur. Only with the passage of time does the patient regress and display further deterioration (Cohen, 1988).

Other reversible causes of mental impairment can include cardiopulmonary and cardiovascular disease, malnutrition and anemia, infection, head trauma, alcoholism, diabetes, dehydration, emphysema, brain tumors, liver failure, thyroid disorders, cancer, vitamin deficiencies, environmental changes, exhaustion, and grief reactions or bereavement. With the increasing use of drug treatments in the medical and psychiatric management of the elderly, drug reactions also are a significant cause of reversible mental disorders (Lipowski, 1983).

Due to multiple chronic conditions, 64% of the elderly are prescribed a variety of different drugs, which leads to *polypharmacy.* Polypharmacy is the concurrent use of two or more medications, particularly in excessive doses or inappropriate combinations. It is because of polypharmacy that *iatrogenic disorders* among the elderly are common. Iatrogenic disorders are those pathological brain conditions that paradoxically result from medications, diagnostic procedures, or therapies and not from any physical dysfunction. There is no substitute for careful monitoring of the individual patient (Butler, Lewis, and Sunderland, 1991; Harper, 1991).

Functional Mental Disorders

Functional mental disorders are those in which behavioral problems or distress are not due to physical disease processes (Edinberg, 1985). Mental illness in the elderly is fairly common. Depressive symptoms have been reported in over 20% of the U.S. adult population, and approximately 20% of all Americans suffer from a mental illness. The majority of elderly persons with mental disorders reside in the community. In nursing homes it is estimated that 50% of elderly clients suffer from some mental disturbance. Since older persons do not frequently seek treatment for mental health disorders, it is difficult to estimate the true extent of the problem (Butler, Lewis, and Sunderland, 1991; Jenike, 1989).

Depression

One type of functional mental disorder is depression. *Depression* is likely to be misdiagnosed and poorly treated in elderly persons. Because depression has such broad effects, there appears to be a range of possible causes. Depression is viewed as a function of genetic and biological factors, environmental stresses, and habitual ways of thinking and acting. For many elderly persons these factors interact in a complex manner that causes or maintains depression (Hinrichsen, 1990). There is considerable evidence regarding a hereditary contribution to depression, however, research has suggested that genetic causation of depressive disorders in late life is weaker than at other stages of the life cycle (Hopkinson, 1964; Mendlewicz, 1976). The desire to restore functioning in spite of the inevitable losses in late life is a major developmental task of aging individuals, but older adults also recognize their declines (Cath, 1965).

Depression impacts many physical and psychological functions. The physical functions of energy, appetite, digestion, sleep, and metabolism are suppressed. Cognitive functions of memory, reasoning, concentration, and problem solving are affected. Disturbances of mood, lack of interest, helplessness, anger, and lowered frustration tolerance are displayed in depressed elderly individuals. Decreased functioning also is exhibited in a lack of meaning in life, pessimism, and hopelessness (Kemp, 1986). Depressed clients generally complain of insomnia and loss of interest in activities such as his or her job, hobbies, social situations, and sex.

Feelings of guilt, lack of energy, the inability to concentrate, confused thinking, and suicidal thoughts also may be present. In order to be diagnosed, a major depressive episode must last for at least a two-week period and represent a change from previous functioning (Jenike, 1989).

Older adulthood often is accompanied by change. The relative stability of middle age may lead to transitions in late life that may or may not have been expected. Late life stresses often involve loss such as loss of one's partner, friends, money, and health. Older persons have had many years to develop attachments, and they also are the most likely to suffer the loss of people and things to which they have become attached. Despite losses during late life, the majority of older people maintain good emotional health. For some older persons, however, the stresses of late life increase their risk for depression (Hinrichsen, 1990).

In older age groups, the depressed patient may not admit to the symptoms of depression, but anxiety, physical symptoms, chronic pain, loss of concentration, memory problems, and pseudodementia are frequent. The most common situation that contributes to depressive symptoms is *bereavement*, a universal human experience and the normal response to the loss of a loved one, a job, economic security, or one's home (Blazer, 1990; Jenike, 1989).

Any medical condition associated with bodily systems and metabolic disturbances can have an impact on the mental functioning of the elderly. The most common are fever, dehydration, and electrolyte disturbances. Cancer, heart failure, strokes, and Alzheimer's disease often are associated with depression. Drugs and medication also may cause depressive symptoms in a great many cases (U'Ren, 1990). There is no substitute for systematic monitoring of the older individual using repeated measures of cognitive performance to identify toxic drug effects (Morrison and Katz, 1990).

The clinical treatment and management of older persons suffering from depression includes *antidepressant drugs, electroconvulsive therapy, counseling,* and *family therapy* (Blazer, 1990). Considerable evidence indicates that antidepressant medication is more effective when used in combination with some type of counseling (Goff and Jenike, 1986). Electroconvulsive therapy, however, may be the only choice of treatment in the elderly depressed patient whose illness is accompanied by self-destructive behavior such as suicide attempts or refusal to eat (Jenike, 1989; Weiner, 1982).

Often older persons do not tolerate antidepressants well. Although heart problems are the most serious side effect from a medical viewpoint, dryness of the mouth, constipation, blurring of vision, and confusion are frequently reported as the most disturbing side effects to the client (Nies et al., 1977). There is a potential for addiction and overdose with several of the antidepressant drugs (Blazer, 1989).

Electroconvulsive therapy is a treatment option for depressed older adults. It involves causing a series of seizures in patients with severe depression. The seizure itself, rather than the electrical stimulation, is the therapeutic agent. Electroconvulsive therapy is more effective and faster-acting than drugs in the treatment of depression, and it is both safe and effective for the treatment of affective illness in the elderly (Jenike, 1989).

Individual *psychotherapy* and *counseling* are the basis of psychological intervention. The themes in psychotherapy with older persons are generally different than
those of younger persons. Older persons frequently deal with cumulative losses,
preparation for life's end, maintenance of personal independence, physical health
concerns, family relations, and the preservation of self-worth and self-esteem
(Kemp, 1986). A final consideration for the treatment of depressive symptoms in
older adults must be their consequences for independent functioning. Without
intervention, those persons who are depressed will stay depressed, and everyday
functioning and adaptation will be limited (Murrell and Meeks, 1991).

Counseling differs from psychotherapy in that it is less focused on maladjusted
behavior. Counseling is concerned with providing information, advice, resources,
and referrals to "normal individuals" in order to attain concrete goals. Examples of
issues that may be addressed in counseling situations include stress management,
relaxation techniques, leisure involvements, and communication skills (Kemp,
1986).

Group therapy approaches to psychological problems are beneficial for several
reasons. They are economical and present opportunities for socialization and
learning from peers. They are more multidisciplinary, often including physical
exercise, psychotherapy, education, and recreation (Kemp, 1986).

The family plays a large role in the well-being of older disabled persons and
cannot be excluded from treatment. Treatment of the whole family is both an
effective and efficient form of therapy (Kemp, 1986). The goal of family intervention is to improve the functioning of the family system. The focus of *family therapy*
is on the physical functioning and relationships of the older person, as well as the
person's support systems (Edinberg, 1985).

Suicide

The seriousness of depression in the elderly is demonstrated by an increase in and
success of suicidal attempts in this age group (Georgotas, 1983). Depression is
involved in two-thirds of the suicides committed by elderly persons (Gurland and
Cross, 1983). The elderly comprise the age group that is most at risk for suicide, and
the rate of suicide among the elderly is 50% higher than that of younger persons.
Elderly suicidal patients tend not to contact crisis intervention workers, but they may
contact physicians or other health service providers (Osgood, 1985). More than 75%
of the elderly who commit suicide visit a physician prior to completing the act
(Foster and Burke, 1985).

Many elderly persons provide clues to their impending suicidal behavior. Clues
to suicide may be classified as verbal, behavioral, situational, or syndromatic.
Verbal clues may be direct or indirect. An example of a direct verbal clue would be
"I am going to kill myself." Direct suicidal threats always should be taken seriously.
Of those persons who threaten suicide, 80% eventually kill themselves (Osgood,
1985).

Indirect verbal clues are more subtle than direct suicidal threats, but they also
should be taken seriously. Indirect verbal clues include statements such as "I'm tired
of life" and "my family would be better off without me." Some verbal clues require

interpretation to detect the self-destructive intent such as "You shouldn't be having to take care of me any longer" (Osgood, 1985).

Behavioral clues also may be either direct or indirect. The most direct behavioral clue is the suicide attempt. Most elderly persons who attempt suicide kill themselves within one to two years after an attempt. Indirect behavioral clues include putting personal and business affairs in order, giving away money and/or possessions, changes in behavior, general confusion, and loss of judgment or memory (Osgood, 1991).

Syndromatic clues consist of the psychological syndromes that often are associated with suicide. Depression, when accompanied by anxiety, appears to be the most important clue to suicide in the aged. Stress, agitation, guilt, isolation, and dependency are other important syndromatic clues (Osgood, 1985; Osgood, Brant, and Lipman, 1989).

Accurate assessment in the aged is crucial to suicide prevention. The key factors in recognizing suicidal elderly persons may be discovered by using the *ASK* approach (Pavkov, 1982):

- **A**ttention to expressed suicidal interests,
- **S**ymptomatic variations, and
- **K**een observation of attitudinal and/or activity change.

In the final analysis, elderly people in the U.S. may kill themselves because old age has nothing worthwhile to offer them. When old age is viewed as a valued status by society, then the number of elderly suicides may be significantly reduced (Osgood, 1985).

Anxiety

Anxiety disorders are among the more common problems experienced throughout the life cycle and may include panic disorders, phobias, posttraumatic stress disorders, physical disorders accompanied by anxiety, and generalized anxiety disorders. Anxiety is a state of inner distress composed of dread, fear, or anticipation of imagined harm that is accompanied by various symptoms including shortness of breath, dry mouth, dizziness, increased heart rate, trembling, sweating, and/or chills. In order to diagnose an anxiety disorder, four or more attacks must have taken place within a four week period or at least a month of persistent fear of having another attack must have occurred. Also, organic factors cannot be established as the cause of the disturbances (Jenike, 1989; Shamoian, 1991).

An estimated 10% to 15% of women over the age of 65 experience severe anxiety symptoms (Turnbull and Turnbull, 1985). The presence of anxiety symptoms alone often does not cause patients to seek help. Even patients with severe anxiety symptoms wait, on the average, a period of 12 years before seeking treatment for the symptoms. Another difficulty is that elderly patients with anxiety disorders often may have physical complaints that hide the underlying disorder (Jenike, 1989).

Unrealistic or excessive worry about problems is a distinguishing characteristic of anxiety disorders. Anxiety symptoms often are a component of many emotional problems that afflict older adults. Anxiety can arise in older persons who reflect upon their lives and their positions in society. Older adults may become aware of a sense of "nothingness" or insignificance in life. This type of anxiety can accompany and exaggerate anxiety from other sources (Blazer, 1990).

Anxiety disorders may be treated with medications. However, manipulation of environmental factors or discussion of the patient's problems is considered when an elderly individual suffers from anxiety. Many older patients respond favorably to counseling techniques (Jenike, 1989).

Coping with stress can provide a means for developing practical knowledge, wisdom, and positive self-esteem (Baldwin, 1992). Stress management techniques such as meditation, relaxation, and exercise or physical activity often prove useful in the treatment of elderly anxiety disorders (Lewis, 1990). Coping skills may be indicated, such as effective communication, assertiveness, and positive thinking. Social support also can provide a sense of competence to anxious and stressed elderly individuals (Gatz, 1992).

Psychosis

Psychosis involves major distortions in reality and is used to describe many general behaviors. Among these behaviors are *hallucinations,* which are psychotic symptoms involving sensory perceptions of sights and sounds that are not actually present. Due to decreased hearing capacities auditory hallucinations are particularly common in the elderly. *Delusions* and *paranoia* also may be present in psychosis. Delusions are false personal beliefs that are firmly upheld despite external reality. Paranoid thoughts involve suspiciousness or the sense of being treated unfairly. The instances of paranoia increase with age. Specific risk factors for paranoia include sensory impairment, brain damage, and social isolation (Butler, Lewis, and Sunderland, 1991).

Schizophrenia

Schizophrenia patients have characteristic disturbances in several of the following areas: content and form of thought, perception, affect, sense of self, behavior, and relationship to the external world. A continuous six-month period of symptoms is required for diagnosis (Jenike, 1989). Onset of schizophrenia most often occurs before age 45; however, late-life schizophrenia does occur. Older schizophrenics generally display differences in symptoms with their delusions focused on sex and personal possessions (Edinberg, 1985). Schizophrenia with a late life onset is termed *paraphrenia* and affects 1% to 2% of individuals over the age of 65 (Almeida, Howard, Forstl, and Levy, 1992). Paranoid behaviors are the prominent symptoms of persons experiencing paraphrenia. The behavior of the paraphrenia sufferer becomes increasingly bizarre and self-neglect is a pronounced feature. The condition usually improves in response to drug treatment (Stokes, 1992). It is estimated that between 56% and 80% of nursing home clients in the U.S. have chronic mental conditions such as schizophrenia and paraphrenia (Frazier, Lebowitz, and Silver, 1986).

Major tranquilizers are used to control psychotic symptoms in all age groups. Commonly used antipsychotic drugs are Haldol, Loxitance, Mellaril, Moban, Navane, Permitil, Prolixin, Serentil, Stelazine, Taractan, Thorazine, Trilafon, and Vesprin (Kaplan and Sadock, 1991). The side effects of major tranquilizers are potentially serious. Side effects include visual problems, vulnerability to heat or cold, sensitivity to the sun, weight gain, seizures, drowsiness, confusion, anxiety, agitation, and movement disorders (Edinberg, 1985; Jenike, 1989).

Tardive dyskinesia is a side effect of antipsychotic drugs and involves involuntary movement that may appear after three to six months of treatment with antipsychotic drugs. It is characterized by involuntary movements of the tongue, face, trunk, and extremities (American Psychiatric Association, 1987). Tardive dyskinesia has been reported in more than 50% of the elderly who are on long-term drug therapy (Kazamatsuri, Chien, and Cole, 1972).

The goals of intervention with older schizophrenics are generally adaptive. Rehabilitation of the patient focuses on behavior and socialization. Exercise and counseling often are employed (Edinberg, 1985; Harper, 1991).

Bipolar Disorders

In *bipolar disorders* the depressive state cannot be distinguished from other types of depression. Bipolar disorder, often termed manic-depressive illness, is characterized by severe mood swings from depression to elation. A history of manic episodes in the patient or in his family is central to the diagnosis (Butler, Lewis, and Sunderland, 1991; Jenike, 1989). Lithium carbonate is widely accepted as the treatment for bipolar illness and is indicated for elderly patients (Cade, 1949; Jenike, 1989; Sheard, 1975). However, anticonvulsants such as Depakene, Depokate, Klonopin, and Tegretol, also are used in the treatment of geriatric bipolar disorders (Kaplan and Sadock, 1991).

Alcoholism and Other Drug Abuse

Alcoholism in the elderly is difficult to diagnose. About 10% of elderly individuals in the U.S. have an alcohol-related problem, with men outnumbering women at the rate of 12 to 1. Older alcoholics tend to avoid contact with agencies or professionals who may notice signs of alcoholism. The signs of alcoholism are similar to those of other physical and emotional problems commonly diagnosed in the elderly. The majority of elderly alcoholics abused alcohol as younger adults and can be viewed as having a lifelong problem that has persisted into older adulthood. Some elderly patients, who are referred to as late-onset alcoholics, did not have problems with alcohol until later maturity (Jenike, 1989).

Criteria for and indications of alcohol abuse include: physical symptoms such as shaking and blackouts, psychological dependence on alcohol, health problems, and difficulties with family and friends. Alcohol generally has a more profound effect on the elderly than on younger persons because of aging-related physical changes that result in slower metabolism of alcohol (Edinberg, 1985). Prolonged alcohol abuse also can lead to a progressive dementia similar to Alzheimer's disease (Stokes, 1992).

Every effort should be made to ensure that the elderly alcoholic patient actually presents himself or herself for treatment (Jenike, 1989). Treatment for alcoholism may include Antabuse, a drug that inhibits alcohol consumption, paired with social support from peers, specifically in Alcoholics Anonymous. Therapeutic intervention with the family also is essential in order to avoid a return to alcohol abuse (Edinberg, 1985; Jenike, 1989). Additionally, Naltrexone is used in the treatment of alcoholism. Naltrexone is a drug that counteracts the mood-altering effects of alcohol (Yoder, 1990).

Although less is known about *drug abuse* in the elderly, it appears that for every five alcoholics there is one elderly person who abuses other drugs (Redick, Kramer, and Taube, 1973; Reifler, Raskind, and Kethley, 1982). Because elderly persons comprise the largest group of drug consumers, the potential for drug misuse and abuse is great (Harper, 1991). Prescription drug abuse is common among the aged. Over-the-counter drugs are frequently abused including laxatives, sedatives, pain relievers, and cold medications. The fact that drugs are easily obtained, generally inexpensive, and perceived as completely safe by many elderly persons frequently promotes abuse (Jenike, 1989).

Of those individuals over the age of 60, 69% report using over-the-counter medications and 40% take drugs on a daily basis (Guttman, 1978; Kofoed, 1984). Additionally, overuse of caffeine with the consumption of coffee, tea, and soft drinks contributes to anxiety, panic disorders, heart irregularities, gastric problems, and osteoporosis (Heaney, 1981; Kofoed, 1984).

Prescription drug abuse may be difficult to detect in the elderly due to the multiple legitimate reasons older persons have for taking medications. Some of the warning signs associated with prescription drug abuse by the elderly include pain disorders, depression, organic cognitive disorders, poor social functioning, changes in tolerance to drugs, proneness to accidents, and defensiveness (Finlayson, 1984).

Substance abuse problems in the elderly can be as difficult to treat as they are to detect. Older persons usually respond quite well to emotional support, encourage-ment, and improvements in their social systems. Family involvement also enhances treatment outcomes (Finlayson, 1984). Once dependence is recognized, hospitaliza-tion will likely be required for management of withdrawal symptoms and observa-tion. Education and correction of associated psychological problems such as anxi-ety, loneliness, grief, and depression usually will improve the situation (Jenike, 1989).

Summary

This chapter provides a general description of the diseases that are associated with cognitive dysfunction in older persons. The psychological and psychiatric conditions that affect older persons are often neglected by care providers. Depression is perhaps the most common condition, and many older persons suffer from organic brain syndrome. These conditions may affect memory function, as well as the emotional state of the individual. A broad range of treatments can be employed to help the older person cope with or recover from emotional disturbance or cognitive dysfunction. Functional mental disorders such as depression, anxiety, and alcoholism are treatable conditions for which the activity specialist may have an important role to play in the treatment process.

In conclusion, it is important to remember that all persons respond on some level to emotional and social support, although they may not respond in the manner that is expected. Although formal contact might seem impossible, presence, touch, favorite music, and quiet affirmation of care and concern all may be received beyond the states of awareness that are normally comprehended or displayed. "The force of love remains eternal, giving of itself in faith and hope with no need of reciprocity" (Karr, 1991, pp. 69–70).

Comprehension Questions

1. Describe dementia in the elderly, including incidence and common symptoms.
2. What are functional mental disorders?
3. Discuss depression in elderly persons.
4. Why is depression common in older persons and what can be done to treat it?
5. Discuss the impact that alcohol and other drug use has on the mental health of elderly persons.

References

Almeida, O. P., Howard, R., Forstl, J., & Levy, R. (1992). Late paraphrenia: Our view. *International Journal of Geriatric Psychiatry, 7*(8), 543-548.

American Psychiatric Association. (1987). *Diagnostic and statistical manual of mental disorders* (3rd ed.). Washington, DC: Author.

Baldwin, B. A. (1992). Stress in the elderly: Environments of care. In M. L. Wykle, E. Kahana, & J. Kowal (Eds.), *Stress and health among the elderly* (pp. 197-208). New York, NY: Springer Publishing Co., Inc.

Belsky, J. K. (1990). *The psychology of aging: Theory, research, and interventions* (2nd ed.). Pacific Grove, CA: Brooks/Cole Publishing Co.

Beresin, E. V. (1988). Delirium in the elderly. *Journal of Geriatric Neurology, 1,* 127-143.

Blazer, D. G. (1990). *Emotional problems in later life: Intervention strategies for professional caregivers.* New York, NY: Springer Publishing Co., Inc.

Blazer, D. G. (1989). Current concepts: Depression in the elderly. *The New England Journal of Medicine, 320*(3), 164-166.

Butler, R. N., Lewis, M. I., & Sunderland, T. (1991). *Aging and mental health: Positive psychosocial and biomedical approaches* (4th ed.). New York, NY: Merrill.

Cade, J. F. J. (1949). Lithium salts in the treatment of psychotic excitement. *Medical Journal of Australia, 36,* 349-352.

Cath, S. H. (1965). Some dynamics of middle and later years: A study in depletion and restitution. In M. A. Berezin & S. H. Cath (Eds.), *Geriatric psychiatry: Grief, loss, and emotional disorders in the aging process* (pp. 21-72). New York, NY: International Universities Press, Inc.

Cohen, G. D. (1989). The interface of mental and physical health phenomena in later life: New directions in geriatric psychiatry. *Gerontology and Geriatrics Education, 9*(3), 27-38.

Cohen, G. D. (1988). *The brain in human aging.* New York, NY: Springer Publishing Co., Inc.

Edinberg, M. A. (1985). *Mental health practice with the elderly.* Englewood Cliffs, NJ: Prentice Hall.

Finlayson, R. E. (1984). Prescription drug abuse in older persons. In R. E. Atkinson (Ed.), *Alcohol and drug abuse in old age* (pp. 61-70). Washington, DC: American Psychiatric Association.

Foster, B. G., & Burke, W. J. (1985). Assessing and treating the suicidal elderly. *Family practice recertification, 71*(11), 33-45.

Frazier, S. H., Lebowitz, B. D., & Silver, L. B. (1986). Aging, mental health, and rehabilitation. In S. J. Brody & G. E. Ruff (Eds.), *Aging and rehabilitation: Advances in the state of the art* (pp. 19-35). New York, NY: Springer Publishing Co., Inc.

Gatz, M. (1992). Stress, control, and psychological interventions. In M. L. Wykle, E. Kahana, & J. Kowal (Eds.), *Stress and health among the elderly* (pp. 209-222). New York, NY: Springer Publishing Co., Inc.

Georgotas, A. (1983). Affective disorders in the elderly: Diagnostic and research considerations. *Aged and Aging, 12*, 1-10.

Goff, D. C., & Jenike, M. A. (1986). Treatment-resistant depression in the elderly. *Journal of the American Geriatrics Society, 34*, 63-70.

Gurland, B. J., & Cross, P. S. (1983). Suicide among the elderly. In M. K. Aronson, R. Bennett, & B. J. Gurland (Eds.), *The acting-out elderly* (pp. 456-465). Binghamton, NY: The Haworth Press, Inc.

Guttman, D. (1978). Patterns of legal drug use by older Americans. *Addiction Disorders, 3*, 337-356.

Harper, M. S. (1991). *Management and care of the elderly: Psychosocial perspectives.* Newbury Park, CA: Sage Publications, Inc.

Heaney, R. P. (1981). Nutritional factors in post-menopausal osteoporosis. *Roche Seminar on Aging, 5*, 8-12.

Hinrichsen, G. A. (1990). *Mental health problems and older adults.* Santa Barbara, CA: ABC-CLIO.

Hopkinson, G. (1964). A genetic study of affective illness in patients over 50. *British Journal of Psychiatry, 110*, 244.

Jenike, M. A. (1989). *Geriatric psychiatry and psychopharmacology.* St. Louis, MO: Mosby.

Kaplan, H. I., & Sadock, B. J. (1991). *Synopsis of psychiatry: Behavioral science clinical psychiatry* (6th ed.). Baltimore, MD: Williams and Wilkins.

Karr, K. (1991). *Promises to keep: The family's role in nursing home care.* Buffalo, NY: Prometheus Books.

Katzman, R. (1988). Alzheimer's disease as an age-dependent disorder. *CIBA Foundation Symposium, 134*, 69-85.

Katzman, R. (1985). Aging and age-dependent disease: Cognition and dementia. In Institute of Medicine and National Research Council, *Health in an older society* (pp. 129-152). Washington, DC: National Academy Press.

Kazamatsuri, H., Chien, C., & Cole, J. W. (1972). Treatment of tardive dyskinesia: Clinical efficacy of a Dopamine-competing agent, methyldopa. *Archives of General Psychiatry, 27*(2), 824-827.

Kemp, B. J. (1986). Psychosocial and mental health issues in rehabilitation of older persons. In S. J. Brody & G. E. Ruff (Eds.), *Aging and rehabilitation: Advances in the state of the art* (pp. 122-158). New York, NY: Springer Publishing Co., Inc.

Kermis, M. D. (1986). *Mental health in late life: The adaptive process.* Boston, MA: Jones & Bartlett Publishers, Inc.

Kofoed, L. L. (1984). Abuse and misuse of over-the-counter drugs by the elderly. In R. M. Atkinson (Ed.), *Alcohol and drug abuse in old age* (pp. 49-59). Washington, DC: American Psychiatric Association.

Leng, N. R. C. (1990). *Psychological care in old age.* London, UK: Hemisphere.

Lewis, C. B. (1990). *Aging, the healthcare challenge: An interdisciplinary approach to assessment and rehabilitative management of the elderly* (2nd ed.). Philadelphia, PA: F. A. Davis Co.

Lipowski, Z. J. (1983). Transient cognitive disorders (delirium, acute confusional states) in the elderly. *American Journal of Psychiatry, 140*(11), 1426-1436.

Liston, E. H. (1982). Delirium in the aged. *Psychiatric Clinics of North America, 5,* 49-66.

McCartney, J. R., & Palmateer, L. M. (1985). Assessment of cognitive deficit in geriatric patients: A study of physician behavior. *Journal of the American Geriatrics Society, 33*(7), 467-471.

McKhann, G. M., Drachman, D. B., & Folstein, M. F. (1984). Clinical diagnosis of Alzheimer's disease. *Neurology, 34,* 939-944.

McPherson, S. (1991). Transient cognitive disorders in the elderly. In M. S. Harper (Ed.), *Management and care of the elderly: Psychosocial perspectives* (pp. 180-188). Newbury Park, CA: Sage Publications, Inc.

Mendlewicz, J. (1976). The age factor in depressive illness: Some genetic considerations. *Journal of Gerontology, 32*(3), 300-303.

Morrison, R. L., & Katz, I. R. (1990). Drug-related cognitive impairment: Current progress and recurrent problems. *Annual Review of Gerontology and Geriatrics, 9,* 232-279.

Murrell, S. A., & Meeks, S. (1991). Depressive symptoms in older adults: Predispositions, resources, and life experiences. *Annual Review of Gerontology and Geriatrics, 11,* 261-286.

Nies, A., Robinson, D. S., Friedman, M. J., Green, R., Cooper, T. B., Ravaris, C. L., & Ives, J. O. (1977). Relationship between age and tricyclic antidepressant plasma levels. *American Journal of Psychiatry, 134*(7), 790-793.

Osgood, N. J. (1985). *Suicide in the elderly: A practitioners guide to diagnosis and mental health intervention.* Rockville, MD: Aspen Publishers Inc.

Osgood, N. J., Brant, B. A., & Lipman, A. A. (1989). Patterns of suicidal behavior in long-term care facilities: A preliminary report on an ongoing study. *Omega Journal of Death and Dying, 19*(1), 69-78.

Pavkov, J. R. (1982). Suicide in the elderly. *Ohio's Health, 34,* 21-28.

Redick, K. R. W., Kramer, M., & Taube, C. A. (1973). Epidemiology of mental illness and utilization of psychiatric facilities among older persons. In E. W. Busse & E. Pfeiffer (Eds.), *Mental illness in later life* (pp. 199-231). Washington, DC: American Psychiatric Association.

Reding, M. J., Orto, L. A., Winter, S. W., Fortuna, I. M., DiPonte, P., & McDowell, F. H. (1986). Antidepressant therapy after stroke. *Archives of Neurology, 43,* 763-765.

Reifler, B. V., Raskind, M., & Kethley, A. (1982). Psychiatric diagnoses among geriatric patients seen in an outreach program. *Journal of the American Geriatrics Society, 30,* 530-533.

Reisberg, B., Ferris, S. H., DeLeon, M. J., & Crook, T. (1982). The Global deterioration scale for assessment of primary degenerative dementia. *American Journal of Psychiatry, 139*(9), 1136-1139.

Sahakian, B. J. (1991). Depressive pseudodementia in the elderly. Special issue: Affective disorders in old age. *International Journal of Geriatric Psychiatry,* *6*(6), 453-458.

Shamoian, C. A. (1991). What is anxiety in the elderly? In C. Salzman & B. D. Lebowitz (Eds.), *Anxiety in the elderly: Treatment and research* (pp. 3-15). New York, NY: Springer Publishing Co., Inc.

Sheard, M. H. (1975). Lithium in the treatment of aggression. *Journal of Nervous Mental Disorders, 160,* 108-118.

Stokes, G. (1992). *On being old: The psychology of later life.* Washington, DC: Falmer.

Stuart-Hamilton, I. (1991). *The psychology of aging.* London, UK: Jessica Kingsley.

Turnbull, J. M., & Turnbull, S. K. (1985). Management of specific anxiety disorders in the elderly. *Geriatrics, 8,* 75-82.

U'Ren, R. C. (1990). Emergency geropsychiatry. In G. Bosker, G. R. Schwartz, J. S. Jones, & M. Sequeira (Eds.), *Geriatric emergency medicine* (pp. 107-118). St. Louis, MO: Mosby.

Weiner, R. D. (1982). The role of electroconvulsive therapy in the treatment of depression in the elderly. *Journal of the American Geriatrics Society, 30,* 710-712.

Yoder, B. (1990). *The recovery resource book.* New York, NY: Simon and Schuster.

Zung, W. W. K. (1980). Affective disorders. In E. Busse & D. Blazer (Eds.), *Handbook of geriatric psychiatry* (p. 357). New York, NY: Van Nostrand Reinhold.

Unit III

The Intervention Process

Activities and rehabilitation, when functional impairment and/or disability are present, are used with older adults to enhance their quality of life. The process of planning and implementing activity intervention programs involves multiple considerations. Activity specialists use assessment, activity analysis, environmental design, motivational techniques, and a systematic program planning process to provide high quality activity intervention to older clients.

Unit III covers information that is central to the development and implementation of good activity intervention programming. The unit is organized according to the central elements of providing therapeutic care. Chapter 7 covers assessment, activity analysis, and the program planning process. Chapter 8 details the role and function of assessment. Chapter 9 addresses issues dealing with motivation and control. Chapter 10 completes the unit with information on the role of environment in supporting the optimal performance of older clients in activity intervention programs. Upon completing the unit, readers should have an understanding of the basic elements of activity intervention with older adult clients.

Key Terms

Activity Analysis
Assessment
Deconditioning
Evaluation
Individual Treatment Plan
Intervention

Maintenance
Planning
Prevention
Promotion
Rehabilitation
Therapeutic

Learning Objectives

1. Describe how therapeutic activity intervention can be used to meet the physical, social, emotional, and cognitive needs of older adults.
2. Identify the phases of systematic therapeutic activity intervention programming.
3. Distinguish between the use of therapeutic activity to attain promotion, preventive, maintenance, and rehabilitative treatment goals.
4. Discuss individual treatment goals and objectives in therapeutic activity intervention.
5. Identify categories of activities used in therapeutic intervention with older adults.
6. Identify barriers to participation in therapeutic activity intervention programs.

Chapter 7

Programming for Therapeutic Outcomes

Introduction

The purpose, content, process, and outcomes of therapeutic activity intervention with older adults are presented in this chapter. The use of activities to reach therapeutic goals and to enhance the overall quality of life of elderly persons is discussed within the context of decline. Losses in functioning may be due to the accumulated effects of normal aging-related changes, the need to preserve remaining abilities, or disablement resulting from disease. The intervention process including assessment, activity analysis, program planning, implementation, and evaluation is outlined. Important principles and sample tools guiding steps in the process are presented. Categories of activities that can be used to reach therapeutic goals are introduced. The chapter concludes with a brief discussion of motivation as a leading barrier to participation in therapeutic activity intervention.

The Purpose of Therapeutic Activity Intervention

As adults age, the accumulated effects of the aging process eventually impress every aged person with the importance of maintaining his or her personal health and functional capabilities. To remain independent in as many areas of functioning as possible is a concern to most older people, especially as they reach their eighth and ninth decade of life or experience impairment from disease or injury. A sense of well-being, perceptions of life satisfaction, and quality of life are often governed by how independent and active the older person is able to be on a daily basis. The use of activities to promote health, prevent impairment and dependence, maintain optimal functional capability, and to remediate in the instance of disablement forms the underlying rationale for therapeutic activity intervention.

The word *therapeutic* distinguishes the use of activities for purposive as opposed to diversionary reasons (Hamill and Oliver, 1980). A therapeutic approach is one that is intended to stimulate a change in behavior which will then be directed by one or more goals in the different areas of functioning (e.g., physical, emotional, mental, social) (Smith and Couch, 1990). The goal might be the *promotion* of optimal health, well-being, and vitality in older adulthood through engagement in a sport skill class, or the goal might be the *prevention* of accelerated declines that result from sedentary living. Activities that are of interest to the participant also can be used to *remediate* when there are functional losses due to injury, disability, disease, or illness. This use is another example of goal-directed intervention that distinguishes therapeutic activity from diversionary activity programs. An illustration of a remediation or *rehabilitation* goal might be the use of bibliotherapy to stimulate memory and to regain communication skills following a stroke. Therapeutic activity intervention, therefore, is fundamentally concerned with the use of activities for the purposes of inducing, facilitating, and maintaining independent functioning in the older adult to the degree that is possible within the individual's immediate environment. Behavioral change may be achieved through promotion, prevention, maintenance, or rehabilitation goals, or any combination thereof.

Figure 7.1 presents a model illustrating the continuum of therapeutic purposes and treatment goals that guide activity intervention. As can be seen in the model, promotion goals at the right end of the continuum are typical in situations where more independent functioning exists and the need for fewer supports characterize the status of the older person. Promotion goal–directed activities are targeted toward fostering and maintaining optimal functioning in the individual. These types of intervention activities may be incorporated into the normal routines of everyday life and are often less clinical in nature.

Prevention and maintenance goal–directed activities are at the mid-range of the continuum. Participants involved in prevention and maintenance activities understand that the behaviors produced through attaining these goals are essential for managing their risk for further decline and increasing dependency. *Deconditioning* is a leading reason underlying the use of prevention and maintenance activities. Deconditioning is the added and accelerated loss in functioning beyond that which is associated with normal aging-related change. Deconditioning is perpetuated by disuse due to illness or sedentary living (Saltin and Rowell, 1980). Deconditioning is reversible whereas the effects of normal aging-related declines are not (Asmussen, 1981). Deconditioning is amenable to therapeutic activity intervention and is most appropriate following extended bed rest due to illness, or in response to the propensity of aging adults to become increasingly sedentary, both mentally and physically. *Reconditioning,* therefore, is a guiding principle for prevention and maintenance goal–directed activity interventions. Deconditioning can be reversed through the prescriptive use of activities that are low impact, progressive in intensity, regular in frequency, and of an adequate duration to cause change or reconditioning. Physical

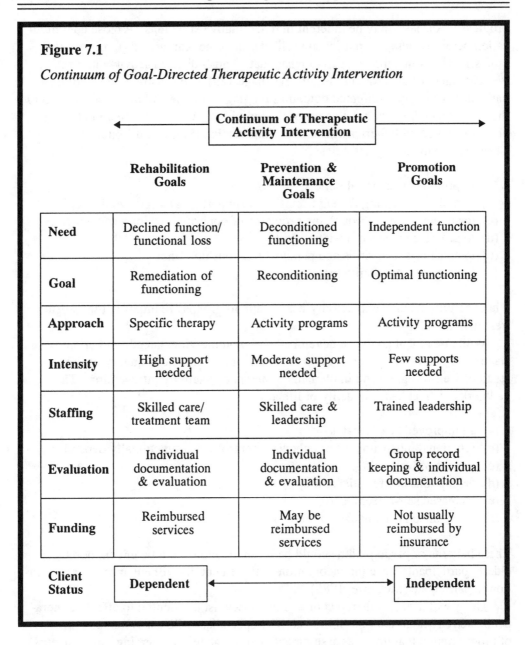

Figure 7.1

Continuum of Goal-Directed Therapeutic Activity Intervention

Continuum of Therapeutic Activity Intervention

	Rehabilitation Goals	Prevention & Maintenance Goals	Promotion Goals
Need	Declined function/ functional loss	Deconditioned functioning	Independent function
Goal	Remediation of functioning	Reconditioning	Optimal functioning
Approach	Specific therapy	Activity programs	Activity programs
Intensity	High support needed	Moderate support needed	Few supports needed
Staffing	Skilled care/ treatment team	Skilled care & leadership	Trained leadership
Evaluation	Individual documentation & evaluation	Individual documentation & evaluation	Group record keeping & individual documentation
Funding	Reimbursed services	May be reimbursed services	Not usually reimbursed by insurance
Client Status	Dependent		Independent

activities typically characterize reconditioning activity interventions, but carry over effects have been demonstrated in other areas of functioning (e.g., increased mental alertness, improved sociability, and greater independence in activities of daily living) (Larson and Bruce, 1986; Vallbona and Batzer, 1984).

Rehabilitation goals are directed by significant functional losses which have resulted in impairment or disablement to the extent that increased support is needed with individual skilled therapy. Progress is closely monitored and is documented from one session to the next. Long-term rehabilitation goals are often broken down into short-term goals that have task-specific components. Maintenance of declined functioning, or the expected continued decline of the individual as in the case of progressive disease, may be inherent in rehabilitative situations. A close communication between therapist, participant (client), and other caregivers (family and/or professionals) is an important part of rehabilitation goal–directed activity intervention.

The intent of the model in Figure 7.1 (page 129) is to illustrate how activities have therapeutic, goal-directed outcomes ranging from one end of the continuum to the other depending upon the needs of the individual. Certainly, other goals have been associated with therapeutic activity intervention (Smith and Couch, 1990). They include the use of activities:

(a) to provide avocational outlets,
(b) to assist in adapting the environment to support greater independence,
(c) to support coping through the provision of opportunities for achievement,
(d) to promote the use of residual skills,
(e) to enhance social skills and personal relationships, and
(f) to promote community membership.

Direct activity therapy and activity-based support groups are important therapeutic treatment modalities.

While treatment goals are developed based on individual needs and circumstances, ultimately all participants will experience an enhanced quality of life as a result of well-designed and implemented therapeutic activity intervention. The hallmarks of an enhanced quality of life are:

(a) an improved health status,
(b) functional independence or enhanced control when functionally dependent,
(c) a sense of well-being,
(d) perceptions of life satisfaction,
(e) increased self-esteem, and
(f) an enhanced personal/social network.

These benefits of participation should be apparent and should be understood by elderly participants since the recognition of these benefits will enhance their motivation to participate (McGuire, 1985).

The use of a skilled therapist or activity specialist is essential to effective therapeutic activity intervention. Skilled activity specialists utilize a systematic process of programming that involves assessment, activity analysis, planning, implementation, and evaluation. Therapeutic activity intervention, or goal-directed activity, is distinctly shaped by the functional status and needs of the individual. Declines in physical, social, emotional, and mental functioning are of immediate concern, as are other aspects of the person's life such as financial resources, social networks, and the design of the individual's daily life environment. Explicit in effective therapeutic activity intervention is the activity specialist's understanding of the programming process and the systematic delivery of intervention services.

Systematic Activity Intervention Programming

Why are activities used to intervene in the lives of older adults? In the preceding section the purposes of goal-directed therapeutic activity intervention were discussed. In this text the authors promote the use of activities to meet therapeutic goals that are normally inherent in the services delivered in a variety of senior service settings. These settings include adult daycare, senior center programs, nursing homes, rehabilitation centers, hospitals, and in-home care. Explicit in these settings are the needs of older adults for support, care, and treatment. Otherwise, the program of activity offerings would serve more diversional purposes and would not be within the purposes associated with therapeutic activity intervention. Diversional activity programs are not included in this text. The material contained in this book specifically addresses the use of activities to meet therapeutic treatment goals.

Once again, the question arises, "Why use activities to meet therapeutic goals?" Activities that are normally pursued in leisure reflect certain characteristics that motivate participation while also producing desired affective and physical states. Activities typically thought of as recreational are associated with pleasurable feelings, creativity, personal choice and preference and thus foster feelings of control. Enjoyable, satisfying, and often physically challenging activities are health promoting. Recreation activities foster positive health and perceived well-being, enhance social and personal relationships, and provide opportunities for human growth and development. Because of these inherent characteristics, the use of activities (recreational in origin) in intervention programming to effect changes in behavior that will produce therapeutic goal–directed outcomes is an appropriate and effective tool in the treatment process with elderly persons.

In this context, therapeutic activity intervention is like therapeutic recreation. The central functions of therapeutic recreation are to promote functional independence and to enable older individuals to attain a higher level of health, well-being, and satisfaction in later life. The use of activities as therapy using a systematic process of program planning parallels the same steps used in the delivery of therapeutic recreation services. In the following sections, a process of systematic program planning and implementation is presented that builds on the programming literature from both therapeutic recreation and gerontology (cf., Austin and Crawford, 1991; Elliott and Sorg-Elliott, 1991; Hamill and Oliver, 1980; Howe-Murphy and Charboneau, 1987; Kraus and Shank, 1992; O'Brien, 1982; Thews, Reaves, and Henry, 1993). Five major steps comprise the process:

(a) assessment,
(b) activity analysis,
(c) program planning,
(d) program implementation, and
(e) documentation and evaluation.

Assessment

Assessment is the critical first step in the process of effective therapeutic activity intervention. Assessment is client focused and is concerned with the environments in which the person functions on a daily basis. Assessment follows specific pragmatic techniques and procedures to construct a precise picture of the older person and his or her environment. Assessment of the individual and the environment allows the activity specialist to plan ahead for the best activities, methods for implementing the activities, and procedures for meeting the individual's need for support.

Multidimensional geriatric functional assessment is covered in detail in Chapter 8. This step in the process provides complete documentation about the person's functional status—physically, socially, emotionally, and mentally. A complete assessment also will include information about past activity participation, specific activity preferences and interests, and other pertinent background information (e.g., financial need, social support, insurance). In treatment facilities such as nursing homes where Medicare and Medicaid are used for service reimbursement, the Minimum Data Set (MDS) will form the first standard assessment to be administered. This tool will be supplemented with other instruments to provide complete client information. Short, easy-to-complete inventories and scales will be used to collect information about skill strengths and special abilities, functional declines, and problem areas in which the individual may need extra assistance. Comprehensive assessment of the individual also includes a medical history, the evaluation of functional competence in activities of daily living (ADLs) and instrumental activities of daily living (IADLs), a social history, and a mental status examination.

The goal of a thorough assessment is to collect and analyze information about the individual that will support the activity specialist in identifying problems, needs, strengths, residual skills, and special abilities. This information is instrumental to selecting, planning, modifying, implementing, and evaluating effective therapeutic activity interventions. The initial assessment begins the programming process but also is an integral part of ongoing intervention as the reassessment of skills, interests, needs, and strengths is used to evaluate progress and make changes in treatment.

Along with individual client assessment, the activity specialist will assess the physical and social environments in which the client functions on a day-to-day basis. Environmental factors that will potentially influence client functioning will be identified and evaluated in regard to their impact on performance (Ferrini and Ferrini, 1993). Architectural barriers and arrangements will be described and evaluated. For example, are the temperature, lighting, walking surfaces, and furniture layout appropriate for the individual's level of functioning, or do they present potential barriers or hazards? A systematic assessment will consider elements of the exterior and interior of the residential environment. Walkways, handrails, step surfaces, lighting, carpeting and walking surfaces are evaluated for safety and needed supports. Living areas also are reviewed for cluttered furniture and the security of any furniture that may be used for additional mobility support. The spatial layout of cabinets and closets, the safety features of appliances, and the overall safety of the bathroom are assessed. In the bedroom, adequate night lighting and a clear pathway to the bathroom should be provided and should be appropriate for the needs of the individual. In general, the mobility, safety, and comfort of the individual in his or her residence and daily activity environments are addressed through a detailed assessment and evaluation.

The social attitudes of family members, significant others, caregivers, and other program participants are assessed to identify potential barriers or problems. The social atmosphere, cultural background (including values, beliefs, and customs), and family functioning (family support) are important and will have a direct impact on the individual's needs and potential success in activity intervention. The social environment can support or detract from success of the individual and, therefore, must be taken into consideration during the assessment phase.

Adaptive devices, environmental redesign or modification, special equipment and materials, and support services each need to be considered since they may be instrumental in the success of activity intervention. As each individual becomes a potential client receiving activity intervention, these aspects of environment are equally important to individual functioning at assessment and in the program planning and implementation phases.

Based upon a thorough individual and environmental assessment, the activity specialist will identify the daily demands placed on the individual's functional competence and on any limitations imposed by the environment. A goal of this step in the therapeutic activity intervention process is to optimize the match between the individual, the environment, and the therapeutic activity intervention. If the demands of the environment exceed the individual's needs and capabilities, negative consequences rather than therapeutic goal attainment may result.

As a result of this initial and important step in the process, the activity specialist is able to identify a list of potential treatment goals and objectives that are appropriate for the individual. Environmental considerations and needs also will be known. The treatment goals may be both long range and short range. Global goals may be further subdivided into smaller, more task-specific objectives. Finally, treatment goals may be grouped according to their primary purpose; for example, rehabilitation, prevention, maintenance, and/or promotion. The grouping process is useful in distinguishing the level of need for skilled individual therapy from group interventions and is helpful to the activity specialist in organizing overall service delivery for a number of clients.

Activity Analysis

Activity analysis is the next step in the systematic process of programming for therapeutic activity intervention. Selecting just any activity to use in reaching a treatment goal is not an effective approach to ensure that the most appropriate activity has been employed. Therefore, activity analysis is a systematic evaluation of activities for their appropriateness and usefulness in attaining individual treatment goals for each client.

Individual activities are identified and analyzed on the basis of psychosocial and physical components and the specific skills required to engage in each activity. The activity specialist is concerned with whether or not the activity can be graduated or modified in order to accommodate the client's physical, mental, and emotional capabilities and residual skills. Is the activity amenable to adaptation? Does the activity present increasing complexity so that skill advancement can be fostered? Will the activity be directly applicable in meeting the individual's treatment goals or several treatment goals? Activities that are analyzed should include those that meet key psychosocial needs such as identity, affiliation, control, autonomy, security, self-esteem, inclusion, and meaningfulness (Zgola, 1987). If these psychosocial needs also are considered, the personal value of the activities to the individual is more likely to be realized. These are pertinent questions that the activity specialist will ask when analyzing activities to meet treatment goals.

Elliott and Sorg-Elliott (1991) developed a simple, efficient, and effective activity analysis form to assist the activity specialist (see Figure 7.2). This tool can be easily applied when conducting an activity analysis at this step of the systematic program planning process. The analysis process examines the demands of the activity on the participant in the following specific areas: physical, cognitive, and social.

Zgola (1987) suggested that activities be graded according to the degree of environmental demand on the participant. Figure 7.3 (page 136) presents the grading hierarchy. Each activity should be evaluated regarding task demand ranging from the lowest level of involvement which is passive attending to the highest level where active planning and implementation are done by the participant. Grading activities will assist the activity specialist in a number of important ways, including:

(a) helping to increase motivation for participation,
(b) assisting in the tracking of progress in treatment, and
(c) enhancing a better client-treatment fit with the selected activities.

In the process of identifying and analyzing activities to meet client need-based treatment goals, the activity specialist is on a constant watch for additional activities that can be used in the treatment plan and in the overall activity program for the facility. Elliott and Sorg-Elliott (1991) pointed out that activity analysis is useful to the professional in helping to assure that a well-rounded, client-oriented activity program is developed.

Program Planning

When client and environmental assessment information is complete and is combined with the activity analysis data, the activity specialist is prepared to engage in the program planning phase. At this step in the process, several tasks are to be accomplished including:

(a) goals and objectives will be stated,
(b) specific activities will be selected,
(c) resources and problems will be identified,
(d) alternative plans of action will be proposed, and
(e) a clear plan of action will be articulated in writing.

Figure 7.2

Recreation Activity Analysis

Activity:_____ Rater:_____

Description:_____

_____

Directions: For each category and item below, evaluate the requirements of participation in the mentioned activity. Use the following scale to mark the appropriate number for each item: 0=None; 1=Very Low/Little; 3=Intermediate/Medium; 5=Very High/Very Much. For example, if no body movements are needed for the activity, mark the [0] at the "sedentary" end.

Physical Aspects

Body Movements:	sedentary [0] [1] [3] [5] bending/stooping	Comments:
Arms/Hands—Range of Motion:	little [0] [1] [3] [5] full	
Dexterity:	little [0] [1] [3] [5] great	
Lifting:	light [0] [1] [3] [5] heavy	
Legs/Feet—Joint Motion:	none [0] [1] [3] [5] much	
Flexibility:	little [0] [1] [3] [5] much	
Coordination—Body Parts:	none [0] [1] [3] [5] precise	
Hand/Eye:	none [0] [1] [3] [5] precise	
Endurance:	little [0] [1] [3] [5] much	

Cognitive Aspects

Concentration:	none [0] [1] [3] [5] great
Memory Retention:	short-term [0] [1] [3] [5] long-term
Verbalization:	none [0] [1] [3] [5] much
Skill Level:	low [0] [1] [3] [5] high
Sensory Discrimination:	
Sight:	low [0] [1] [3] [5] high
Smell:	low [0] [1] [3] [5] high
Touch:	low [0] [1] [3] [5] high
Hearing:	low [0] [1] [3] [5] high
Taste:	low [0] [1] [3] [5] high

Affective/Social Aspects

Interaction:	low [0] [1] [3] [5] high
Physical Contact:	low [0] [1] [3] [5] high
Competition:	low [0] [1] [3] [5] high
Emotional Response:	low [0] [1] [3] [5] high

Source: Modified from Elliott & Sorg-Elliott, 1991, pp. 14–15

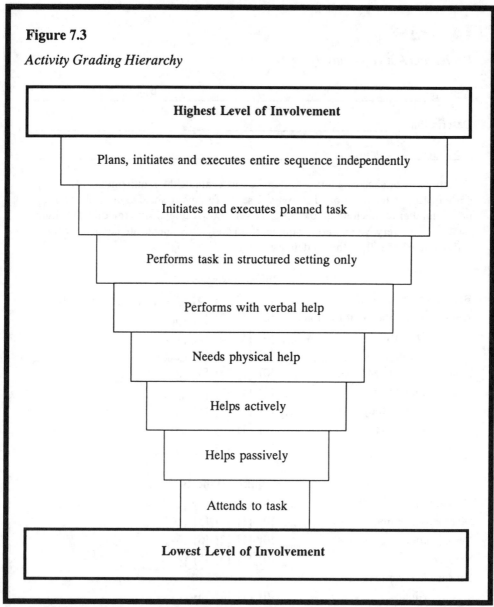

Figure 7.3

Activity Grading Hierarchy

Highest Level of Involvement
Plans, initiates and executes entire sequence independently
Initiates and executes planned task
Performs task in structured setting only
Performs with verbal help
Needs physical help
Helps actively
Helps passively
Attends to task
Lowest Level of Involvement

Source: Modified from Zgola, J.M. (1987). *Doing things: A guide to programming activities for persons with Alzheimer's disease and related disorders,* p. 35. Reprinted by permission of the Johns Hopkins University Press.

It is important that careful consideration be given to each of these aspects of the plan. The focus will be on the individual, the environment, and the overall program. An individual treatment plan and an overall activity program are developed in writing. At this stage, the activity specialist is still engaged in planning what and how therapeutic activity intervention will be provided.

In developing the individual treatment plan, defining specific treatment goals and objectives will be matched with selected intervention activities. Treatment objectives will have three parts:

(a) the target behavior,
(b) the conditions under which the target behavior will be facilitated, and
(c) how progress or change will be measured on the target behavior (Zimmerman, 1988).

Clear, measurable treatment goals and objectives are placed within a target time frame for accomplishment. Conditions, therefore, are the kinds of supports that the client will need in order to attain the target behavior, and measurement is the documented evidence that the behavior has been attained.

Specified treatment goals and objectives with target behaviors form the basis of the written individual treatment plan. For example, a treatment goal for Mrs. A could be to improve her ability to transfer independently from her wheelchair to the toilet by engaging in regular upper body strength training. A target behavior under this goal might be that Mrs. A will perform the "hands to shoulders" exercise independently for a minimum of 10 repetitions on three separate occasions per week following a six-week treatment program. This target objective could be further graded to a series of smaller, task-specific objectives with specified conditions for measuring progress. To illustrate this grading, Mrs. A will perform the "hands to shoulders" exercise at five repetitions with 75% assistance for three different occasions during the first week of therapeutic activity. This task-specific objective can be graded by changing the assistance over the six-week program, eventually eliminating assistance. The number of repetitions can be increased, also. The goal of the treatment program is that Mrs. A will have attained adequate upper body strength to transfer independently from her chair to the toilet after the six-week intervention.

As can be seen in this brief example, the objectives are measurable, and they progressively move the client toward attaining the long-range treatment goal. Objectives have clearly specified performance criteria, whereas goals specify the outcome expected by meeting the treatment objective(s) (O'Brien, 1982). Specific activities are selected as they match treatment goals and provide the best conditions for meeting individual needs. A processing form for organizing and utilizing the results from the analysis of individual activities is recommended (see Figure 7.4, page 138).

As activities are selected to meet individual treatment goals, the activity specialist considers the resources that are needed and available for delivering the activities. Problems and possible constraints (e.g., inadequate space, money, staff) will be identified and carefully evaluated for potential impact on the delivery of the program. Often the activity specialist discovers that problems and constraints are resolvable by considering them at this step in the process and seeking solutions. However, in the instance where a potential consequence provides a formidable barrier (e.g., legal liability risks) and is not readily resolvable, it may be appropriate to redesign the program to reflect a more feasible plan of activities. This also is the appropriate time to make backup or alternative written plans to safeguard against circumstances (e.g., inclement weather) that will prevent the original plan of activities. Trouble shooting in advance can help to assure implementation of a rewarding and successful therapeutic activity intervention program.

Figure 7.4

Therapeutic Intervention Activity Program Analysis

Activity												
Physical Aspects:												
Bending												
Range of Motion												
Dexterity												
Lifting												
Leg/Feet												
Flexibility												
Coordination of Body Parts												
Hand/Eye Coordination												
Endurance												
Cognitive Aspects:												
Concentration												
Memory Retention												
Verbalization												
Skill Level												
Sight												
Smell												
Touch												
Hearing												
Taste												
Affective/Social Aspects:												
Interaction												
Physical Contact												
Competition												
Emotional Response												

Source: Modified from Elliott & Sorg-Elliott, 1991, p. 16

It is important to build consensus and commitment to the treatment plan among all those persons who will be involved in insuring its success. First and foremost, the client must be consulted, and ideally should approve his or her individual treatment plan. Other staff and activity leaders also can be involved in this phase. Often it is also appropriate to involve family members and other caregivers by informing and involving them in the decisions that are made at this point in planning. With a developed and agreed upon plan in place, the activity specialist is ready to move on to the implementation phase.

Program Implementation

When the activity specialist has completed the planning phase with careful consideration given to client needs, therapeutic goals, activity selection, and program design, it is time to implement the plan. During the implementation phase, the activity specialist engages in the process of:

(a) staffing,
(b) scheduling,
(c) supervising or directing the delivery of therapeutic activities,
(d) managing the environment where service delivery is occurring,
(e) attending to safety and the management of risk, and
(f) managing the funding aspects of the program.

Each of these tasks is an important component of successful program implementation.

Staffing entails selecting, training, and supervising all staff (paid professionals and volunteers) who are in leadership roles, or who provide support services that are needed to insure participant participation (e.g., aides), or who are associated with program management (e.g., clerical). Staffing is critical to program success. Selecting and hiring staff with the necessary qualifications for the direct delivery of therapeutic activity intervention is a special consideration. Hiring professionals with a college degree and/or certification, specifically in therapeutic recreation, gerontology, or general recreation programming, will help to insure high quality service delivery. There is no substitute for professional leadership. However, many programs also rely on volunteer staff in addition to qualified professionals. Beyond the hiring of qualified staff, such as the Certified Therapeutic Recreation Specialist (CTRS), the development of leadership skills is incorporated into staff training.

The activity staff will benefit from in-service training to learn about different disabling conditions and the effects of these conditions on behavior. Technical skills training should be routinely offered. The following topics are examples of technical skill training areas: transferring from bed to wheelchair and chair to toilet as well as safety procedures for handling wheelchairs and other assistive devices. Other topics that can be regularly included in staff training are: motivation and control in elderly persons, environmental design and modification, activity intervention techniques, communication skills, and caregiving strategies. Regular staff meetings and educational sessions will help to insure a well-trained, smooth working staff. Technical skills plus leadership preparation are critical components of a quality program.

A well-designed program plan is one with structure but not rigidity. Scheduling is an important step in matching the daily life routines of individuals with their treatment plans and management considerations (e.g., staffing). Balancing treatment plans while considering personal daily rhythms plus the overall program and facility schedule can be challenging. A clearly defined schedule is the goal of a well-developed and implemented plan. The schedule of a well-developed and implemented plan should cover:

(a) individual needs,
(b) program and group structure,
(c) staff and program resources, and
(d) facility time, space, resources, and operation.

The ability to be flexible is part of balancing the structured schedule with unexpected circumstances that quite frequently arise.

Solid program implementation and management means being attentive to participants, staff, the environment, and the overall atmosphere created with the merging of these elements during activity intervention. The activity specialist is responsible for ensuring that the environment is accessible, spacious, stimulating to the senses, safe, and organized for maximum ease of use. Is the activity area arranged to foster socialization and to provide a quiet place for privacy or rest? Are participants involved in how the environment is arranged or used? Are there an adequate number of staff immediately available if needed? The management of participants, staff, environment, and program are all important aspects, as is fiscal management. Maintaining program funds and resources is essential to full program implementation.

Finally, as the program plan moves into full implementation, the activity specialist will attend to the evaluation phase. In reality, evaluation is inherent in all phases of programming from beginning to end. In addition to ongoing evaluation at the end of a program or a specific activity intervention, an overall program evaluation is completed as a distinct step in the process of service delivery.

Evaluation

The successful operation of a therapeutic activity intervention program is the ultimate goal of using a systematic programming process. Evaluation provides feedback through the documentation, recordkeeping, and decision making that is necessary to measure success at each phase, and at the end of the program. Evaluation is concerned with appropriateness, effectiveness, acceptability, efficiency, adequacy, efficacy, and impact. Did the client receive the benefits expected from the activity intervention? Were staff adequately trained to provide skilled care and intervention? Was the environment appropriately designed and managed to support the client's participation and progress? These and other questions will form the evaluation phase and a feedback loop to assessment, activity analysis, planning, and implementation. Because this systematic approach to programming is intended to be dynamic and ongoing, the feedback gained through evaluation is essential in the ongoing programming process.

Evaluation as it relates to assessment and intervention will focus on a careful appraisal of client needs, treatment goals and objectives, progress measurement, and the overall efficacy of the intervention in terms of bringing about the targeted behaviors specified in the individual treatment plan and in the overall program goals and objectives. In addition to staff progress notes and the documentation of client performance on standard assessment measures, the activity specialist also will seek interview data from the client. The interviewer will request feedback on aspects of the program and will include the individual's perceptions of social and psychological benefits of participation in therapeutic activities. This careful documentation of client progress and feedback is essential in program evaluation and for service reimbursement purposes. In addition to these sources of information, observational data from activity leaders and volunteers regarding psychosocial benefits of participation can be utilized in program evaluation. These observations may be found in staff meeting minutes, staff log books, or in anecdotal recollections after the program or activity intervention has ended.

In addition to the essential evaluation of client treatment goals and progress, the activity specialist will want to appraise other aspects of the program including:

(a) staff performance,
(b) the cost-effectiveness of the program,
(c) environmental quality and management,
(d) risk management and safety, and
(e) scheduling.

Staff meeting minutes, administrative records, critical incident documentation, and cost-benefit statistical information serve as evaluation indicators.

Evaluating the quality of the program helps to assure accountability of the activity staff and facility. It is a measurement process that should be guided by stated programmatic goals and objectives beyond those that are client specific. Therefore it is the responsibility of the activity specialist to state overall programmatic and administrative goals at the beginning of the programming process in order to insure that adequate and appropriate evaluative data are collected. Salamon (1986) suggested that five broad questions shape and direct evaluation efforts:

1. *What* is to be evaluated? If it is to be staff, program/activities, scheduling, management, or participants, be certain to clearly and operationally define both the long-term goals and specific program objectives.
2. *Who* will be evaluated—staff, program participants, volunteers? Be certain that the role and expectations associated with the "who" are clear and specific.

3. *Where* will the evaluation information or data come from? Does the data already exist or does it need to be collected, and from what sources—people, documents, records, observations?
4. *When* will the evaluation information be collected—when the program begins, during, or after? Are there multiple times when evaluation should take place?
5. *How* will the evaluation information be analyzed—statistically, qualitatively, or both?

Evaluation is the phase in systematic program planning that binds the process together. The resulting information is used in a feedback loop that sustains the programming cycle. Figure 7.5 illustrates this systematic process and the dynamic nature of the relationship among all the phases.

Activity Categories and Barriers to Participation

Prospective activities that are being considered for meeting individual and group intervention goals can be organized according to the major areas of functioning (i.e., physical, cognitive, and psychosocial). This organizational scheme can help give direction to the systematic programming process described in the previous section. Activities within these categories subsequently can be analyzed for their contribution to attaining therapeutic intervention goals and objectives in the activity analysis and planning phases. Based on the outcome of client assessment, activity analysis, and individual treatment program planning, some activities over others will emerge as having the best potential for meeting the intentions of therapeutic intervention.

The authors of the present text present these three major categories of activities, physical, cognitive and psychosocial, in Chapters 12, 13, and 14. A chapter on leisure education (Chapter 11) is also included as an integral service function associated with therapeutic activity intervention. The rationale for including leisure education is that activity intervention embraces more than direct skilled intervention using activities. Therapeutic activity intervention can impact the development of awareness, values, attitudes, knowledge, and skills that are related to the daily leisure behavior and quality of life for all older adults. The systematic process of teaching the decision-making and problem-solving skills associated with the wise use of leisure is central to any activity intervention that is used for attaining prevention and promotion goals. As clients move along the continuum from rehabilitation to prevention and promotion goals, leisure education will enhance their progress and satisfaction.

Leisure education focuses on the use of task analysis, learning, and motivating behaviors that support an active, healthy lifestyle. Another purpose for providing leisure education, therefore, is to enable elders to develop and maintain independent, healthy, socially acceptable, and satisfying leisure pursuits after leaving the intervention program.

Activity interventions in the physical, cognitive, and psychosocial areas, along with leisure education, are collectively aimed at promoting optimal functioning, preventing further decline, and rehabilitating functional losses. Physical activities

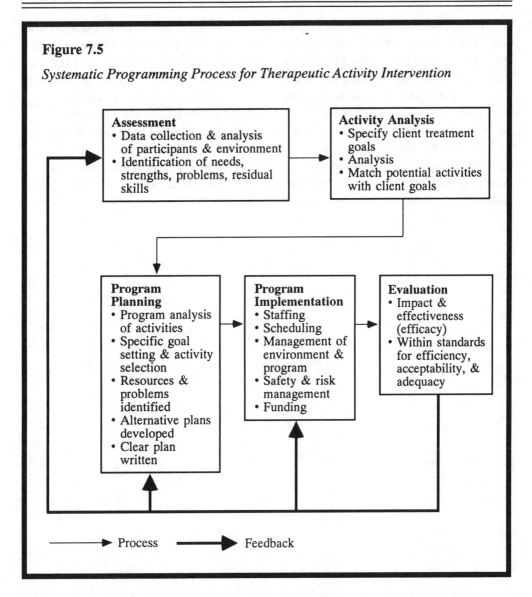

Figure 7.5

Systematic Programming Process for Therapeutic Activity Intervention

include games, sports, outdoor pursuits, exercise, and fitness-related movement. Cognitive activities are directed toward memory skills and learning. They include games, bibliotherapy, debate groups, reading, and others. Psychosocial activities are those that address adjustment, socialization, social relationships, and community membership. They include such activities as parties, visiting, reminiscencing, remotivation, relaxation, and others.

One of the most formidable barriers to activity participation among elders is motivation. It is so important that an entire chapter in this book is devoted to motivation and control (Chapter 9). To help insure the participation of elders in activity intervention programs, several factors will need to be considered. A leading factor is the individual's personal motivation for behavior change. If the activity program is perceived to be meaningful to the individual, enjoyable, and within the person's capabilities, motivation to participate will be heightened.

How an activity intervention is structured also is important to participant motivation. The removal of social and physical barriers is crucial. Making the participant feel welcome and part of the group is the first step. Providing adequate time for the individual to become oriented to the other participants, the place, and the structure of the activity intervention also is instrumental in motivating or demotivating the participant. Sharing and building commitment are necessary for staff to attain motivation with more hesitant participants. Learning when and how to approach, as well as when to step back when working with older adults, are part of the overall therapeutic activity intervention process. Understanding motivation is central to achieving program success. It must not be overlooked in the process of planning and implementing successful therapeutic activity interventions.

Summary

Therapeutic activity intervention is aimed at meeting prevention, health promotion, and rehabilitative purposes depending upon the client's functional status and the nature of his or her impairment or disability. Activity intervention follows a systematic process which includes the following steps: assessment, activity analysis, planning, implementation, and evaluation. Activity specialists develop goal-directed interventions using activities from four main categories: physical, cognitive, social, and leisure education. This chapter sets the stage for Chapters 8, 9, and 10 which provide greater detail about assessment, motivation and control, and environmental considerations in therapeutic activity intervention.

Comprehension Questions

1. Describe how therapeutic activity intervention can be used to meet promotion, prevention, rehabilitation (remediation), or maintenance goals.
2. Explain three categories that can be used for grouping therapeutic activities and why these categories are pertinent to the functional status of older adults.
3. Identify barriers to successful activity intervention with older clients.
4. What are the major phases in developing and implementing systematic therapeutic intervention programming?

References

Asmussen, E. (1981). Aging and exercise. In S. M. Horvath & M. K. Yousef (Eds.), *Environmental physiology, aging, heat and altitude: Proceedings of light, heat, and altitude conference* (pp. 419-428). New York, NY: Elsevier Science Inc.

Austin, D. R., & Crawford, M. E. (Eds.). (1991). *Therapeutic recreation: An introduction.* Englewood Cliffs, NJ: Prentice Hall.

Elliott, J. E., & Sorg-Elliott, J. A. (1991). *Recreation programming and activities for older adults.* State College, PA: Venture Publishing, Inc.

Ferrini, A. F., & Ferrini, R. L. (1993). *Health in the later years* (2nd ed.). Madison, WI: Brown & Benchmark.

Hamill, C. M., & Oliver, R. C. (1980). *Therapeutic activities for the handicapped elderly.* Rockville, MD: Aspen Publishers Inc.

Howe-Murphy, R., & Charboneau, B. G. (1987). *Therapeutic recreation intervention: An ecological perspective.* Englewood Cliffs, NJ: Prentice Hall.

Kraus, R., & Shank, J. (1992). *Therapeutic recreation service: Principles and practices* (4th ed.). Dubuque, IA: Wm. C. Brown.

Larson, E. B., & Bruce, R. A. (1986). Exercise and aging. *Annals of Internal Medicine, 105,* 783-785.

McGuire, F. A. (1985). Recreation leader and co-participant preferences of the institutionalized aged. *Therapeutic Recreation Journal, 19*(2), 47-54.

O'Brien, C. L. (1982). *Adult daycare: A practical guide.* Belmont, CA: Wadsworth Inc.

Salamon, M. J. (1986). *A basic guide to working with elders.* New York, NY: Springer Publishing Co., Inc.

Saltin, B., & Rowell, L. B. (1980). Functional adaptations to physical inactivity and activity. *Federal Proceedings, 39*(5), 1506-1513.

Smith, J., & Couch, R. H. (1990). Adjustment services and aging. *Vocational Evaluation and Work Adjustment Bulletin, 23*(4), 133-138.

Thews, V., Reaves, A. M., & Henry, R. S. (1993). *Now what? A handbook of activities for adult day programs.* Winston-Salem, NC: Bowman Gray School of Medicine, Wake Forest University.

Vallbona, C., & Batzer, S. B. (1984). Physical fitness prospects in the elderly. *Archives of Physical Medicine and Rehabilitation, 65,* 194-200.

Zgola, J. M. (1987). *Doing things: A guide to programming activities for persons with Alzheimer's disease and related disorders.* Baltimore, MD: The Johns Hopkins University Press.

Zimmerman, J. (1988). *Goals and objectives for developing normal movement patterns.* Rockville, MD: Aspen Publishers Inc.

Key Terms

Active Rehabilitation Program
Activities of Daily Living (ADLs)
Assessment
Environmental Assessment
Formal Functional Assessment
Functional Assessment
Health/Wellness Status Assessment
Informal Functional Assessment
Instrumental Activities of Daily
 Living (IADLs)
Leisure Activity Assessment

Medical Assessment
Multidisciplinary Assessment
Multidisciplinary Team
Observation
Preventive/Maintenance Programs
Psychiatric Assessment
Screening
Skill Performance
Social-Role Performance
Sociocultural/Socioeconomic
 Assessment

Learning Objectives

1. Understand the purpose and function of multidimensional geriatric assessment in the care of elderly persons.
2. Describe how a functional assessment in conjunction with a medical history can assist in the identification of specific problems that interfere with daily life functioning.
3. Explain how information from a multidimensional geriatric assessment may be used for program planning and evaluation purposes.
4. Discuss the differences between a functional assessment and a medical assessment.
5. Describe several assessment instruments suitable for use with elderly persons.

Chapter 8

The Role and Function of Assessment

Introduction

The care and daily life functioning of elderly persons may be enhanced through the knowledgeable use of assessment techniques. This chapter provides a rationale for the provision of ongoing assessment services to older individuals. Information about the objectives and functions of the assessment process with elderly persons also is included.

The chapter describes the elements of a multidimensional geriatric assessment including medical, psychiatric, sociocultural/socioeconomic, activity, and environmental evaluation. Functional assessment and its components such as activities of daily living (ADLs) and instrumental activities of daily living (IADLs) are defined. Information is offered regarding several assessment instruments. The chapter concludes with some general guidelines for the implementation of assessment procedures.

Rationale for Assessment

Aging may be viewed according to two basic principles. First, specific aging-related changes occur at various intervals in the physical, psychological, and social areas of an individual's life. The progression of aging from the physical, psychological, and social perspectives, however, is not uniform from one individual to the next. The second basic principle of aging indicates that there is a significant degree of hetero-geneity among members of the elderly population regarding the rate and progression of aging-related change. Assessment of elderly persons, therefore, requires gathering information from several sources on a variety of characteristics while focusing upon the individual and his or her circumstances. A comprehensive assessment will take into consideration the interrelationship between a declining functional status and its impact upon the daily and basic living skills of the elderly individual (Teague, 1987).

Typically, the older person's functional status is positively correlated with a sense of well-being and is also a useful predictor of health service consumption (Teague, 1987). Assessment information is useful in decreasing the inappropriate use of healthcare services, preventing the waste of resources, and contributing to a reduction in the diagnosis of disability when early declines are detected and treated. Proper assessment will lead to improved diagnosis, more appropriate placement of persons within the healthcare system, less dependency on skilled nursing facilities, improved functional status of the elderly, and more appropriate use of medications (Koff, 1988).

Professionals who engage in assessing elderly persons include social workers and health service workers (e.g., physicians, nurses, and therapists of various types, including activity specialists) (Teaff, 1985). Assessment of the elderly has an individual focus, as well as a community or public health perspective. These two approaches are complimentary. The first approach is intended to meet the needs of individuals who have applied for, or have been referred for, service. The second approach is useful in uncovering other elderly persons in the community who are in need of assistance (Biegel, Shore, and Gordon, 1984).

Assessment Defined

Assessment represents a systematic approach to identifying and describing client problems (Edinberg, 1985). Assessment is a method of viewing the problems of older people, deciding what is wrong, and determining what can be done to alleviate or eliminate these problems (Butler, Lewis, and Sunderland, 1991). Competent care of older persons requires a broad outlook because often they are vulnerable to disability from a variety of perspectives such as disease states or economic conditions (Gallo, Reichel, and Andersen, 1988).

According to Kane and Kane (1981), a careful assessment will accomplish several objectives and functions:

- documentation of an individual's problems,
- determination of conditions that need additional services or support,
- documentation of minor changes in functioning,
- provision of accurate diagnosis of problems,
- provision of an efficient monitor of progress,
- assistance in the prediction of outcomes or decisions, and
- obtaining critical information in an efficient manner.

Many problems in the elderly are hidden; they are problems that are not frequently mentioned because of embarrassment, negativity, modesty, or ignorance. Professionals who assess elderly persons should possess sufficient knowledge concerning common health problems of older adults (e.g., arthritis, high blood pressure, diabetes, heart disease). They must not only be good listeners, but they also must ask the right questions in order for the geriatric assessment to achieve its fullest potential in the identification and clarification of problems (Ham, 1989).

A thorough and appropriate assessment constitutes the basis for any rational, systematic, and effective treatment program for older persons. For the majority of frail elderly, comprehensive assessment should initially be undertaken and repeated at intervals. According to Kemp and Mitchell (1992), geriatric assessment is pursued for one or more of the following reasons:

- to establish a diagnosis;
- to determine the personal, social, and environmental dynamics that maintain, control, and influence behavior;
- to establish baseline measures and information from which to assess the effects of treatment or natural changes in the client's status; and
- to assess the ability to care for oneself and to function in various environments.

Assessment also is a tool for encouraging the maintenance of good health and well-being. Assessment information can aid in the identification of resources within the individual, the family, and the environment that can contribute to the life quality of the elderly individual. Because frail elderly persons are highly vulnerable to adverse changes in their environments, the available resources of family, home, social network, formal care system, and access to transportation are important components of both individual assessment and care plans (Koff, 1988).

Multidimensional Assessment

Assessment is at the heart of geriatric practice, and activity specialists utilize the information that results from a *multidimensional assessment* to assist in the development of appropriate activity interventions. Assessment of the problems and needs of the elderly person may be directly translated into the appropriate plan for therapeutic activity intervention and caregiving. Because of the nature of many elderly persons' problems coupled with the frequent presence of multiple interacting medical and functional conditions, comprehensive evaluation can be a time-consuming and costly process. Multidimensional assessment broadens the traditional medical approach to also include the assessment of mental status and affect, functional status, social situations, economic circumstances, values assessment, and preventive strategies (Gallo, Reichel, and Anderson, 1988; Kane, Kane, and Rubenstein, 1989).

The use and coordination of the *multidisciplinary team* may allow for minimal redundancy in the assessments that are conducted. The value of assessment exists in its subsequent actions and strategies that make the process more efficient (Kane, Kane, and Rubenstein, 1989). Geriatric assessment usually involves professionals working together, a distinct set of criteria for evaluating the elderly, and three levels of intensity for the assessment—brief, intermediate, or comprehensive—based upon the individual's needs (Butler, Lewis, and Sunderland, 1991). The more frail older person usually will require many different services if optimal functioning and independence are to be achieved. Therefore, it is appropriate to make the comprehensive assessment of the elderly client a collaborative, information-sharing experience. Such a multidisciplinary approach can assist in the creative use of existing health services and the active development of such services in areas where they are lacking (Ham, 1989).

The principles that are applied in rehabilitation of the aging client depend upon the nature of the intervention to be performed. The information derived from the multidisciplinary assessment is instrumental in decisions concerning appropriate intervention approaches. *Active rehabilitation programs* involve the performance of skilled therapy. *Preventive/maintenance programs* utilize interventions that are integrated into the everyday life of the client. Multidimensional geriatric assessment can assist in guiding and selecting active rehabilitation interventions and in monitoring medical and preventive/maintenance interventions (Feinstein, Josephy, and Wells, 1980; Germain, 1987; Robinson, 1989).

Multidimensional geriatric assessment may be accomplished through the use of broadly designed scales such as the Older Americans Resources and Services (OARS) Functional Assessment Questionnaire (Fillenbaum, 1988). The OARS assessment was designed to assess the overall functional status and service use of elderly adults. Because older adults tend to experience chronic impairments, concern must focus less upon cure and more on the maintenance of personal welfare and independence (Fillenbaum, 1988). The OARS assessment was developed for a diverse group of practitioners and service providers; therefore, it may serve multiple purposes including program evaluation, needs assessment, and resource allocation decision making (Kemp and Mitchell, 1992).

Another broad-based tool, the Comprehensive Assessment and Referral Evaluation (CARE) (Gurland et al., 1977), was developed to provide extensive, reliable, multidimensional information on older people in urban communities. The assessment of psychiatric, medical, nutritional, economic, and social problems are embraced by the scale. Shorter versions of the scale also are available (Gurland and Wilder, 1984).

Screening and Observation

A distinction should be made between screening and assessment. *Screening* is a preliminary assessment based upon quick and often observational measures. Screening is used to identify people who need a more thorough assessment. *Formal assessment* is a longer process conducted with the identified "at risk" client. Formal assessment is used in the diagnosis and treatment process to identify the full range of problems and functional abilities/deficits, as well as to monitor progress during treatment (Kane and Kane, 1981).

The basis of assessment of human behavior is *observation* and *evaluation*. Although a care provider may feel that he or she knows a person well, the systematic and formal observations that are used in assessment are necessary to confirm the actual functional and health status of the individual. Another important reason for observation is to assess a person's ability to engage in activities that may be used in the treatment/intervention process (Barrowclough and Fleming, 1986).

General Guidelines for Assessment

The practitioner who conducts a geriatric assessment needs to establish rapport and a trusting relationship with the client. Older people may feel uncomfortable or anxious during assessment sessions which can lead to poor or decreased performance. Establishment of rapport plus explanation of the purposes of testing to the elderly client have added meaning for accurate assessment (Edinberg, 1985).

Another concern regarding assessment should involve keeping the sessions short, especially for ill or heavily-medicated clients. The phrasing of questions can be critically important. Discrepancies also may arise between different informants (i.e., between the client's responses and family members' responses). Tests should not be used by themselves to make decisions about the care and living arrangements of older persons. Rather, they should be considered as a part of the assessment process (Edinberg, 1985; Kane, Ouslander, and Abrass, 1989).

Elements of Basic Geriatric Assessment

Typically, a basic assessment will include:

(a) general personal information,
(b) physical health/medical assessment,
(c) mental status/psychiatric assessment,
(d) sociocultural/socioeconomic assessment,
(e) leisure activity assessment,
(f) evaluation of living environment and resources, and
(g) functional assessment.

A completed assessment provides baseline information and measurement of the individual's present status as well as a standard against which to evaluate future changes. Many older adults, particularly frail persons, will need various services for the remainder of their lives, and the collection of assessment information provides useful information in the current and future implementation of treatment interventions. An incomplete or haphazard approach to assessment is neither timesaving nor is it considered appropriate care (Butler, Lewis, and Sunderland, 1991).

Medical Assessment

A physical health/medical evaluation of the elderly individual focuses particular attention upon present illness and chronic conditions and on past medical problems. Medical assessments involve the examination and evaluation of all body systems including:

(a) vital signs;
(b) analysis of the skin, head, mouth and teeth, eyes, ears, nose, and throat;
(c) inspection of the neck;
(d) testing of the heart, lungs, and musculoskeletal system;
(e) exploration of the abdominal area, breasts, gastrointestinal system, and genitourinary tract; and
(f) neurologic assessment.

Laboratory analysis will include information about hematologic values, renal function, thyroid capacity, and glucose intolerance (Gallo, Reichel, and Anderson, 1988). *Medical assessment* should be comprehensive, multiphasic, and repeated on a regular basis. It is usually completed by a physician or a nurse. It should be emphasized that Medicare programs do not cover routine checkups which makes it extremely difficult for older persons to take advantage of early detection and prevention through regular physical examinations (Butler, Lewis, and Sunderland, 1991; Clark, 1984; U.S. Department of Health and Human Services, 1993).

Psychiatric Assessment

In the *psychiatric assessment,* the mental health professional must be aware of the possible presence of reversible delirium, functional disorders, and reactions to stress (e.g., situational depression). Much of what is viewed as "old age" may have a psychiatric component that deserves proper diagnosis and treatment. Both adaptive and maladaptive characteristics accompany adults into old age. Only through careful evaluation of the client's life history can differences be distinguished between those qualities possessed by the individual throughout life and those that first occurred in old age due to personality reorganization (Butler, Lewis, and Sunderland, 1991). When judging the adaptation of older persons, it should be remembered that the elderly commonly deal with more stresses than any other age group. Maintenance of the status quo may be all that is possible, and pride in present accomplishments is both significant and appropriate (Butler, Lewis, and Sunderland, 1991).

The psychiatric assessment often is termed a mental status examination. A traditional mental status assessment adapted from Strub and Black (1985) encompasses an evaluation of behaviors and mental capability over a range of intellectual functions. Assessment may include:

(a) level of consciousness,
(b) attention,
(c) language and communication skills,
(d) short-term and long-term memory,
(e) interpretation of proverbs,
(f) perception of similarities and differences,
(g) calculations,
(h) writing ability, and
(i) the capacity for construction.

Other mental status assessment instruments that can be utilized with older persons are the Short Portable Mental Status Questionnaire (Pfeiffer, 1975), the Folstein Mini-Mental State Examination (Folstein, Folstein, and McHugh, 1975), and the Kokmen Short Test of Mental Status (Kokmen, Naessens, and Offord, 1987). The Geriatric Depression Scale (Yesavage and Brink, 1983) and the Beck Depression Inventory (Beck and Beck, 1972) are appropriate in psychiatric assessment.

Psychiatrists are not the only persons who are qualified to do psychiatric evaluations. In community mental health centers, psychiatric hospitals, and other environments serving older persons, a team of professionals from many disciplines may conduct a joint mental status evaluation. Also, paraprofessionals with appropriate training often can assess the psychiatric condition of older persons (Butler, Lewis, and Sunderland, 1991).

Sociocultural/Socioeconomic Assessment

A *sociocultural/socioeconomic assessment* includes information concerning family structure, housing, work or retirement, friendship patterns, economic circumstances, social roles, activities, and interests. An evaluation of the family is crucial because the onset and maintenance of disorders often can be identified from the family context. It is inappropriate to routinely judge all older persons as helpless or fragile. Many elderly individuals still retain substantial influence over family and friends (Butler, Lewis, and Sunderland, 1991).

It is important to assess the support system of the older adult client. The informal social network, the formal support system, and semiformal supports are considered elements of the elderly person's total support system. These categories are reciprocal in nature. The informal support system includes family and friends. Formal supports are comprised of the Social Security Administration, Medicaid, and other social welfare agencies. Semiformal supports refer to neighborhood organizations such as churches and senior citizen centers (Berkman, 1983; Rzetelny and Mellor, 1981).

An adequate evaluation of social support will also determine the older person's healthcare coverage and economic circumstances. It is usually necessary to determine the individual's ability to pay for treatment. Personal financial responsibility, however, is generally not very useful because of the escalating costs in healthcare, the denial of adequate income programs, and the availability of job opportunities for older persons (Butler, Lewis, and Sunderland, 1991).

Sociocultural or socioeconomic assessment generally is completed by a social worker or other members of the social services staff. However, therapeutic activity specialists also can be involved in this type of assessment because of its relevance for activity programming. The Family or Friends APGAR (Adaptation, Partnership, Growth, Affection, and Resolve) (Smilkstein, Ashworth, and Montano, 1982) and the Social Resources component of the OARS assessment (Duke University Center for the Study of Aging and Human Development, 1988) are useful in conducting the sociocultural assessment of older adults. Additionally, the OARS assessment can be used to estimate the economic resources of older adults.

Activity Assessment

Activity assessment may be separated into two distinct components. Both of these appraisals, health/wellness status and leisure-time use skills, are completed by the activity specialist or in conjunction with other members of an interdisciplinary team (Hawkins, 1988).

The purpose of the *health/wellness status assessment* is to identify strengths and weaknesses of the older adult in order to enhance the leisure or recreation needs of the individual to the optimum. The basic components of a comprehensive health and wellness assessment include:

(a) general health status evaluation, completed by or with the guidance of a physician;
(b) physical fitness appraisal;
(c) nutritional analysis, which is usually accomplished by a dietitian; and
(d) stress or emotional adjustment appraisal (O'Donnell and Ainsworth, 1984; Teague, 1986).

The assessment of physical fitness typically involves:

(a) an exercise history,
(b) body composition,
(c) flexibility,
(d) muscle strength and endurance,
(e) balance and equilibrium,
(f) cardiopulmonary capacity, and
(g) contraindications for exercise (Teague, 1986).

A qualified activity specialist and an exercise physiologist generally can conduct an assessment of the physical fitness of older adults. Examples of physical fitness assessment instruments may be found in Ford (1985), and Katch and McArdle (1983).

A stress or emotional adjustment appraisal is generally useful in activity programming with older persons. This assessment includes documentation of the events that have produced stress in the individual's life and how he or she reacts to anxiety-producing circumstances. By developing an understanding of the older person's responses to stress and the phenomena that elicit stress reactions, more effective management of behaviors and social milieus can be facilitated. In addition, activities often are the logical intervention when stressful situations occur (Hawkins, 1988).

Leisure activity assessment is essential in the development of an appropriate therapeutic activity program for elderly persons. Leisure activity assessment involves gathering a variety of information (Wehman and Schleien, 1981). The activity specialist, as well as other interdisciplinary team members, will solicit information concerning the older person's repertoire of activities, interests, preferences, desires, and specific skills that support independent functioning (Hawkins,

1988). These data can be accumulated by using qualitative methods and/or standardized instruments such as the Linear Model for Individual Treatment in Recreation (Compton and Price, 1975), the Recreation Therapy Assessment (Cousins and Brown, 1979), and the Leisure Assessment Inventory (Hawkins, Eklund, and Martz, 1992). Leisure activity assessment clearly provides a picture of the individual's leisure activity participation patterns, his or her independent leisure decision-making, barriers to activity involvement, and some assessment of the overall satisfaction that leisure provides in his or her daily life.

Environmental Assessment

Environmental assessment is closely related to sociocultural/socioeconomic assessment. Typically, the social worker will initiate an evaluation of the older person's community resources. Available community services are appraised in order to improve the appropriate utilization of community-based services and professionals (e.g., visiting nurses, occupational therapists, and senior service volunteers) in the ongoing care and evaluation of elderly clients (Butler, Lewis, and Sunderland, 1991). The identification of supports that are needed in order to maintain community involvement may become the deciding factor between enabling the older person to remain at home or placement in an institutional setting such as a nursing home (Kane, Ouslander, and Abrass, 1989).

An important goal in the care and treatment of older persons is the restoration and/or maintenance of an optimal level of independent functioning in the most personally desired environmental setting (Clark, 1984). Because chronic functional impairment becomes more prevalent in old age with 50% of all elderly individuals living at home having some functional limitation in performing daily living activities and 80% having at least one chronic condition (e.g., high blood pressure, diabetes, heart disease, arthritis), personal independence becomes a primary concern to the elderly client. Due to the substantial burden of functional impairment in older persons, reliable objective assessment of the role of environmental support and design in relationship to functional loss is critical for the delivery of preventive, maintenance, and rehabilitative services to the elderly (Teague, 1987).

Functional Assessment

An assessment of functional competence or independence is an important part of any diagnostic process. It is relevant to assess functional status because physical health/medical diagnosis alone do not predict final outcome or the ability to live independently. The capacity of the individual to function independently or with assistance in the home is poorly described or predicted by medical condition alone. It is not enough to diagnose medical problems and treat them in isolation from the other aspects of the individual's life (e.g., family members, social constraints). When medical illness is determined, it affects the older person's total life including his or her functional capacity and underscores the dynamic relationship between functional competence and health status (Gallo, Reichel, and Anderson, 1988).

The functional assessment informs all members of the caregiving team (including aides and activity specialists) as to the elderly person's performance and need for support. Allied health professionals who conduct a functional assessment will:

(a) provide detail of the individual's overall functional status,
(b) define all factors interfering with or modifying normal function,
(c) identify all correctable factors in order to optimize functioning,
(d) judge appropriateness of current and future environments,
(e) objectively chart mental status,
(f) evaluate rehabilitation potential,
(g) define existing support services,
(h) evaluate overall prognosis, and
(i) construct a plan for the future (Gallo, Reichel, and Anderson, 1988; Ham, 1989).

Functional assessment is both formal and informal in nature (Robinson, 1989). *Formal functional assessment* is useful in determining health status, insurance compensation for health benefits, level and amount of social services required, and the most beneficial type of living arrangements or environments for the individual. Further, the planning of treatment interventions and the prediction of treatment outcomes are enhanced through accurate formal functional assessment (Feinstein, Josephy, and Wells, 1980; Germain, 1987).

Informal functional assessment involves the collection and integration of functional data that complement traditional formal assessment procedures. The older adult and his or her support persons are asked questions in a simple, open-ended manner. The questions address survival skills, the support system, barriers to optimal functioning, stress-related problems, and other issues of concern (Robinson, 1989).

The functional assessment is targeted at measuring and quantifying human behavior in regard to the performance of survival skills in day-to-day living. It focuses upon what clients can do and what they desire to do. It also provides data upon which to base and evaluate therapeutic activity intervention recommendations to older clients and their families (Mezey, Rauckhorst, and Stokes, 1993). Routine functional assessment of persons over 65 years of age can be incorporated into the annual physical examination. Functional assessment also is indicated when the individual's status suddenly changes, as well as at regular intervals for *at-risk populations* such as individuals with Parkinson's disease, frequent falls, or severe arthritis (Mezey, Rauckhorst, and Stokes, 1993).

Functional assessment usually includes *activities of daily living* (ADLs) and *instrumental activities of daily living* (IADLs). Assessment includes skill performance and social-role performance. ADLs are generally divided into seven tasks: eating, dressing, grooming, toileting, bathing, transferring, and mobility (Kemp and Mitchell, 1992). These seven abilities constitute the skills of self-maintenance or basic self-care activities, and are recognized as including the basic independence-promoting activities that are progressively lost in the declining elderly person. Other ADLs may include communication, continence, vision, and the use of the upper extremities. The functional abilities necessary for basic ADL performance include endurance, strength, range of motion or flexibility, and coordination (Kemp and Mitchell, 1992).

IADLs are the more complex activities that are necessary to lead an independent life. IADLs refer to the skills and behaviors that are needed to survive in the community. IADLs include the following: money management, household chores, use of transportation to access the community, shopping, taking care of one's health, communicating with others, and safety preparedness (Kemp and Mitchell, 1992).

Social-role performance is another component of functional competence and ability. This area consists of role performance as a member of society as well as interpersonal functioning. Factors related to social-role performance include the following: job performance, friendships, intimacy, parenthood/grandparenthood, recreation, assisting others, and self-maintenance. These abilities also include the skills of self-preservation (Kemp and Mitchell, 1992). *Skill performance* is another area included under functional status and located between IADLs and social-role performance in terms of complexity and the level of skills. These skills involve intellectual, motor, and personality traits (Kemp and Mitchell, 1992).

Although the use of instruments to assess the functional status of older persons is frequently ignored by physicians, it is highly relevant to activity specialists. Functional assessment is critical because the ability of elderly individuals to remain independent may depend upon their competence to perform essential ADLs. There are many geriatric functional assessment instruments available for use in this area (Gallo, Reichel, and Anderson, 1988). The Katz Index (Katz, Ford, Maskowitz, Jackson, and Jaffe, 1963) is one of the most well-known and widely-used of the ADL instruments (Kane and Kane, 1981). It is so popular that it has been used as a guide for the development of other ADL scales. The Barthel Index and Barthel Self-Care Ratings also are widely known and often used scales with demonstrated reliability and validity (Mahoney and Barthel, 1965).

The Performance Test of Activities of Daily Living (Kuriansky and Gurland, 1976) is a structured performance test of ADLs based upon actual observation of the individual's performance. Observation of the person's performance and reaction to various tasks provides information regarding mental status and its effect upon ADL activity. The Physical Self-Maintenance Scale and Instrumental Activities of Daily Living Scale measure ADLs and IADLs among community and hospitalized older adults (Lawton and Brody, 1969).

The Blessed-Roth Dementia Rating Scale (Blessed, Tomlinson, and Roth, 1968) and the Direct Assessment of Functional Status Scale (Lowenstein et al., 1989) were designed to measure the ADL and IADL status of clients with cognitive impairments such as Alzheimer's disease and other forms of dementia. These scales rely on information from a caregiver, relative, or other persons who are in close contact with the elderly individual. Information from these scales is best interpreted when used in conjunction with other measures of cognitive status (Kemp and Mitchell, 1992).

Summary

Multidimensional assessment of the elderly is a challenging but essential aspect of the treatment process. Professionals who assess the physical, mental, social, activity, economic, and ethical conditions that impact the well-being of older persons can become more effective and knowledgeable through the utilization of standard evaluation techniques. Assessment is a valuable tool for the preservation of health status, well-being, and quality of life of older persons. It also is useful in the identification of individual, family, and environmental resources that are instrumental in the care and treatment process. Assessment offers important benefits to the elderly and their family members. It can assist in understanding the value and significance of the environment for the maintenance of well-being and provide goals for improvement. Assessment also may define a plan for realistic expectations of family members' participation in the care of their elderly relatives.

Comprehension Questions

1. Discuss why a multidisciplinary geriatric assessment is desirable when planning the care and treatment of older persons.
2. What are the components of a functional assessment? Name an assessment tool that can be used in each assessment area.
3. What is the difference between a functional assessment and medical evaluation?
4. Describe the assessment information that activity specialists will utilize in planning a therapeutic activity intervention with an elderly client.

References

Barrowclough, C., & Fleming, I. (1986). *Goal planning with elderly people: How to make plans to meet an individual's needs.* Dover, UK: Manchester University.

Beck, A. T., & Beck, R. W. (1972). Screening depressed patients in family practice: A rapid technique. *Postgraduate Medicine, 52,* 81-85.

Berkman, L. (1983). The assessment of social networks and social support in the elderly. *Journal of the American Geriatrics Society, 31,* 743-749.

Biegel, D. E., Shore, B. K., & Gordon, E. (1984). *Building support networks for the elderly: Theory and applications.* Newbury Park, CA: Sage Publications, Inc.

Blessed, G., Tomlinson, B., & Roth, M. (1968). Association between quantitative measures of dementia and of senile change in the cerebral gray matter of elderly subjects. *British Journal of Psychiatry, 114,* 797-811.

Butler, R. N., Lewis, M. I., & Sunderland, T. (1991). *Aging and mental health: Positive psychosocial and biomedical approaches* (4th ed.). New York, NY: Merrill.

Clark, G. S. (1984). Functional assessment in the elderly. In T. F. Williams (Ed.), *Rehabilitation in the aging* (pp. 111-124). New York, NY: Raven.

Compton, D., & Price, D. (1975). Individualizing your treatment program: A case study using LMIT. *Therapeutic Recreation Journal, 9,* 127.

Cousins, B., & Brown, E. (1979). *Recreation therapy assessment.* Jacksonville, FL: Amelia Island ICF/MR.

Duke University Center for the Study of Aging and Human Development. (1988). *Older Americans Resources and Services (OARS) methodology: Multidimensional functional assessment questionnaire* (2nd ed.). Durham, NC: Author.

Edinberg, M. A. (1985). *Mental health practice with the elderly.* Englewood Cliffs, NJ: Prentice Hall.

Feinstein, A. R., Josephy, B. R., & Wells, C. K. (1980). Scientific and clinical problems in indexes of functional disability. *Annals of Internal Medicine, 105,* 413-420.

Fillenbaum, G. G. (1988). *Multidimensional functional assessment of older adults: The Duke Older Americans Resources and Services procedures.* Hillsdale, NJ: Lawrence Erlbaum Associates Inc.

Folstein, M. F., Folstein, F. E., & McHugh, P. R. (1975). Mini-mental state: A practical method for grading the cognitive state of patients for the clinician. *Journal of Psychiatry Research, 12,* 189-198.

Ford, R. (1985). *Health assessment handbook.* Springhouse, PA: Springhouse.

Gallo, J. J., Reichel, W., & Andersen, L. (1988). *Handbook of geriatric assessment.* Rockville, MD: Aspen Publishers Inc.

Germain, P. S. (1987). Measuring functional disability in the elderly population. *American Journal of Public Health, 71,* 1197-1199.

Gurland, B., Kuriansky, J., Sharpe, L., Simon, R., Stiller, P., & Birkett, P. (1977). The comprehensive assessment and referral evaluation (CARE): Rationale, development, and reliability. *International Journal of Aging and Human Development, 8,* 9-42.

Gurland, B. J., & Wilder, D. E. (1984). The CARE interview revisited: Development of an efficient, systematic, clinical assessment. *Journal of Gerontology, 39,* 129-137.

Ham, R. J. (1989). Functional assessment of the elderly patient. In W. Reichel (Ed.), *Clinical aspects of aging* (3rd ed.) (pp. 26-49). Baltimore, MD: Williams and Wilkins.

Hawkins, B. A. (1988). Leisure and recreational programming. In M. P. Janicki, M. W. Krauss, & M. M. Seltzer (Eds.), *Community residences for persons with developmental disabilities* (pp. 217-227). Baltimore, MD: Paul H. Brookes Publishing Co.

Hawkins, B. A., Eklund, S. J., & Martz, B. L. (1992). *Detecting aging-related declines in adults with developmental disabilities: A research monograph.* Cincinnati, OH: Research and Training Center Consortium on Aging and Developmental Disabilities.

Kane, R. A., & Kane, R. L. (1981). *Assessing the elderly: A practical guide to measurement.* Lexington, MA: D. C. Heath & Co.

Kane, R. A., Kane, R. L., & Rubenstein, L. Z. (1989). Comprehensive assessment of the elderly patient. In M. D. Petersen & D. L. Wilhite (Eds.), *Healthcare of the elderly.* Newbury Park, CA: Sage Publications, Inc.

Kane, R. L., Ouslander, J. G., & Abrass, I. B. (1989). *Essentials of clinical geriatrics* (2nd ed.). New York, NY: McGraw-Hill.

Katch, F. I., & McArdle, W. D. (1983). *Nutrition, weight control, and exercise.* Philadelphia, PA: Lea & Febiger.

Katz, S., Ford, A., Maskowitz, R., Jackson, B., & Jaffe, M. (1963). Studies of illness in the aged. The Index of ADL: A standardized measure of biological and psychosocial function. *Journal of the American Medical Association, 185,* 914-919.

Kemp, B. J., & Mitchell, J. M. (1992). Functional assessment in geriatric mental health. In J. E. Birren, R. B. Sloane, G. D. Cohen, N. R. Hooyman, B. D. Lebowitz, M. Wykle, & D. E. Deutchman (Eds.), *Handbook of mental health and aging* (2nd ed.) (pp. 671-697). San Diego, CA: Harcourt, Brace, Jovanovich.

Koff, T. H. (1988). *New approaches to healthcare for an aging population.* San Francisco, CA: Jossey-Bass.

Kokmen, E., Naessens, J. M., & Offord, K. P. (1987). A short test of mental status: Description and preliminary results. *Mayo Clinic Proceedings, 62,* 281-288.

Kuriansky, J., & Gurland, B. (1976). Performance test of activities of daily living. *International Journal of Aging and Human Development, 7,* 343-352.

Lawton, P., & Brody, E. (1969). Assessment of older people: Self-maintaining and instrumental activities of daily living. *Gerontologist, 9,* 179-186.

Lowenstein, D., Amigo, E., Duara, R., Guterman, A., Hurwitz, D., Berkowitz, N., Wilke, F., Weinberg, G., Black, B., Gittleman, B., & Eisdorfer, C. (1989). A new scale for the assessment of functional status in Alzheimer's disease and related disorders. *Journal of Gerontology, 44*(4), 114-121.

Mahoney, F., & Barthel, D. (1965). Functional evaluation: The Barthel index. *Maryland State Medical Journal, 14,* 61-65.

Mezey, M. D., Rauckhorst, L. H., & Stokes, S. A. (1993). *Health assessment of the older individual* (2nd ed.). New York, NY: Springer Publishing Co., Inc.

O'Donnell, M. P., & Ainsworth, T. H. (1984). *Health promotion in the workplace.* New York, NY: John Wiley & Sons, Inc.

Pfeiffer, E. (1975). A short portable mental status questionnaire for the assessment of organic brain deficit in elderly patients. *Journal of the American Geriatrics Society, 23,* 433-441.

Robinson, K. M. (1989). Module 2.B: Rehabilitation services. In B. A. Hawkins, S. J. Eklund, & R. Gaetani (Eds.), *Aging and developmental disabilities: A training inservice package* (pp. 1-44). Bloomington, IN: Indiana University Institute for the Study of Developmental Disabilities.

Rzetelny, H., & Mellor, J. (1981). *Support groups for caregivers of the aged.* New York, NY: Community Service Society.

Smilkstein, G., Ashworth, C., & Montano, D. (1982). Validity and reliability of the family APGAR as a test of family function. *Journal of Family Practice, 15,* 303-311.

Strub, R. L, & Black, F. W. (1985). *The mental status examination in neurology* (2nd ed.). Philadelphia, PA: F. A. Davis Co.

Teaff, J. D. (1985). *Leisure services with the elderly.* St. Louis, MO: Times Mirror/ Mosby.

Teague, M. L. (1987). *Health promotion programs: Achieving high-level wellness in the later years.* Indianapolis, IN: Benchmark Press.

Teague, M. L. (1986). Comprehensive health assessment: An algorithmic model. *Therapeutic Recreation Journal, 20,* 39-50.

U.S. Department of Health and Human Services. (1983). *Medicare.* SSA Publication No. 05-10043. Washington, DC: Author.

Wehman, P., & Schleien, S. (1981). *Leisure programs for handicapped persons: Adaptations, techniques, and curriculum.* Baltimore, MD: University Park Press.

Yesavage, J. A., & Brink, T. L. (1983). Development and validation of a geriatric depression screening scale: A preliminary report. *Journal of Psychiatry Research, 17,* 37-49.

Key Terms

Amotivation	Extrinsic Motivation
Antecedents of Behavior	Independence
Autonomy	Intrinsic Motivation
Blocks to Communication	Motivation
Compliance	Nonverbal Techniques
Consequences of Behavior	Objective Autonomy
Control	Physical Restraint
Designated Autonomy	Privacy
Direct Autonomy	Rapport
Disruptive Behavior	Self-Determination
Elderly Mystique	Subjective Autonomy
Environment	Wandering Behavior

Learning Objectives

1. Understand the importance of autonomy, motivation, and control for elderly persons in treatment settings.
2. Differentiate between independence and autonomy.
3. Describe the concepts of motivation and control as they apply to elderly persons.
4. Examine the problems associated with a lack of motivation or control.
5. Explain techniques to improve motivation among elderly persons.
6. Identify common behavior management techniques.

Chapter 9

Motivation and Control

Introduction

Perceptions of autonomy and control can positively influence the physical and psychological well-being of elderly persons. Uncontrollable situations may have detrimental effects on thinking and behavior. This chapter discusses the importance of autonomy, motivation, and control for elderly clients. The issue of independence also is reviewed.

This chapter explores various motivational techniques—improvement of rapport and nonverbal skills—and behavioral strategies including environmental management, relaxation, and communication. By examining disability programs, one is able to consider problems associated with the infringement of individual rights. The chapter concludes with the suggestion that complex matters of autonomy should be resolved jointly by elderly individuals and their caregivers.

Importance of Autonomy, Motivation, and Control for Elderly Persons

Older individuals who reside in restrictive settings (e.g., nursing homes) are often alienated, less satisfied, and more dependent upon other persons. Real or perceived *autonomy* and *control* are central concerns. Opportunities for clients to make choices and control events that influence outcomes should be promoted (Langer and

Rodin, 1976). It has been demonstrated that belief in one's control over an undesirable event can reduce aversion to that situation (Glass and Singer, 1972). Perceptions of control also may have a positive effect on psychological functioning, performance, and physical well-being (Rodin, 1983). At the same time, uncontrollable situations can have detrimental effects on thoughts and behaviors and may create severe stress and anxiety (Geer, Davison, and Gatchel, 1970).

Perceptions of control are expected to change with age. The loss of valued social roles, the normal biological changes associated with aging, and the occurrence of major life events such as retirement and bereavement may challenge one's sense of control. These events also can alter the explanations and interpretations of less significant occurrences which further may erode feelings of competency and self-worth for many older persons (Rodin and Langer, 1980). For elderly clients in restricted environments, choices about clothing, diet, and other aspects of daily living have the potential to enhance perceptions of control and mastery over the environment (Newcomer and Caggiano, 1976).

Privacy is another aspect of environmental control that is related to autonomy and self-concept. When personal space is unavailable, many individuals withdraw from social interaction. Privacy can be provided through the use of physical room dividers, a decrease in noise levels, the closing of room doors, rearrangement of furniture, and use of private areas or rooms where confidential conversations may occur (Moos, 1976; Windley and Scheidt, 1976).

Motivation is comprised of those sources that energize behavior in general and in particular situations. Motivation helps to maintain a person's goal-directed behavior and to contribute to the continuity and persistence of certain behaviors (Blazer, 1985). Motivation refers to a prompt for action or a desire that makes an action pleasant or necessary. In psychology, motivation is viewed in terms of a physiological or psychological need or drive which stimulates behaviors that attempt to reduce the drive or need. Motivation is considered to be an important factor in performance with the implication that if motivation is improved, performance might also improve (Carroll and Gray, 1981).

Independence and Autonomy

Independence

The issue of *independence* can be viewed as the right to flourish. The right to flourish implies that there are many routes to independence which may exist, even in what may seem like inconsequential areas of choice (Cohen, 1992). The independent living movement views services for older persons as either encouraging or limiting independence. Services can be controlled and directed by consumers or by agencies. Consumer-directed services accept risk-taking and uncertainty and are directed at a level of involvement that gives meaning to life. The independence striven for by the independent living movement means more than mere survival with the limited goal of preventing institutionalization (Berkowitz, 1987).

Most elderly persons with disabilities have approached late life free of disability. It is not until the age of 80 or 90 that many older individuals must learn to cope with the disabling effects of arthritis, osteoporosis, cardiovascular disease, blindness, diabetes, and other ailments. However, the *elderly mystique* as described by Rosenfelt (1965) is apparent in the common myth that disability in old age indicates inevitable decline and demise and a significant end to skill and mastery. According to the elderly mystique, elderly persons who become disabled are no longer able to travel, to eat the foods they prefer, to engage in physically demanding activities, to maintain schedules, or to exercise authority. The elderly mystique is one that many disabled elderly individuals have come to accept as the inevitability of aging (Cohen, 1992).

Government assistance, such as Social Security disability disbursements and Medicare reimbursements, requires dependence. Older individuals' awareness of their own potentials for autonomy has made Social Security disability ineffective for many. Disability does not suggest the inability to participate in life, and receiving disability benefits does not imply abdicating responsibility for oneself or for one's community (Beedon, 1992; Rubinstein, Kilbride, and Nagy, 1992).

An increase in beliefs that powerful others control elderly intellectual functioning indicates that older persons consider themselves to be less competent than many persons and therefore more dependent upon particular individuals to complete various cognitive tasks. Even if an elderly adult is not influenced by the stereotypes of aging, the older individual may believe that adaptation requires relinquishing primary control in favor of assuming control through secondary sources (Rothbaum, Weisz, and Snyder, 1982; Schulz, 1987).

All too frequently, policymakers, program planners, and practitioners commonly support and encourage the elderly mystique. Programs for the elderly often utilize and promote activities based upon a model of incompetence (Minkler, 1990). Because independence cannot be easily measured, it is often considered to be without meaning. Healthcare, rehabilitation, and social service program providers must explore the similarities and differences between and among younger and older persons with regard to their attitudes toward rehabilitation, decision making, independence, control, activities, and role expectations (Cohen, 1992).

Autonomy

Autonomy refers to self-rule or self-determination and includes the attributes of liberty, independence, and freedom of choice. The feeling of autonomy is similar to a sense of control; that is, feeling in control rather than believing that one is controlled by others. Autonomy includes both an objective and a subjective component. The objective aspect refers to the enhancement of self-determination through the removal of apparent barriers, while the subjective portion includes the more personal experience of self-determination—the feeling of control over one's life (Tobin, 1991).

Objective autonomy is most often the focus in the care of elderly persons—the presence of barriers (choice of clothing, bed times, types of food, etc.) should be minimized. However, the concept of autonomy must be expanded to incorporate a personal sense of autonomy within each individual. This enhancement of *subjective autonomy* is more difficult to achieve than merely removing objective barriers. An increased subjective sense of personal autonomy for the elderly often may involve the maintenance of interdependent relationships with other individuals (Tobin, 1991).

The justification for autonomy of elderly persons is based in law. All persons must receive due process and equal protection even though they may be elderly and/ or chronically impaired. A second justification for older adult autonomy is intrinsic to medical ethics which require health professionals to utilize their knowledge and skill to find the greater balance of good over harm in treatment and care. This responsibility may lead to parent-like behaviors that impose on the autonomy of elderly individuals. A third justification is concerned with how to modify policies and practices when a cure is not possible or probable. In such a situation the relationship of the client with physicians and other healthcare professionals is clearly different. The client often exhibits a greater degree of awareness of his or her adaptation to the disease or disability than do "expert" health professionals. The challenge then is to modify professional judgments to include greater sensitivity to the potential adverse consequences of treatment, policies, and practices (Hofland, 1988; Tobin, 1991).

Likewise, it is unclear why there is a tendency to turn every decision in the lives of older persons into a healthcare decision. Elderly nursing home clients generally desire more control over many areas of their lives. However, many older persons state that they currently possess little control (Kane, Caplan, Freeman, Aroskar, and Urv-Wong, 1990). A solid commitment to the value of human life provides insurance against discrimination, repression, and murder (Thomasma, 1991).

Autonomy should be promoted because it advances individual welfare and generally, most individuals know how to further their own interests better than anyone else (Buchanan and Brock, 1986). However, many individuals do not have the capacity to act on their decisions. These persons must be encouraged to make decisions for themselves and be provided assistance in implementing the decisions even in difficult or nearly impossible situations. Also, far too little attention is given to understanding older persons as they really are and assisting them in being themselves; an omission that occurs even with the best of intentions (Collopy, 1988).

Direct versus designated autonomy means making decisions and acting on one's own or granting the authority to others to decide or to act. It is often necessary to combine both with explicit, mutually-accepted responsibilities. The inability of many mentally-impaired elderly persons to make rational decisions should be considered. The reasoning of elderly individuals whose choices may appear unreasonable demands respect. In many instances, there is no simple answer regarding professionally responsible behavior (Collopy, 1988). Autonomy may be promoted, but that does not insure that client satisfaction is guaranteed. Certainly, no one person receives everything that he or she desires. Autonomous elderly individuals must have the right to exercise at least some small amount of choice and control (Kane, Caplan, Freeman, Aroskar, and Urv-Wong, 1990).

Autonomy is not merely an end state. It also comprises the use of particular skills, abilities, desires, and preferences that are the products of past efforts and interactions. One's abilities and capacities are subject to interpretation by others in a complex and dynamic manner. Autonomy means freedom to experience the world within the framework of personal habit, choice, necessity, insight, and validation. Autonomy exists and is best understood on an individual basis with no preset standards or criteria. It is spontaneous within events and environments in which caregivers are responsive to being a part of a true community (Agich, 1993; Tulloch, 1990).

Motivation

Motivation causes one to initiate, direct, and sustain behavior. *Intrinsic motivation* refers to behaviors that are engaged in for their own sake—for the pleasure and satisfaction that are to be gained. *Extrinsic motivation* refers to behaviors that are performed in order to acquire or to avoid some consequence and are not performed merely for the experience of engaging in them (Deci, 1971, 1975; Deci and Ryan, 1985).

In addition to intrinsic and extrinsic motivation, *amotivation* also can be considered. Amotivated behaviors are neither intrinsically nor extrinsically motivated. They are nonmotivated behaviors in which individuals perceive a lack of dependence or interconnection between their behaviors and outcomes. For example, a nursing home client may state that he or she really does not know why he or she plays cards—that playing cards does not accomplish anything for him or her. There are no intrinsic or extrinsic rewards, and participation in the activity will decline and eventually cease. Learned helplessness can be a consequence of amotivation. Amotivated behavior is the least self-determined. There is no sense of purpose, no expectation of reward, nor the chance to change the progression of events (Deci, 1971, 1975; Deci and Ryan, 1985).

Motivation is central in the management of older persons in congregate care environments. It represents a quality and an attitude of mind that provide a sense of direction and purpose, a desire and willingness to participate. Chronically ill elderly persons often do not possess the necessary resources or skills to remain active and involved in everyday life. These clients generally want to remain independent while maintaining both physical and mental activity (Clark, 1978; Hunt, 1988). Motivation, or the lack of it, possibly is the most frequently used explanation for success and failure in rehabilitation settings and clinical practice (Kemp, 1986).

There are several theories of motivation. Humanistic theory is useful and relevant for explaining mature adult behavior. A hierarchy of needs is associated with humanistic theory and includes physical concerns, safety, belonging, love, esteem, self-actualization, desire for knowledge and learning, and aesthetic or beauty interests. Humanistic needs are motivating, and elderly persons with impairment or degeneration may feel threatened at any or all levels of need (Dreher, 1987; Klausmeier, 1975).

In motivating the elderly, the caregiver will consider the circumstances that encourage or support behavior and the conditions that discourage or prevent behavior. Motivation is most desirable when:

(a) the person knows what he or she wants and expects that it can be obtained,
(b) the associated rewards are meaningful and timely, and
(c) the consequences of the behavior are not negative or substantial.

To improve motivation, strategies are undertaken that will maximize the chances of the individual receiving what he or she wants, promote his or her belief and expectation that what is wanted can be obtained, reward progress toward that goal, and minimize any undue costs of the behavior (Kemp, 1986).

Age-related differences in motivational levels may affect the rehabilitation of older persons. Older adults require more and different reinforcement than do younger individuals. Rehabilitation activities are usually harder for elderly persons. It is, therefore, generally less useful to promise benefits that are far in the future because the emergence of disability can indicate the approach of life's end (Riley and Foner, 1968). Older individuals respond best to concrete goals that affect the functions of daily living. A concern for safety and security are more significant than career, future achievement, financial compensation, and materialism (Neugarten, 1968).

Self-determination is a necessary condition for the enhancement of motivation. Self-determination allows the elderly individual to try new activities, to explore unfamiliar territories or arrangements, and to experience satisfaction from the exploration (Deci, 1980).

Elderly persons need to be supported in their attempts to engage in enjoyable and challenging activities of their own choosing. Participation in elected activities can heighten motivation and is related to positive consequences. A focus upon the nature of encouragement for participation in the activities of daily living will be a concern. If elderly persons feel compelled by others to engage in particular activities, intrinsic or self-determined extrinsic motivation toward certain activities may be reduced (Vallerand and O'Connor, 1989). Many elderly persons have decreased expectations concerning their abilities and potentials. Without a positive belief in oneself, behavior can be undecided and easily suppressed. Older individuals, as well as the younger persons who offer them treatment, must truly believe that improvement is possible (Kemp, 1986).

Control

A fear of a loss of *control* over one's environment often is a concern of the elderly. A loss of control frequently is associated with a loss in independence (Feingold and Werby, 1990). A person's beliefs concerning control may be a result of an ability to engage in and to complete various tasks (Cornelius and Caspi, 1986). The idea of control over the environment is a powerful force that also serves as a motivator. Yet, caregivers generally do not trust the decision-making capabilities of older clients (Chowdhary, 1990). It also has been demonstrated that restricted opportunities for control will limit the positive effects of interventions designed to increase the perceived control and competence of elderly clients (Timko and Moos, 1989).

Behavior that increases control in a manner which is mutually beneficial to both the client and the staff has been shown to result in positive outcomes. However, nursing home staff members often reinforce dependent rather than independent behavior (Hutchison et al., 1983). Personal choice increases perceived control, and, as a consequence, motivation and performance also are enhanced. Attempts to encourage self-determination must take into account the amount of control desired by the individual because there is much diversity in preferences for control among the elderly. Too much choice or control can sometimes be as overwhelming and detrimental as too little (Perlmuter, Monty, and Chan, 1986; Rodin, 1987).

Individuals who have experienced more negative life events and those persons who are more functionally impaired often display a greater decline in perceived control (Arling, Harkins, and Capitman, 1986). A significant number of the oldest nursing home clients are more likely to have the desired amount of control when compared to younger nursing home clients. Clients of nursing homes with high degrees of desired control also are generally in poorer health with decreased functional abilities (Mullins, 1985).

Lack of control can cause increasingly poor mental and physical health. Control is likely to be an issue in old age because of the accumulated losses related with the aging process. It has been confirmed that control directly affects health status by altering an individual's physiological processes (Rodin, 1986). A pattern of reliance upon one's own efforts or skills to attain goals can facilitate the development of a variety of efficient coping strategies that enable one to deal more directly and successfully with the many problems identified with old age. Aging may simply become another obstacle for which effective coping strategies are determined and then utilized (Die, Seelbach, and Sherman, 1987). Enhancement of elderly clients' perceptions of control can include:

(a) promotion of choice and the elimination of helpless stereotypes,
(b) encouragement of positive accomplishments and a sense of responsibility,
(c) provision of successful experiences and modification of unrealistic goals, and
(d) the utilization of communication skills that reinforce control (Teitelman and Priddy, 1988).

Physical Restraint

In any discussion of control the issue of *physical restraint* of elderly clients must be addressed. It has been confirmed that restrained elderly persons are likely to be ill, frail, and at risk of death during hospitalization or institutionalization (Frengley and Mion, 1986; Robinson, Boyko, Lane, Cooper, and Jahnigen, 1987; Strumpf and Evans, 1988). The reasons offered by staff members for restraint of the elderly include prevention of falls, impaired mental status, and facilitation of treatment. In contrast, clients rarely cite the need for restraints to prevent falls or for other safety reasons. A strong emotional response to the application of restraint may be explained by the fact that so few older persons perceive the need for restraints (Strumpf and Evans, 1988).

Responses to the experience of restraint vary in intensity and reflect feelings of denial, discomfort, anger, and resistance. Yet, many staff members often are unable to propose alternatives to physical restraint. Elderly persons can provide several practical suggestions. When restraints are used, they must be considered as a special treatment requiring further assessment, intensive monitoring, and consultation with healthcare team members. Alternative interventions should be attempted. The possible elimination of restraining devices except under the most extreme, short-term circumstances is recommended (Strumpf and Evans, 1988).

Motivational Techniques

The extent to which decisions are made about activities, the nature of participation in activities, and the progression of the activities determines individuals' success in adaptation. Elders will become discouraged and less satisfied with their lives if they perceive themselves as lacking control. Older persons may then perform less well and become increasingly at risk for illness and injury (Blazer, 1990). Individuals who work with elderly persons will consider the factors that influence motivation. Providing opportunities for autonomy and choice are strongly recommended because self-determination is necessary for the increase of motivation (Vallerand and O'Connor, 1989).

Activity leaders maximize a sense of control and freedom by offering activities in which choice is promoted. Through experiencing personal control and competence, elderly clients will overcome a fear of failure and learn to more realistically assess the demands of their environments (Dowd, 1984).

The development of trust is essential to a group leader's success in the encouragement of participation. As much time as is necessary should be spent in the establishment of *rapport*. An especially useful motivational technique is the provision of snacks. Refreshments can be used as a means to secure additional interest and to provide a period of relaxation during activities that require a high degree of mental, emotional, or physical involvement (Salamon, 1986).

Motivation may be based upon giving participants recognition. The participation of a visitor in an activity also can be a powerful motivator. The importance of motivation must not be minimized. Imagination and creativity are required for thoughtful programming which attracts the greatest number of participants (Salamon, 1986).

Elderly individuals who have received control-enhancing interventions (e.g., instruction in self-responsibility, stress-management, physical fitness, nutritional awareness, and spirituality) have experienced significant improvements in their levels of perceived control and well-being (Slivinske and Fitch, 1987). The practitioner's challenge is to assess accurately the elderly individual's need for therapy, leisure education, or voluntary recreation participation and then to provide relevant activities that have the potential for the emergence of freedom within the activity. Respect for individual human rights and dignity should be the standard in all activity programs. Individual differences must be considered with an emphasis upon previous lifestyles, leisure interests, former roles, individual personality, and personal values when programming relevant activity interventions (Iso-Ahola, 1980; Robertson, 1988).

Additionally, elderly clients should not be overstimulated. Older persons tend to perform less well when arousal is too great. When the arousal states caused by anxiety and stress are reduced however, the performance of elderly individuals tends to improve. Meaningful material will be remembered more often, and the material is also more motivating if it is relevant. Unique experiences also may be remembered well. However, individuals can more clearly remember if they realize that the information to be recalled has some priority (Carroll and Gray, 1981).

Motivation for involvement is influenced by several factors including a desire for change. Hamill and Oliver (1980) noted other relevant aspects of motivation to be the desire to please others, the need for approval, associations between past experiences and the present, social rewards gained from sharing, a sense of creativity, curiosity, achievement and recognition, and the need to improve competence.

Elderly participants will be more highly motivated when they are related to as adults. "They deserve respect and will respond to it" (Hamill and Oliver, 1980, p. 30). Activities should be offered that are age-appropriate and based on goals determined by and shared with participants. The recognition of any degree of progress also can be rewarding. Ongoing staff-participant interaction must occur in order to ensure that needs and goals are met (Hamill and Oliver, 1980).

Although nonverbal techniques may be as effective as verbal motivational techniques, *nonverbal techniques* often are neglected. A shoulder touch, a gentle hand squeeze, or a hug, will make an individual feel welcome. Smiles and laughs are also motivational cues. Sincerity is essential when utilizing verbal and nonverbal techniques. It is important to remember that elderly persons of different cultural/ ethnic backgrounds may respond differently to the various nonverbal techniques (Leitner and Leitner, 1985).

The specific benefits of an activity and how those benefits relate to the particular needs of an individual should be emphasized. Personal invitations and the provision of leadership roles for clients can assist in motivating them to participate in an activity. Another practical technique concerns the use of peer influence as a motivator of participation. Further, the enhancement of self-image is important in motivating client involvement and also is a significant outcome of participation in activities (Leitner and Leitner, 1985).

Participation in a broad range of challenging activities within one's capabilities should be encouraged (Steinkamp and Kelly, 1985). However, the elderly client's capacity for self-direction will remain underutilized as long as the idea of providing more and more directed activities is maintained. Value must be assigned to a person's own accomplishments, but encouragement and recognition are always necessary (Hamill and Oliver, 1980; Kiernat, 1987).

Behavioral Techniques and Strategies

The appropriate assessment of behavior problems in older persons may lead to treatment planning that utilizes reinforcement, the shaping of desired behaviors, and/ or new learning and skills. *Antecedents of behavior* require evaluation before behavioral interventions can be applied. Antecedents of behavior are the events and circumstances that immediately precede the problem behavior. Antecedents are related to location—the behavior occurs at a certain place. Some antecedents are cognitive; that is, they reflect certain thought patterns or feelings within the client.

Additional antecedents are social—other persons can trigger problem behavior. Any or all antecedents can be related to the maintenance of problem behavior (Edinberg, 1985).

The *consequences of behavior* also must be determined. It is critical to examine the positive rewards that result from client behavior and to alter the outcomes until the problem behavior is discontinued (Edinberg, 1985). Positive reinforcement is necessary for every client. Elderly persons who are apparently unmotivated to attend activities may become involved when small activity groups meet in the clients' rooms. There is a tendency for elderly individuals to avoid association with clients who function at lower levels than themselves. It is apparently too great a reminder of the decline associated with aging and the additional care that is required (Elliott and Sorg-Elliott, 1991).

The terms motivation and compliance are often confused. *Compliance* refers to obedience or submission to the desires of another person. *Motivation* refers to self-directed behavior. Persons who appear to be unmotivated often are described as passive, indecisive, and easily frustrated. When an elderly individual does not perform or respond in the way that someone else believes is appropriate, or when others cannot understand or control the behavior of an older person, the individual often is labeled as unmotivated (Kemp, 1986). In fact, nothing could be further from the truth. These apparently *unmotivated* persons must work hard at attaining their goals even though they may be entirely different from the goals that staff members have established for them.

Relaxation

Relaxation is a technique that can be utilized in corrective, adaptive, enrichment, and preventive interventions. It is focused on the moderation of individual internal feeling states such as anxiety and anger. Relaxation may be viewed as a natural way of being, a stage of self-awareness, or simply the absence of excessive anxiety.

Relaxation has been utilized as a treatment intervention with a wide range of older persons. With certain adaptations, relaxation techniques can be used with persons of limited cognitive abilities and with those who function independently. However, with cognitively impaired elderly individuals, instructions must be clear and simple while not requiring significant memory for detail. The strengths of relaxation are its flexibility and proven effectiveness in combination with other forms of treatment. Relaxation techniques also may be practiced on the client's own time and in his or her own environment as a reinforcer of previously learned skills (Edinberg, 1985).

Environmental Management and the Confused or Disruptive Client

The physical *environment* should be organized so that impaired individuals have access to relevant information without having to ask for assistance from others. A variety of aids such as calendars, clocks, names on doors, and posted activity schedules are helpful. It also is useful to maintain a consistent daily routine. Major daily events (i.e., group meetings and activities, meals, and everyday living functions) should occur at the same time each day. A *reality board* can serve as a valuable aid.

These boards commonly provide information regarding time, place, date, weather conditions, and, perhaps, the next meal. To be most effective, reality boards should be positioned at eye level (for wheelchair users and ambulant clients) and in a conspicuous location. Boards are frequently referred to during daily reality orientation to reinforce their use (Edinberg, 1985).

The provision of an environment in which achievement is possible can be extremely significant when working with disabled elderly clients. Clients who are confused often display great frustration or restlessness and appear worried again and again over the same problem. Refocusing their efforts and attention should provide troubled clients with something else to think about and with a sense of purpose. The challenge for staff members is to assign a task before the elderly client reaches a state of agitation and unrestraint. The idea is not practical with all confused clients; however, it has proven useful with many impaired individuals. The most appropriate tasks are those which are familiar or comfortable, and the client must feel that the task is helpful. Some examples of repetitive tasks that have been used successfully include: dusting, polishing shoes or silverware, sorting silverware, cleaning tables, folding towels or other laundry items, and rolling yarn into balls (Elliott and Sorg-Elliott, 1991).

Disruptive behavior, such as angry outbursts or throwing things, should be deterred by assisting the agitated individual to express emotion in a more socially acceptable manner. After a direct response to the distressed behavior, quiet and nonthreatening activities such as listening to music or eating a snack may be attempted. Other activities to which it might be appropriate for some disturbed individuals to transfer their emotions include: carpentry, creating with clay, or physical exercise (Hamill and Oliver, 1980).

Many confused elderly clients remain ambulatory and are at risk for *wandering behavior.* In the past, the solution to wandering has been the use of physical restraints. Restraints have been used to detain the wandering older client. However, the use of restrains almost always results in the deterioration of older clients to a point of little or no responsiveness.

Following their request, clients may be permitted short walks on the facility grounds or within the facility when accompanied by a staff member. When older clients realize that a walk can be taken at most any time, wandering may decrease. Activity staff and nursing personnel join efforts in the provision of a walking program. Many patients regress because they are forced to refrain from an activity that apparently provides enjoyment (Elliott and Sorg-Elliott, 1991).

Communication

Staff attention also should focus upon the skills necessary for the exchange of information. *Blocks to communication* may include the following partial list:

- ordering, directing, commanding;
- warning, reprimanding, threatening;
- inciting, preaching, moralizing;
- providing solutions;

- lecturing or arguing;
- judging, criticizing, blaming, ridiculing; and
- interpreting, analyzing, diagnosing, and probing.

Active listening attends to the feelings of others and to one's own feelings or reactions. Active listening is useful when communicating with elderly clients. The genuineness of the staff member is critical to the success of this approach. A great number of problems encountered by elderly clients will require more direct intervention. However, due to a lack of meaningful roles and relationships, active listening and genuine behavior can provide much needed emotional support to elderly individuals (Corey, 1982; Edinberg, 1985; Gordon, 1970).

Summary

Although many elderly persons maintain their independence, they do so in a society that cares little for their dilemma, for their quality of life, or for human nurturance. Independence has often been emphasized in legal terms, yet physicians, social workers, therapists, other healthcare personnel, and adult children of elderly persons continue to assume dependence. Independence and autonomy issues should not be considered as conflicts, but as complex circumstances that elderly individuals, caregivers, and most healthcare providers resolve together. It is imperative that public policy be influenced in a manner which is consistent with an individual's right to pursue his or her full potential, regardless of age or disability.

The importance of autonomy, motivation, and control for elderly persons is considered in this chapter. Independence is recognized as existing in many areas of choice. The existence of the elderly mystique is verified as the belief that disability in old age indicates an unavoidable decline in functioning. The elderly mystique is acknowledged as frequently being supported by policymakers, program planners, and practitioners.

Motivational techniques such as the development of rapport and the implementation of nonverbal approaches are reviewed. Behavioral techniques and strategies including relaxation, environmental management, and effective communication also are described. In conclusion, the independence of elderly persons is determined to be contingent on elders and their caregivers working together to maximize the potentials of all involved.

Comprehension Questions

1. Distinguish between autonomy and independence.
2. Why is motivation important when working with elderly clients?
3. Discuss techniques that can be used to enhance motivation in older persons.
4. Why are some older people not motivated?
5. What is meant by amotivation?

References

Agich, G. J. (1993). *Autonomy and long-term care.* New York, NY: Oxford University Press Inc.

Arling, G., Harkins, E. B., & Capitman, J. A. (1986). Institutionalization and personal control: A panel study of impaired older people. *Research on Aging, 8*(1), 38-56.

Beedon, L. (1992). Autonomy as a policy goal for disability and aging. In E. F. Ansell & N. N. Eustis (Eds.), *Aging and disabilities: Seeking common ground* (pp. 157-164). Amityville, NY: Baywood Publishing Co., Inc.

Berkowitz, E. D. (1987). *Disabled policy: America's programs for the handicapped.* Cambridge, UK: Cambridge University Press.

Blazer, D. G. (1990). *Emotional problems in later life: Intervention strategies for professional caregivers.* New York, NY: Springer Publishing Co., Inc.

Blazer, D. G. (1985). Depressive illness in late life. In United States Institute of Medicine and National Research Council, *Health in an older society* (pp. 105-128). Washington, DC: National Academy Press.

Buchanan, H., & Brock, D. W. (1986). Deciding for others. *Milbank Quarterly, 64*(Suppl. 2), 17-94.

Carroll, K., & Gray, K. (1981). Memory development: An approach to the mentally impaired elderly in the long-term care setting. *International Journal of Aging and Human Development, 13,* 15-35.

Chowdhary, U. (1990). Notion of control and self-esteem of institutionalized older men. *Perceptual and Motor Skills, 70*(3), 731-738.

Clark, A. N. G. (1978). Morale and motivation. *Practitioner, 220,* 735-737.

Cohen, E. S. (1992). What is independence? *Generations: The Journal of the Western Gerontological Society, 16*(1), 49-52.

Collopy, B. J. (1988). Autonomy in long-term care: Some crucial distinctions. *The Gerontologist, 28*(Suppl.), 10-17.

Corey, G. (1982). *Theory and practice of counseling and psychotherapy* (2nd ed.). Belmont, CA: Wadsworth Inc.

Cornelius, S. W., & Caspi, A. (1986). Self-perceptions of intellectual control and aging. *Educational Gerontology, 12,* 345-357.

Deci, E. L. (1980). *The psychology of self-determination.* Lexington, MA: D. C. Heath & Co.

Deci, E. L. (1975). *Intrinsic motivation.* New York, NY: Plenum Press.

Deci, E. L. (1971). Effects of externally mediated rewards on intrinsic motivation. *Journal of Personality and Social Psychology, 18,* 105-115.

Deci, E. L., & Ryan, R. M. (1985). *Intrinsic motivation and self-determination in human behavior.* New York, NY: Plenum Press.

Die, A. H., Seelbach, W. C., & Sherman, G. D. (1987). Achievement, motivation, achieving styles, and morale in the elderly. *Psychology and Aging, 2,* 407-408.

Dowd, E. T. (Ed.). (1984). *Leisure counseling: Concepts and applications.* Springfield, IL: Charles C. Thomas, Publisher.

Dreher, B. B. (1987). Communication skills for working with elders. *Springer Series on Adulthood and Aging, 17.* New York, NY: Springer Publishing Co., Inc.

Edinberg, M. A. (1985). *Mental health practice with the elderly.* Englewood Cliffs, NJ: Prentice Hall.

Elliott, J. E., & Sorg-Elliott, J. A. (1991). *Recreation programming and activities for older adults.* State College, PA: Venture Publishing, Inc.

Feingold, E., & Werby, E. (1990). Supporting the independence of elderly residents through control over their environment. *Journal of Housing for the Elderly, 6*(1, 2), 25-32.

Frengley, J., & Mion, L. (1986). Incidence of physical restraints on acute general medical wards. *Journal of the American Geriatrics Society, 34,* 565-568.

Geer, J. H., Davison, G. C., & Gatchel, R. I. (1970). Reduction of stress in humans through nonveridical perceived control of aversive stimulation. *Journal of Personality and Social Psychology, 16,* 731-738.

Glass, D., & Singer, J. (1972). *Urban stress.* New York, NY: Academic Press.

Gordon, T. (1970). *Parent effectiveness training.* New York, NY: Peter Wyden.

Hamill, C. M., & Oliver, R. C. (1980). *Therapeutic activities for the handicapped elderly.* Rockville, MD: Aspen Publishers Inc.

Hofland, B. (1988). Autonomy in long-term care: Background issues and a programmatic response. *The Gerontologist, 28*(Suppl.), 3-9.

Hunt, L. (1988). Continuity of care maximizes autonomy of the elderly. *The American Journal of Occupational Therapy, 42*(6), 391-393.

Hutchison, W., Carstensen, L., Silberman, D., O'Keefe, J., Thomassen, J., Pomeranz, J., Reilly, J., Shoenfeld, S., Pezzoli, K., Ohringer, K., Suleiman, J., Diviney, B., & Goodman, M. (1983). Generalized effects of increasing personal control of residents in a nursing facility. *International Journal of Behavioral Geriatrics, 1*(4), 21-32.

Iso-Ahola, S. E. (1980). Perceived control and responsibility as mediators of the effects of therapeutic recreation on the institutionalized aged. *Therapeutic Recreation Journal, 14*(1), 36-43.

Kane, R. A., Caplan, A. L., Freeman, I. C., Aroskar, M. A., & Urv-Wong, E. K. (1990). Avenues to appropriate autonomy: What next? In R. A. Kane & A. L. Caplan (Eds.), *Everyday ethics: Resolving dilemmas in nursing home life* (pp. 306-317). New York, NY: Springer Publishing Co., Inc.

Kemp, B. J. (1986). Psychosocial and mental health issues in rehabilitation of older persons. In S. J. Brody & G. E. Ruff (Eds.), *Aging and rehabilitation: Advances in the state of the art* (pp. 122-158). New York, NY: Springer Publishing Co., Inc.

Kiernat, J. M. (1987). Promoting independence and autonomy through environmental approaches. *Topics in Geriatric Rehabilitation, 3*(1), 1-6.

Klausmeier, H. (1975). *Individually guided motivation.* Madison, WI: Wisconsin Research Center.

Langer, E. J., & Rodin, J. (1976). The effects of choice and enhanced personal responsibility for the aged: A field experiment in an institutional setting. *Journal of Personality and Social Psychology, 34,* 191-198.

Leitner, M. J., & Leitner, S. F. (1985). *Leisure in later life: A sourcebook for the provision of recreational services for elders.* Binghamton, NY: The Haworth Press, Inc.

Minkler, M. (1990). Aging and disability: Behind and beyond the stereotypes. *Journal of Aging Studies, 4*(3), 245-260.

Moos, R. H. (1976). *The human context: Environmental determinants of behavior.* New York, NY: John Wiley & Sons, Inc.

Mullins, L. C. (1985). An examination of the locus of desired control among young-old and old-old nursing home patients. *Sociological Spectrum, 5,* 107-117.

Neugarten, B. L. (1968). Perspectives of the aging process. *Psychiatric Research Reports, 23,* 42-48.

Newcomer, R. J., & Caggiano, M. A. (1976). Environment and the aged person. In I. M. Burnside (Ed.), *Nursing and the aged.* New York, NY: McGraw Hill.

Perlmuter, L. C., Monty, R. A., & Chan, F. (1986). Choice, control, and cognitive functioning. In M. M. Baltes & P. B. Baltes (Eds.), *The psychology of control and aging* (pp. 207-236). Hillsdale, NJ: Lawrence Erlbaum Associates Inc.

Riley, M. W., & Foner, A. (1968). *Aging and society.* New York, NY: Russell Sage Foundation.

Robertson, R. D. (1988). Recreation and the institutionalized elderly: Conceptualization of the free choice and intervention continuums. *Activities, Adaptation & Aging, 11*(1), 61-73.

Robinson, L., Boyko, E., Lane, J., Cooper, D., & Jahnigen, D. (1987). Binding the elderly: A prospective study of the use of mechanical restraints in an acute care hospital. *Journal of the American Geriatrics Society, 35,* 290-296.

Rodin, J. (1987). Personal control through the life course. In R. P. Abeles (Ed.), *Life-span perspectives and social psychology* (pp. 103-119). Hillsdale, NJ: Lawrence Erlbaum Associates Inc.

Rodin, J. (1986). Health, control, and aging. In M. M. Baltes & P. B. Baltes (Eds.), *The psychology of control and aging* (pp. 139-165). Hillsdale, NJ: Lawrence Erlbaum Associates Inc.

Rodin, J. (1983). Behavioral medicine: Beneficial effects of self-control training in aging. *Revue Internationale, 32,* 153-181.

Rodin, J., & Langer, E. J. (1980). Aging labels: The decline of control and the fall of self-esteem. *Journal of Social Issues, 36,* 12-29.

Rosenfelt, R. (1965). The elderly mystique. *Journal of Social Issues, 21,* 37-43.

Rothbaum, F., Weisz, J. R., & Snyder, S. S. (1982). Changing the world and changing the self: A two-process model of perceived control. *Journal of Personality and Social Psychology, 42,* 5-37.

Rubinstein, R. L., Kilbride, J. C., & Nagy, S. (1992). *Elders living alone: Frailty and the perception of choice.* Hawthorne, NY: Aldine De Gruyter.

Salamon, M. J. (1986). *A basic guide to working with elders*. New York, NY: Springer Publishing Co., Inc.

Schulz, R. (1987). Successful aging: Balancing primary and secondary control. *Adult Development and Aging News, 13*, 2-4.

Slivinske, L. R., & Fitch, V. L. (1987). The effect of control-enhancing interventions on the well-being of elderly individuals living in retirement communities. *The Gerontologist, 27*(2), 176-180.

Steinkamp, M. W., & Kelly, J. R. (1985). Relationships among motivational orientation, level of leisure activity, and life satisfaction in older men and women. *The Journal of Psychology, 119*(6), 509-520.

Strumpf, N. E., & Evans, L. K. (1988). Physical restraint of the hospitalized elderly: Perceptions of patients and nurses. *Nursing Research, 37*(3), 132-137.

Teitelman, J. L., & Priddy, J. M. (1988). From psychological theory to practice: Improving frail elders' quality of life through control-enhancing interventions. *The Journal of Applied Gerontology, 7*(3), 298-315.

Thomasma, D. C. (1991). From ageism toward autonomy. In R. H. Binstock & S. G. Post (Eds.), *Too old for healthcare? Controversies in medicine, law, economics, and ethics* (pp. 138-163). Baltimore, MD: The Johns Hopkins University Press.

Timko, C., & Moos, R. H. (1989). Choice, control, and adaptation among elderly residents of sheltered care settings. *Journal of Applied Social Psychology, 19*(8), 636-655.

Tobin, S. S. (1991). *Personhood in advanced old age: Implications for practice*. New York, NY: Springer Publishing Co., Inc.

Tulloch, G. J. (1990). From inside a nursing home: A resident writes about autonomy. *Generations: The Journal of the Western Gerontological Society, 14*(Suppl.), 83-85.

Vallerand, R. J., & O'Connor, B. P. (1989). Motivation in the elderly: A theoretical framework and some promising findings. *Canadian Psychology, 30*(3), 538-550.

Windley, P. G., & Scheidt, R. J. (1976). Person-environment dialectics: Implications for competent functioning in old age. In L. W. Poon (Ed.), *Aging in the 1980s: Psychological issues* (pp. 407-423). Washington, DC: American Psychological Association.

Key Words

Individual Competence
Environmental Press
Prosthetic Approach
Therapeutic Approach

Learning Objectives

1. Describe Lawton's ecological model of aging.
2. Describe Kahana's congruence model.
3. Explain the importance of home in later life.
4. Discuss problems related to relocation.
5. Discuss how aging-related physical changes impact the need for environmental modifications.
6. Discuss how the environment can be modified to facilitate positive results with patients with Alzheimer's disease.

Chapter 10

Environmental Considerations

Introduction

Aging, like all other human experience, does not occur in a vacuum. The effect of environment on the aging adult can be profound. Consequently, it is necessary for activity specialists, therapists, and other helping professionals who give care to the elderly to understand the social and physical context in which aging occurs and the behavioral changes that may be expected. The purpose of this chapter is to acquaint the reader with environmental considerations in planning therapeutic activity interventions. The first part of this chapter introduces the readers to conceptual approaches to understanding the impact of the environment on the aging experience. The remainder of the chapter is devoted to discussion of pragmatic, environmental considerations for activity programmers.

Conceptual Approaches to Understanding Aging and the Environment

Lawton's Model

An ecological model of aging as developed by Lawton (1982) proposes that behavior is a product or function of individual competence in interaction with the environmental press (or demands) of the situation. Individual competence refers to the theoretical upper limit of a person's ability to function. Environmental press refers to the demands placed on the individual by the environment—both socially and physically. When individual competence does not meet the demands of environmental press, maladaptive behavior may occur.

According to Lawton (1982), there are five components of individual competence. The first is biological health or physical health status that reflects the absence of disease. Individual sensory and perceptual capacities compose the second category. Common functional losses in this area include diminished abilities in hearing and vision. The third area of competence is motor skills. Older adults with arthritis, kyphosis (osteoporotic curvature of the spine), Parkinson's disease, and other diseases that affect mobility will typically show decline in this area. Cognitive capacity, the fourth competence area, refers to intelligence, learning, and memory (Hooyman and Kiyak, 1991). Depression and irreversible, as well as reversible, dementia are common disease-related causes of cognitive decline among older adults. The final area of competence indicated by Lawton is ego strength. This concept refers to the ability of the individual to accept the realities of aging. While ego strength is certainly the most challenging to assess, all of the components of competence are quite difficult to assess separate from environmental factors.

Maladaptive behavior due to a lack of congruence between environmental press and personal competence can be modified through maneuvers which are directed at reducing environmental stress and thus, elevating personal competence. Environmental stress may be changed with or without the participation of the older person. Often, a social worker, family member, or care provider will take steps to modify the environment. Activity specialists also may use techniques to adjust the environment to provide greater congruence between individual competence and environmental press. For example, the activity specialist can disguise the exits which confused clients should not use in an activity room (Zgola, 1987). Another method of reducing environmental stress involves an active effort by the individual to produce change.

Older individuals also can assume a passive or active role in efforts to raise their competence levels. Many types of rehabilitation and treatment programs do not require participants to initiate any action. Lawton (1982) described active programs as those that elevate competence such as self therapy or growth experiences. Therefore physical therapy programs in which participants follow the instructions of a therapist tend to be more passive programs. Activity specialists, however, can initiate programs to elevate personal competence. For example, an older adult with signs of cognitive decline may benefit from participation in a guided autobiography program (Birren and Deutchman, 1991). Even though a group leader is providing the writing theme, it is the participant who must explore his or her own thoughts and feelings in such an autobiography program.

Regardless of the approach, the goal of an environmental intervention is to create a situation in which the environmental demand is slightly above the older person's accustomed performance level (Lawton and Nahemov, 1973). One of the most useful aspects of the ecological press model is that it can be applied to almost any intervention situation. Only older adults with the most profound disabilities do not respond to the environment in some discernible way. Lawton (1982) outlined the benefits of improving participants' ability to respond to the environment. These include:

(a) utilization of unrecognized potential,

(b) increase in self-esteem consequent to seeing oneself handle an increase in environmental press, and

(c) affirmation of self in having control over the nature and intensity of environmental press.

Benefits such as these are often central goals in activity programs, and this model is helpful in understanding the role of environment in producing positive behavioral gains for older persons who are engaged in therapeutic activity intervention.

Kahana's Congruence Model

Kahana's (1982) congruence model is another useful approach for understanding the behavior of older adults in the context of their environment. Under Kahana's model, it is proposed that it is more likely that older individuals will be situated in environments that match or are consistent with their needs. When a situation arises in which environmental press and personal needs are not in congruence, the individual will typically modify the press or leave the environment. For example, if an older individual signs up to take an exercise class at the local YMCA which is not sufficiently challenging, he or she will most likely modify the environmental press by attending a more difficult class or leaving the environment to pursue other options elsewhere. Problems arise when individuals do not display the ability to modify or leave environments under these circumstances (e.g., nursing home placements). In these situations, stress and discomfort may follow.

Many older adults with disabilities, especially those who are residing in institutions, have little opportunity to modify or change their environments. In fact, institutional control has been found to play a significant role in explaining morale in long-term care facilities (Kahana, 1982). Consequently, interventions designed to improve the person-environment fit in long-term care facilities should enhance individual feelings of control, thus facilitating congruence. Two types of interventions are included in Kahana's model. The first is the prosthetic approach. This approach assumes that the disability cannot be modified and that environmental supports are needed. The therapeutic approach, on the other hand, seeks to create change in the individual and in his or her ability to negotiate the environment.

The lack of control over who has access to clients and when constitutes an important aspect of the environment in most long-term care facilities (Hooyman and Kiyak, 1991). It is difficult to retain a sense of autonomy when one has no control over when one will be bathed, fed, or allowed to engage in activities. Privacy also is needed in order to retain self-identity and engage in self-reflection (Hooyman and Kiyak, 1991).

Activity specialists should be aware of and respect the need for privacy of older adults. Even though the activity professional believes that participation in social activities is in the best interest of the client, that individual's rights to spend time alone and not to participate must be respected.

Willcocks, Peace, and Kellaher (1987) studied the lives of clients in a variety of long-term care facilities. The results of the study demonstrated that a lack of privacy was an important concern. According to the research results, older adults expect to exercise control in their homes and not have outsiders violate this autonomy by assuming control. The ability of older adults to maintain control was found to be a source of personal power.

Hooyman and Kiyak (1991) discussed the special case of person-environment congruence caused by relocation. Moving from one environment to another requires some adjustment for people of all ages. Typically, successful adjustment is achieved within a relatively brief period of time. For older adults with multiple or severe disabilities, this may not be the case. New floor plans and features in the environment may be a source of great stress for the disoriented individual. The need to adjust to the rules and regulations associated with institutional living, as well as reluctance to move into an institution, may compound the stress. Simple floor plans, easy-to-follow signs, adequate lighting, and enhanced accessibility can contribute to successful environmental adaptation. The elimination of extraneous stimuli (excessive noise, bright colors, extra furniture) also is an important consideration for confused clients (Zgola, 1987).

Preference for Home in Later Life

The vast majority of older adults prefer to remain in their homes for as long as possible. Sixsmith and Sixsmith (1991) indicated that older adults with disabilities prefer to remain in their homes even when negotiating aspects of that environment becomes difficult. In fact, older adults with disabilities view the home as a haven of rest, not a place that "traps" them. Older adults also may find that they can "conceal" their declining abilities better in the home compared with other environments such as institutional care (Willcocks, Peace, and Kellaher, 1987). Sixsmith and Sixsmith (1991) also found that the home is the best place for preserving independence. Further, as maintaining independence becomes more significant, so does the importance of the home.

The home provides a source of personal power beyond that which is promoted through physical independence. While remaining in the home, the individual is able to control what events and activities happen, as well as who enters and when (Willcocks, Peace, and Kellaher, 1987). Outsiders are not expected to make major decisions that control the individual's future.

The home often provides an important link to the past for older adults (Rubinstein and Parmelee, 1992). Pictures of loved ones, valued possessions accumulated throughout life, and symbols of the individual's family and cultural heritage are contained in the home. All of these home environment attributes contribute to the older adult's sense of identity. In one study by Sixsmith and Sixsmith (1991), older adults expressed a strong association between home and the past. This association was so strong for some persons that they felt the "presence" of the deceased partner in the house.

Impact of Relocation

In spite of the fact that the majority of older adults wish to remain in their homes indefinitely, many eventually will have to relocate to a new residence. In many cases, the new place of residence will be a long-term care facility. Relocation, especially if it is not desired, can be very stressful. As a consequence, service providers, including activity specialists, need to be prepared to assist persons in making a positive adjustment to the new residence.

The long-term care facility environment is not viewed as desirable by our society. Attempts by staff to create a warm and welcoming atmosphere may go unnoticed by new clients of the facility due to their perception that they were pushed out of their own homes and into the facility (Rubinstein and Parmelee, 1992). Negative feelings toward relocation to a nursing home also may be created by the perception that the nursing home represents disengagement from the mainstream of society.

The control and power older adults have in their own homes typically does not exist in long-term care facilities (Rubinstein and Parmelee, 1992). While the home serves as a link to the older adults' personal and cultural past, nursing homes are "collectively defined spaces" which are not personally meaningful. Willcocks, Peace, and Kellaher (1987) found the following factors to be important in the social environment: choice/freedom, privacy, involvement, and engagement/stimulation. Each of these need to be considered when facilitating the relocation of an older person to a long-term care facility.

The choice/freedom factor refers to the extent that older adults have freedom to make choices about their lifestyle. Within a nursing home setting, there may be very little opportunity for decision making. Scheduling and staffing restrictions may prohibit clients from making even the most routine decisions including when to get up, when to go to bed, when and what to eat, when to get dressed, and who can enter the client's personal living space.

Privacy refers both to personal privacy and to interactions with others. The need to share a room with another client, as well as the need for assistance with personal care, make it difficult to retain privacy in nursing homes. The public nature of long-term care facilities also makes it difficult to maintain private relationships. For example, a married client may have great difficulty in finding times for intimacy with a nonclient spouse.

Involvement refers to the extent that the client is participating in the operation of the nursing home. Long-term care facilities tend to have strict rules and policies that must be followed for legal, ethical, and financial reasons. This type of structure allows little opportunity for client participation in decision making. In some cases, clients may not even understand the rationale behind facility rules and policies.

Engagement/stimulation refers to the degree to which staff encourage client autonomy and independence. Taking the time to encourage clients to make decisions may not be a priority in a facility that has a small staff working with a large number of clients. It may be much easier for a staff member to make decisions for a client than to explain options in order to support client initiated decision making. Unfortunately, this type of an arrangement can lead to learned helplessness, which is clearly not in the best interest of older adults.

Environmental Modifications

Many older adults experience physical changes that directly impact their ability to successfully negotiate their environments. Earlier in this chapter, the importance of person-environmental fit was discussed. A great part of this book is devoted to teaching people strategies for implementing therapeutic interventions with older adults. The remainder of this chapter will focus on a prosthetic approach and suggestions for environmental modifications to enhance person-environmental fit within activity programs.

Mobility Changes

Arthritis, osteoporosis, Parkinson's disease, and other diseases limit the mobility of many older adults, thus placing them at risk for falling. A well-designed facility for older adults incorporates accident prevention modifications and provides for ease of movement for its participants. Surfaces in such facilities should be level and have a nonslip surface. Stairs should be uniform in size and a handrail must be provided. All program areas should be accessible to individuals who use wheelchairs, canes, or walkers.

Facilities that provide services for older adults, unless affiliated with a church or private club, must be designed in compliance with the Americans with Disabilities Act. If a facility is in compliance, participants with disabilities will have full access to the facility and its programs. To obtain more information about the Americans with Disabilities Act, readers are encouraged to contact the U.S. Department of Justice, Civil Rights Division, Coordination and Review Section, P.O. Box 66118, Washington, DC, 20035-6118.

Visual Changes

Changes in vision are normal in aging adults. The decreased ability of older adults to adapt to changes in light is a crucial factor for facility planners and activity programmers to understand. Cataracts are prevalent among the older adult population so that they also should be of concern when designing program environments. It is necessary to carefully evaluate and design activity environments to match the visual support needs of older adults in order to ensure participant safety and comfort. According to Fogg and Fulton (1994), visual clarity considerations in environmental design include: (a) evenness of light; (b) legibility of graphic information; and (c) understandability of design.

Evenness of light can be achieved by providing several indirect sources of light that utilize a higher watt level than normal. It is also important to design the entrances and exits from facilities so that the slower light-to-dark adaptation of older adults is accommodated. For example, on a bright, sunny day it would not be appropriate to have older adults come from the outdoors into a dimly lit entrance of a building. It would be more helpful to have the entrance slightly less bright than the outside, the hall slightly less bright than the entrance, and the program area at the desired level of illumination.

Signs and other types of graphic information are important orientation tools in any facility or program environment. The most effective signs have large letters and use simple terminology. High contrast colors should be used for signs and printed materials; activity staff should be especially careful to avoid using blues and violets together. Signs need to be located so that both adults who walk and those who use wheelchairs can read them. Finally, the use of nonglare glass is highly recommended.

There are several steps that can be taken to enhance the understandability of a facility. Extra orientation aids can be useful. Many facilities use color-coded doors and walls to assist with orientation to location and layout. In this type of a plan, color lines on a wall lead from a central area, such as a front desk, to different parts of the facility such as the cafeteria or activity room. Color coding also can be used to mark changes in elevation on the walking surfaces.

Hearing Changes

Loss of hearing is another physical change that is normal for the older population. In crowded areas it is often difficult for older adults with hearing loss to distinguish between different frequencies of sound. In some cases, background noise is not distinguishable from the immediate conversation. In such a situation, effective participation in a program may be quite difficult. Activity specialists can help to minimize the impact of hearing loss in a number of ways. It is important that background noise be reduced during programs that involve conversation. The following are some recommendations:

1. Program areas should be located in spaces where participants will not be distracted by noise from another source such as a busy street or a main reception area for the building.
2. Soundproof rooms are costly but useful for offices, conference rooms, or other rooms in facilities that older adults frequently use.
3. Carpeted floors and textured wall coverings absorb sound better than do other surfaces and, consequently, these building materials can be used to reduce background noise.

Environmental Considerations for Persons with Alzheimer's Disease

The design of program spaces is of particular concern to agencies and activity specialists who serve older adults with Alzheimer's disease. Throughout this chapter, the need to provide choice to older adults has been emphasized; however, for patients with Alzheimer's disease or other types of dementia, free choice is usually not appropriate (Bell, Fisher, Baum, and Green, 1990). Consequently, in recent years, nursing homes and adult day programs have developed specialized Alzheimer's programs or units that are designed with the specific needs of older adults with dementia.

Traditionally, the erratic or wandering behavior of many adults with Alzheimer's disease has been treated with chemical or physical restraints (Bell, Fisher, Baum, and Green, 1990). In more recent years, however, federal policies have discouraged the use of restraints and increased research of behavior management techniques. The result has been the development of less restrictive environments for this special client group. Programmatic changes have focused on adjusting environments to behavior rather than attempting to alter the person's behavior to fit the environment. In many cases, the results have been substantial and reflect a positive move forward in the care of persons with Alzheimer's disease.

Older adults with Alzheimer's disease are less likely to be confused or disoriented in environments that are free of ambiguities (Zgola, 1987). Environments that are not overly stimulating and that are consistent tend to promote lower levels of disruptive behavior. The following are several suggestions from Zgola from her guidebook on adult day programs for persons with dementia:

1. Floors and walls should be distinct from each other and steps should be clearly marked. Persons with diminished perceptual capabilities may have difficulty judging distances if the floors, walls, and furniture all meld together. The use of contrasting colors can help clients to negotiate their surroundings.
2. Floors should be free of markings, such as lines or figures, that could be perceived as obstacles. Changes in the texture of the floor also may be perceived as obstacles. For example, a person with the disease may not want to enter a room with a tile floor, walk on a brick sidewalk, or cross over the metal threshold of a door.
3. When an effective arrangement of the facility has been found, it should be kept permanent. Also, it is important to dedicate certain spaces for certain activities. Consistency is important if the client is to feel comfortable in his or her surroundings.
4. The ambiance of the facility should be neutral and subdued. Many bright colors or graphic designs on the wall can be overstimulating and cause agitation.
5. Background noise should be minimized. Techniques for reducing background noise as discussed earlier in this chapter can be used.
6. Washrooms should be marked clearly. Signs that use stick figures or alternative terms for men and women may confuse clients and should be avoided.
7. Large open spaces may be intimidating to persons with dementia. For example, a client may not be willing to cross to the other side of a large activity room. Groups of tables or chairs arranged in small sitting areas within a larger room can help with this problem.

Wandering is a behavior that is exhibited by many people who have Alzheimer's disease. This behavior can be especially problematic for staff charged with ensuring client safety, as it is not uncommon for individuals to try to walk out of their programs. As a result, many Alzheimer's units in nursing homes are locked. If it is not possible or desirable to lock the facility, other options are available. Providing a space within the facility for clients to wander is one option. Long hallways or fenced outdoor areas also may be suitable options. Staff may find it helpful to simply take a client on a walk outside if he or she seems agitated or upset. Disguising exits from the facility also has been found to be useful. Doors can be covered with fabric or paper, or painted to match the wall. One monitored exit should be left apparent.

Working with Alzheimer's Patients in the Home

Most families prefer to keep their older relatives with Alzheimer's disease at home as long as possible. This can be a trying task for any family. Fortunately, there is support available from local chapters of the Alzheimer's Association. Family members may also find the book, *The 36 Hour Day* (Mace and Rabins, 1991), helpful. Mace and Rabins offer several suggestions for modifying homes to accommodate persons with Alzheimer's disease. The following are helpful suggestions for therapists and activity specialists who are serving this client group:

1. Power tools, knives, small appliances, car keys, medicines, and household chemicals should be locked in a cabinet.
2. The water heater should be turned down so no one can be scalded. Exposed water pipes should be covered.
3. Security locks should be installed on balcony windows and doors.
4. Radiators and furnaces should be blocked.
5. Poisonous houseplants should not be used in any type of program. Pins and buttons should be kept out of reach to prevent choking. Some people with Alzheimer's disease may also try to eat chipped paint.
6. A switch should be installed on the back of the stove to prevent it from being turned on or the control knobs should be removed.
7. Gates should be installed at the top of stairs.
8. Patio doors should be marked and storm doors should have grills.
9. Automatic windows in a car may be dangerous. It is also important that the driver of a vehicle be able to control the door locks. Some patients may try to get out of a moving car.
10. Smoking can be very dangerous for the patient with Alzheimer's disease. It is possible that the cigarettes can be taken away from the person without incident. If not, smoking should only be allowed under supervision.
11. "Burglar alarms" or gadgets that monitor sound may help the caregiver monitor behavior at night.

It is important to remember that each individual with Alzheimer's disease will respond differently. Some individuals may need a very simple, structured environment, while others are able to function relatively well in an environment with minimum modifications. If aspects of the current environment do not create a safety hazard or serve as a source of distress, modifications are not necessary.

Summary

This chapter stresses the impact of environment on the functional competence of older adults. Two models are commonly used to explain and understand the dynamic relationship between environmental demand and personal performance—Lawton's environmental press model and Kahana's congruence model. These models can be used to guide the design and implementation of activity interventions and program environments for the maximal performance of older adult clients. Pragmatic environmental modifications include lighting, noise, physical layout, and behavioral supports.

Comprehension Questions

1. Compare and contrast Lawton's ecological model with Kahana's congruence model regarding the impact that environment has on the older person's behavior and competence in daily activities.
2. Discuss why home is important to older persons and how a residential relocation influences personal competence.
3. How can activity specialists modify the environment to accommodate changes in vision, hearing, and mobility in older adults?
4. Describe the special environmental support needs of persons who have Alzheimer's disease.

References

Bell, P. A., Fisher, J. D., Baum, A., & Green, T. C. (1990). *Environmental psychology* (3rd ed.). Austin, TX: Harcourt, Brace, Jovanovich College Publishers.

Birren, J. E., & Deutchman, D. E. (1991). *Guiding autobiography groups for older adults: Exploring the fabric of life.* Baltimore, MD: The Johns Hopkins University Press.

Fogg, G. E., & Fulton, R. F. (1994). *Leisure site guidelines for people over 55.* Arlington, VA: National Recreation and Park Association.

Hooyman, N. R., & Kiyak, H. A. (1991). *Social gerontology: A multidisciplinary perspective* (2nd ed.). Needham Heights, MA: Allyn & Bacon.

Kahana, E. (1982). A congruence model of person-environment interaction. In M. P. Lawton, P. G. Windley, & T. O. Byerts (Eds.), *Aging and the environment* (pp. 97-121). New York, NY: Springer Publishing Co., Inc.

Lawton, M. P. (1982). Competence, environmental press, and the adaptation of older people. In M. P. Lawton, P. G. Windley, & T. O. Byerts (Ed.), *Aging and the environment* (pp. 33-59). New York, NY: Springer Publishing Co., Inc.

Lawton, M. P., & Nahemov, L. (1973). Ecology and the aging process. In C. Eisdorfer & M. P. Lawton (Eds.), *The psychology of adult development and aging* (pp. 619-674). Washington, DC: American Psychiatric Association.

Mace, N. L., & Rabins, P. V. (1991). *The 36 hour day* (rev. ed.). Baltimore, MD: The Johns Hopkins University Press.

Rubinstein, R. L., & Parmelee, P. A. (1992). Attachment to place and the representation of the life course by the elderly. *Human Behavior and Environmental Advances in Theory Research, 12,* 139-163.

Sixsmith, A. J., & Sixsmith, J. A. (1991). Transitions in home experience in later life. *The Journal of Architectural and Planning Research, 8*(3), 181-191.

Willcocks, D., Peace, S., & Kellaher, L. (1987). *Private lives in public places.* New York, NY: Tavistock Publications.

Zgola, J. M. (1987). *Doing things: A guide to programming activities for persons with Alzheimer's disease and related disorders.* Baltimore, MD: The Johns Hopkins University Press.

Unit IV

Activity Intervention

Activities that are used in the therapeutic care of older persons can be grouped under four broad categories. In Unit IV the following activity areas are presented: leisure education, physical activity intervention and health promotion, cognitive activities, and psychosocial activities. Treatment modalities that are used in the rehabilitation of conditions common among the elderly will fall into one or more of these broad categories.

Each chapter in this unit is organized to address the basic goals and purposes of activity intervention within the particular area of functioning (e.g., physical, cognitive, psychosocial) or, as in the case of leisure education, the usefulness of this process in meeting the activity needs of the elderly. Common treatment modalities are described, a sample program is presented, and additional resources are provided to the reader for use in program development. This unit directly addresses the application of aging and impairment knowledge within best practices that use therapeutic activity intervention as the treatment modality.

Key Words

Education
Leisure
Leisure Education
Lifestyle
Recreation

Learning Objectives

1. Become familiar with leisure education and describe its applicability in meeting the activity needs of older adults.
2. Define the content that forms the basis of leisure education and the processes used for delivering leisure education to older adults.
3. Describe the goals of leisure education.
4. Describe sample lessons that are used in leisure education.
5. Identify resources that are useful in developing a leisure education intervention program for older adults.

Chapter 11

Leisure Education

Introduction

Educating adults for leisure-centered living, or the wise use of leisure time, is an appropriate concern of professionals who are providing activity programs to elders in a variety of service settings. As life expectancy increases and the prospects for healthier lives continue to improve, the need for leisure education also can be expected to expand. Adults who reach later maturity will have increased opportunities to continue lifelong leisure pursuits, to explore new activities, and, in some cases, to experience a rebalancing of life as their available hours for leisure increase, especially after retirement.

The life changes associated with later maturity are often both instrumental (i.e., retirement) and sudden (e.g., loss of one's partner or spouse) (Kelly, 1993). These life changes bring on new challenges, one of which is the common experience of increased "free" time or leisure time. The meaningful and constructive use of leisure to enhance one's quality of life and to improve one's overall health, is a desired outcome associated with successful aging. The high quality use of leisure time is also an explicit goal of leisure education.

In this chapter, the meaning of leisure and the purpose of leisure education in the lives of older adults is explored. The scope of content covered in educating for leisure-centered living is discussed. Processes that may be used to structure and deliver leisure education programs are outlined. A sample leisure education program with suggested activities clustered under five primary content areas is included. The chapter concludes with reference and resource information for consultation in developing leisure education programs for older adults.

Educating for Leisure-Centered Living

Brightbill and Mobley (1977) observed that leisure may well be:

> that part of life that comes nearest to allowing us to be free in a regi-
> mented and conforming world, which enables us to pursue self-expres-
> sion, intellectual, physical, and spiritual development, and beauty in
> their endless forms. (p. 7)

These words express some of the hopes and desires that many older adults feel as retirement approaches. However, rarely does the transition from work to retirement happen so smoothly that the "perfect life" is realized.

For many older Americans, there is little preparation for the ideal use of free time when it becomes abundant. The expansion in "free" hours may be especially challenging when life has been filled with work, family responsibilities, and a general sense of the need to be occupied with a task that will either benefit others or produce material possessions. Learning to appreciate leisure, with all its potential, is a vital first step in preparing for an increase in the number of hours that are available for leisure.

Real leisure is not enforced free time; rather, it is the opportunity to choose freely from a wide variety of experiences that promote self-expression and the pursuit of self-development—intellectually, physically, socially, and spiritually (Brightbill and Mobley, 1977). Over the years, scholars who philosophize about and study leisure have identified key characteristics of leisure to be time, activity, and a state of mind. Embraced by the wide array of definitions of leisure are the ideals of:

(a) personal freedom to choose what to do,
(b) freedom to carry it out, and
(c) freedom from obligatory responsibilities (i.e., work, family, school, self-care).

Freedom is what makes leisure distinct from work and other obligatory activities of life. Based on these ideals, participation in leisure is expected to produce feelings of personal satisfaction, pleasure, happiness/joy, fulfillment, creativity, and self-actualization. Perceived freedom, activities that are motivating in and of themselves (i.e., not associated with external rewards such as financial gain), and affective states that embody personal satisfaction and self-actualization are the central ingredients of leisure (Kelly, 1990; Murphy, 1975; Neulinger, 1974).

If leisure is personally directed activity during free time which produces a state of mind that is personally satisfying, then why the need for leisure education? Presently in America, it is expected that most adults by age 65 will retire from lifelong occupations, their families will be grown and living on their own, and later life will be the time to embrace a lifestyle that reflects expanded free time for engaging in leisure. As shown throughout this text, older adulthood also may present many challenges. These challenges may be associated with physical declines due to disease, illness, impairment, or just growing older. Additionally, older persons may confront changes in their social networks due to the death of their spouse, other family members, and friends. Often, retirement from lifelong work may be seen as a loss by older persons. A sense of identity for many adults is closely woven into work roles and family responsibilities throughout the younger and middle adult years. Adapting to this new phase in life (e.g., retirement) may be a significant challenge. The process of adjusting to these changes can be greatly assisted by appropriately designed leisure education programs.

Leisure education is intended to assist older adults in making a positive transition to retirement and into old age. The process and content of leisure education focuses on developing knowledge, attitudes, and beliefs about the value of leisure in enhancing life quality in older adulthood. Leisure education involves a systematic program of learning about:

(a) what leisure is and the instrumental role that it can play in later maturity;
(b) the benefits of leisure in human growth and well-being, especially during the senior years;
(c) the availability of leisure resources and opportunities in one's community; and
(d) how to overcome barriers in developing a fulfilling leisure lifestyle in later life.

In this context, leisure education is a program to develop the knowledge and skills necessary to make a smooth and effective transition to the older adult life stages. Leisure education is learning across the life span into older adulthood about how to shape a healthy, positive lifestyle, especially when leisure time is abundant.

Definitions that have been used to describe leisure education stress the following key ideas:

- enhancing one's quality of life through wholesome use of free time;
- developing knowledge, attitudes, beliefs, and skills that promote constructive use of leisure;
- learning to use leisure to promote self-development and self-actualization;
- learning to accept, appreciate, and enjoy leisure, as well as achieve a sense of personal freedom to pursue leisure;
- recognizing personal needs and abilities that can be satisfied through leisure;
- establishing personal leisure goals and repertoire; and
- empowering the individual to develop his or her own leisure lifestyle (Bender, Brannan, and Verhoven, 1984; Mundy and Odum, 1979).

Leisure education, therefore, is a process through which activity specialists assist elders to discover the benefits of leisure, as well as to develop the necessary skills for pursuing an appropriate leisure lifestyle during the retirement years. In the next section, the basic content and processes of leisure education is described. The section is followed by a sample leisure education program with suggested activities and selected resources.

Leisure Education Content and Process

Successful leisure education programs are developed through careful consideration of both program content and the processes used to deliver the content (Dattilo and Murphy, 1991; Howe-Murphy and Charboneau, 1987; Mundy and Odum, 1979). Typically, the content of a leisure education program will be developed in the following areas:

(a) leisure appreciation,
(b) self-awareness and leisure,
(c) self-determination and leisure choices,
(d) knowledge of leisure opportunities and resources, and
(e) decision-making and activity skills (Dattilo and Murphy, 1991; Mundy and Odum, 1979).

The leisure education process moves participants through each of the five content areas toward the goal of an independent and satisfying leisure lifestyle. The exploration of self-awareness through leisure in later life begins the process of preparing for retirement. Learning about one's preferences, interests, and specific needs enables movement toward seeking leisure experiences that are personally relevant and rewarding.

In order for leisure to provide opportunities for self-development, an understanding of the concept of leisure, as well as related concepts (i.e., recreation, play, entertainment, learning), is essential. Placing the individual's understanding of leisure into the context of changing situations in later life is part of enhancing leisure awareness. Cultivating an appreciation of leisure, coupled with promoting a sense of freedom and control over one's actions and environment, forms the essential building blocks for self-determination in later life with regard to leisure. A guided process for learning to take control over one's destiny, especially when the context of everyday life may be changing dramatically (e.g., as in retirement), is an essential step in the leisure education process. Recognizing that a range of leisure choices exists and that one has certain personal preferences is the beginning of the process. These learning objectives constitute the first steps in the process of educating for leisure-centered living.

Knowledge of the resources available to fulfill one's leisure needs is necessary in order to act on stated activity preferences. Typical settings and resources that were associated with work schedules and work companions fade in prominence on retirement. New connections need to be built in order to prevent social isolation or the development of a sedentary lifestyle. The changing social context of older adults may necessitate learning about new outlets in the community that are available to retirees. Leisure education programs provide the opportunity to learn about the resources and social opportunities that may not have been known by the individual prior to his or her retirement. Knowledge of the range of leisure opportunities, facilities, resources, and programs that exist will help make a smooth and successful transition to retirement. Awareness of resources and social networks also is important to seniors who are making a transition from a healthcare facility back to community-based living.

In addition to knowing about leisure resources, it is important to be familiar with social support networks and services. Leisure education programs can serve a critical support function by assisting older adults in learning about individuals, groups, organizations, and social services that are available to them for meeting social interaction needs. Preventing social isolation or, conversely, promoting a feeling of being connected with a social support network, can be an important component of a well-designed leisure education program. Learning about social resources is a necessary part of most leisure education programs for older adults.

The last area of content that leisure education programs typically embrace is learning leisure decision-making and activity skills. Decision-making skills are often directly taught when leisure education is being provided to individuals who have impaired cognitive abilities. In this situation, the individual is coached to recognize:

(a) what resources are needed in order to act on leisure interests,
(b) the consequences associated with making one leisure choice over another, and
(c) how to proceed once a leisure activity is selected.

The teaching of leisure decision-making skills is frequently associated with leisure education programs that are being delivered in rehabilitative or long-term care settings.

The learning of new leisure activity skills is the component of leisure education in which participants make personal activity choices. The selection of new activities may require learning how to do the activity. This skill development phase often can be one of the most exciting and rewarding points in the program for participants who are building or reconstructing their leisure lifestyles. The discovery and learning of new activities with which to satisfy personal interests can be a capstone experience in life. Further, the development of new skills can be highly motivating and can be a reinforcement of the value of the program to participants.

The success of leisure education programming depends upon age-appropriate and need-based content, as well as on effective processes for delivering the content. A general programming process that encompasses the following steps is recommended:

(a) delineate the overall purpose of the program,
(b) specify the program goals and objectives,
(c) identify specific content with implementation procedures and performance measures, and
(d) document progress and evaluate program outcomes.

For each content area of leisure education, specific goals with learning objectives are developed. Appropriate activities are identified to match the learning objectives. The leisure education activities can be adapted from existing materials or developed for the specific group being served. The activities are matched with performance measures that help the program leader to recognize and document when participants have mastered the specific leisure education content and have thus attained the learning objectives. Finally, the program leader is responsible for structuring activities in a manner that is appealing and socially valued by older adults.

Planning the processes for delivering the leisure education content is important to the overall success of the program. Adult learners appreciate learning experiences that utilize their life experiences and personal abilities. Involving program participants into the planning of activities to meet the specific learning objectives associated with the different content areas is an effective strategy for motivating and sustaining participant investment in the program. In situations where leisure education is part of the overall treatment plan/program (e.g., nursing facilities, adult daycare), it is incumbent on the activity specialist to develop and lead a stimulating program format. As with all programming, documenting individual progress and evaluating the outcomes of the leisure education program are essential steps. Documentation and evaluation will enable the program leader to identify successful components of the program, as well as areas that need to be modified or changed.

In summary, the process of planning and delivering an effective leisure education program for older individuals involves:

(a) identifying educational goals and objectives based upon the target content areas and individual needs,
(b) planning and implementing age- and ability-appropriate learning experiences, and
(c) evaluating learning outcomes.

The next section provides a brief example of a leisure education program that focuses on preretirement preparation. The program embraces the five leisure education content areas of leisure appreciation, self-awareness and leisure, self-determination and leisure choices, knowledge of leisure opportunities and resources, and decision-making and activity skills.

A Sample Program

Preretirement Education for Leisure-Centered Living

The following brief program example illustrates the use of leisure education to help older persons prepare for the major life change of retirement. The goals, objectives, and suggested activities have been adapted from general literature on leisure education and the authors' practical experience with elders (Bender, Brannan, and Verhoven, 1984; Dattilo and Murphy, 1991; Mundy and Odum, 1979; Joswiak, 1989). Suggested activities are provided under five leisure education content areas:

(a) leisure appreciation,
(b) awareness of self and leisure,
(c) self-determination and leisure choices,
(d) knowledge of leisure opportunities and resources, and
(e) decision-making and activity skills.

In each area, information is provided according to:

(a) target goal,
(b) enabling objectives for attaining the goal,
(c) activity format (content and process suggestions), and
(d) ideas for implementation and resource materials.

Leisure education programs are typically organized to contain several activities for each content area. Activities may be developed to reflect incremental steps toward attaining an overall learning goal for each content area. Activity leaders will develop more detailed program plans than what is provided here including: specific information regarding activity format, activity implementation plans, materials list, evaluation methods and procedures, and follow-up activities for participants and/or staff. This chapter, outlines the basic content of a program including its purpose, target goals, enabling objectives, activity suggestions, and implementation ideas.

Program Purpose

The purpose of this leisure education program is to assist adults who are preparing for a near future retirement in the following key ways:

1. To facilitate an understanding of the role of leisure in meeting personal interests and needs in retirement.
2. To explore the possible impact that a change in job/work status may have on personal lifestyle.
3. To investigate ways in which leisure can be instrumental in promoting self-development and adaptation in retirement.
4. To explore potential new leisure interests and activities in the community.

Content Area I: *Leisure Appreciation*

Target Goal

Participants will be able to describe a personal definition of leisure within the context of personal life course and life circumstances.

Enabling Objectives

- To distinguish leisure from associated concepts (play, recreation, relaxation, sports, entertainment, cultural events and activities).
- To compare personal definitions of leisure with definitions held by significant others and those found in literature.
- To understand the role of leisure across the life span, from birth to death.
- To identify personal peak leisure experiences and explain why they were peak experiences.

Activity Suggestion: *Autobiographical Sketch of Leisure in My Life*

This activity is completed over several sessions spanning three to six meetings of one to two hours each. The completed autobiographical sketch includes information about the participant's major work/job experiences, personal relationships and responsibilities, and leisure involvements across the life course. Through the process of developing the autobiographical sketch, the participants explore and construct their definitions for several key concepts including work, family, personal responsibilities, and leisure. They discover how their personal life has unfolded and then place these perspectives within a developing appreciation of the value of leisure, especially in older adulthood. Each session begins with a focus topic which is introduced by the group leader and is processed through group discussion. The topical discussion is followed by a period of personal reflection and writing time. Participants may wish to continue the reflection and writing process between sessions, and should be encouraged to do so.

Focus topics can be arranged according to major periods of life starting with childhood and include memories pertaining to work roles, relationships, and leisure activity patterns. Another strategy is to use people, places, and events as the focal points for the day. The leader will select the focus topic for each session. The leader will organize topics so that the completed project will result in meeting the enabling objectives specified above.

Implementation and Materials Suggestions

This activity is recommended for groups of four to eight. A series of three to six incremental sessions are needed to complete the activity. The activity leader may use guest speakers, slides or video materials, magazines, family photo albums, or genealogical records to assist in focusing the participants on the topics discussed and chronicled each week.

Participants will need a journal, paper for jotting notes, pens, and pencils at each session. They should be encouraged to write in their autobiographical journals between sessions. Birren and Deutchmann's *Guiding Autobiography Groups for Older Adults* (1991) may be helpful to the leader in terms of assisting participants with writing personal biographies.

Suggested Session Sequence

Session 1

At the first session following a preliminary meeting that outlines the objectives of the activity, participants will focus on reconstructing their personal leisure activity patterns from a life span perspective. Participants will be requested to bring photos, memorabilia, diaries, memories, and any other personal artifacts that can be used to help them reconstruct their major leisure activity patterns across the life course. The leader may wish to use his or her own leisure history or a visual time line as an example of leisure across the life course.

In this session, the group leader will start the session by drawing a life-cycle line and segmenting it into the following major life stages: birth through to preteen years (ages 1–10), preteen and teenage years (ages 10–18), college and young adult years (ages 18–25), early adulthood (ages 25–40), middle adulthood (ages 40–55), the transition years (ages 55–65), later maturity (ages 65 and older). Group discussion will facilitate recollection of the major lifestyle patterns associated with each broad life stage. The second half of the session will be spent in preparing notes and recollections from the brainstorming/recollection discussion period.

The group leader will determine whether participants are able to prepare their written journals for this session during the time between the first and second sessions. In the case where participants do not wish to work on writing between sessions, the second session should be reserved for the completion of the personal leisure history.

Session 2

For the second session, the leader will invite an expert in the area of recreation and leisure service delivery to come to the group to talk about what leisure means from different perspectives—historically, in contemporary society, and from a developmental/life span perspective. The speaker should be requested to cover primary conceptualizations of leisure as they are presented in the literature. Part of the session should be reserved for discussion of common meanings, questions, summarizing prevalent conceptualizations for leisure, and for allowing participants to share with each other their own personal definitions.

The second half of the session is used for each participant to write notes, reflections, and insights into a journal. The journal, when completed, will be used in the development of the autobiographical sketch.

Once again, the leader will need to determine whether or not an additional session is needed to complete the writing related to the content presented in the second session. It is recommended that participants be encouraged to continue writing on topics that are presented during sessions one and two so that they can focus their attention on new topics for discussion during the ensuing sessions.

Session 3

In this session, participants will explore memories of their *peak leisure experiences* from a life span perspective. The leader facilitates the session by beginning with a group exploration of the concept of peak leisure experience. All participants will be requested to recall a leisure experience that was the best they had ever experienced. Participants will proceed to define what makes a peak experience. The group leader may use word association techniques to assist the group in developing the definition. For example, the leader may ask participants to use adjectives to describe their peak experiences. By listing the adjectives on a flip chart or blackboard, the leader can ask participants to group the adjectives into categories and to follow this categorization process with identification of the key components of a peak experience. Using this process the group will be facilitated in developing their own definition of peak leisure experience.

Next, participants will list their own personal peak experiences across the life course. For each experience, participants will identify the reasons why each experience was a peak experience for them. Using a grid composed of each experience listed down the left hand side of the page and followed by several columns labeled *why, what, where, with whom,* and *how.* Each participant will process each experience in regard to identifying the reasons under each column that may have contributed to the high quality of the experience.

Following this evaluation process, each participant will be asked to share a peak experience, as well as to provide the reasons he or she listed for why, what, where, with whom, and how it came to be that this experience was perceived as a peak experience. The leader will record notes from group discussion on a blackboard, flip chart, or overhead projection in order to guide participants in discovering what makes selected leisure activities peak experiences.

Following the group discussion, participants will recollect those experiences across their life that have been peak experiences. They will modify or develop brief explanations or descriptions of these experiences. Finally, each participant will prepare journal notes regarding what kind of activities have constituted peak experiences for him or her. An effective close to this activity is to have participants identify activities that they will want to pursue in the near future in an attempt to recapture and reexperience the peak experience.

Session 4

Based on the notes and passages prepared in the previous three or more sessions, this session will be used to prepare a draft version of a autobiographical sketch entitled "My Leisure Life." Participants will be encouraged to use self-directed time frames and focal points for their autobiographical essays. The role of the group leader is to encourage individual expression and choice of content. The entire session will be spent composing the autobiographical sketch. At the end of the session, participants will be asked if they wish to share or do anything more with their autobiographies. Some participants may wish to put all group members' autobiographies together in an anthology; for others the final results are private and should remain as a personal product of participating in the group exploration activity.

Content Area II: *Leisure and Self-Awareness*

Target Goal

The participant will explore the meaning of work and leisure to one's self.

Enabling Objectives

- To identify personal needs that are fulfilled through work and leisure.
- To classify daily activities into self-defined categories.
- To identify values and benefits received from leisure experiences.
- To compare leisure benefits with those received from work-related activity and personal responsibilities.

- To recognize barriers to leisure involvement and resources necessary to negotiate barriers.

Activity Suggestion: *Leisure and Work Values Debate*

This activity will consist of only one session of about one to two hours. The session is structured to facilitate discussion and debate of the values, benefits, and constraints associated with work and leisure activities. In the first half of the session, participants engage in small group discussion followed by a debate in the second half. The session uses values clarification as a process for attitude change and development. This activity is one example of exercises that can be used to assist participants in exploring their own values, attitudes, and beliefs regarding the roles of work, leisure, and personal responsibilities in their lives.

Implementation and Materials Suggestions

This session is structured into two distinct components, the preparatory discussion segment followed by the debate. The leader requests that participants form into round-table discussion groups of three to four members in size. Each round-table group is given a flip chart for recording the group's ideas and discussion.

Each round-table discussion group is instructed to develop a grid on its flip chart. Across the top are three columns labeled *work activities, leisure activities,* and *personal responsibility activities.* Down the left side of the page are listed *values, benefits,* and *barriers.* Each group is then instructed to go around the table with each participant naming an activity that he or she does and classifying it as work, leisure, or personal responsibility. Then the participant, along with other group members, identifies the personal values associated with the activity, benefits gained from engaging in the named activity, and any barriers that constrain his or her participation in the activity (Figure 11.1). This process is continued for 30–45 minutes of discussion so that each round-table group has several activities under each category (work, leisure, personal responsibility) that it has discussed in terms of values, benefits, and barriers to participation.

In preparation for the debate segment of the session, each round-table is given a set of value statements. If there are two round-table discussion groups, they both receive the same set. If there are four or more groups, the statements are subdivided with different sets being distributed to paired groups. In the case of an odd number of discussion groups, one group should divide itself up with members evenly distributing themselves among the other groups.

Round-table discussion groups will work in pairs to debate value statements according to whether they were randomly assigned by the leader as

Figure 11.1

Example of Round-Table Discussion Grid

	Work Activities	Leisure Activities	Personal Responsibility Activities
Example Activity	Mowing the lawn Delivering meals to home bound	Golfing with friends Listening to the radio	Exercising Preparing meals for self and spouse
Personal Values Associated with the Activity	Helping others makes me feel good, useful Contributing to the quality of life in my community by being a productive member	Maintaining my social network Providing for the aesthetic qualities of my life	Maintaining my health Improving my personal appearance Keeping the social part of eating meals in my daily life
Benefits from Doing the Activity	Maintaining my home in good condition	Good health, good friends, good times, pleasure Continuing my learning of music types	Lower healthcare costs Higher functional status and lower risk for impairment or disability in late life
Barriers that Constrain Personal Participation in this Activity	Sometimes I am too tired to feel motivated for these activities Transportation	Money Available friends	Too tired Living alone No motivation Poor lifelong habits

either assuming the pro or con position for each statement. Participants should be given approximately 10 minutes to discuss among themselves each value statement in preparation for stating a convincing position for or against the statement. Participants should be encouraged to use the previously discussed values, benefits, and constraints associated with their own activity involvements to help them in structuring their debate.

The following statements are examples of values that can be used in the debate (the leader may wish to develop his or her own statements based on knowledge of the participants or other issues that have surfaced during previous sessions in the leisure education program):

- Idle hands are the devil's workshop.
- All work and no play makes Jack a dull boy (or Jill a dull girl).
- Winning at all costs is the only thing that counts in a game.
- Anything worth doing is worth doing well.
- Work first, play later.
- Play is children's work.
- Families that play together, stay together.

At the end of this session, participants should have experienced a growing awareness of the importance and benefits of leisure to themselves as well as to the other participants in the leisure education program. Through the discussion and debate, some participants may recognize that they have built-in attitudes and biases against leisure and for work. If the leader discovers that this situation exists, additional activities may be developed to enhance positive attitudes and values for leisure.

Content Area III: *Self-Determination and Leisure Choices*

Target Goal

The participant will be able to pursue his or her personal interests and preferences through leisure.

Enabling Objectives

- To understand that pursuing one's interests and preferences through making independent choices in leisure is vital.
- To recognize one's personal decision-making style and how it affects personal leisure.
- To identify one's personal leisure preferences, interests, and barriers to participation in leisure.

Activity Suggestion: *Time Diary and Lifestyle Analysis*

This activity will cover two to three sessions of one to two hours each. The activity is intended to move participants through the process of keeping a time diary of their major life activities and conducting an analysis of their lifestyles for the purpose of planning change or maintaining continuity in life activity. The time diary and analysis take about two to three weeks to complete due to the need for:

(a) preliminary instructions,
(b) a time frame in which to conduct the diary recording process, and
(c) debriefing sessions for analysis and change planning.

The time diary process and analysis include maintaining a record of activities plus analysis of activity patterns in regard to major categories and personal needs.

Implementation and Materials Suggestions

Each participant will need a time-incremented 10–14 day diary that is organized into hourly periods. Preliminary instructions are to log in the major activities by time blocks and to complete the diary at the end of each day before retiring to bed. For each activity logged, the participant will also record major attributes associated with the activity (Figure 11.2, page 216). The key attributes will be determined during the first session as a group activity.

Session 1

During the initial session, the leader will introduce the participants to the activity. The leader will explain the purpose and process for developing the 10–14 day diary of daily activities.

The leader will work with participants to decide what criteria will be used to code key characteristics for each activity. For example, each activity can be rated on the following attributes:

- I do this activity because I *want to* (WT) or because I *have to* (HT).
- I do this activity *with others* (WO) or *alone* (A).
- This activity is *physically active* (PA) or *sedentary* (S).
- This activity is done at *home* (H) or in the *community* (C).
- I would classify this activity as **primarily** *recreation* (R), *leisure* (L), *work* (W), *education* (E), *personal maintenance* (PM), *family responsibility* (FR), or *civic involvement* (CI).
- If I had the choice, I *would do* (Y) this activity or I *would not do* (N) this activity.

Figure 11.2

Sample Page from a Time Diary

Day #1 Time:	Activity	WT/ HT	WO/ A	PA/ S	R/L/W/ E/PR/CI	H/ C
7:00 a.m.	Exercise	HT	WO	PA	PM	C
8:00	Breakfast	WT	WO	S	PM	H
9:00	Read paper	WT	A	S	L	H
10:00	Grocery shop	HT	A	PA	FR	C
11:00	Grocery shop	HT	A	PA	FR	C
Noon	Snack lunch	HT	A	S	PM	H
1:00 p.m.	Senior Center —cards	WT	WO	S	R	C
2:00	Senior Center —cards	WT	WO	S	R	C
3:00	Senior Center —cards	WT	WO	S	R	C
4:00	Television and nap	WT	A	S	R	H
5:00	Prep dinner	HT	A	PA	FR	H
6:00	Dinner and news	HT	WO	S	FR	H
7:00	Television	WT	WO	S	R	H
8:00	Television	WT	WO	S	R	H
9:00	Televsion	WT	WO	S	R	H
10:00	Televsion	WT	WO	S	R	H
11:00	Bed	WT	WO	S	PM	H
Mid-night	Bed	WT	WO	S	PM	H
1:00 a.m. to 6:00 a.m.	Bed	WT	WO	S	PM	H

Key: WT—want to, HT—have to, WO—with others, A—alone, PA—physical activity, S—sedentary, R—recreation, L—leisure, W—work, E—education, FR—family responsibility, PM—personal maintenance, CI—civic involvement, H—home, C—community.

While the leader should have a set of characteristics in mind that can be used to analyze major activities and life patterns, the group should be encouraged to develop and agree on the set that will be used for this activity.

Session 2

The second session is intended as follow-up after a 10–14 day cycle of maintaining the activity diary. Participants will bring their diaries to the session for review, discussion, and self-evaluation.

Each participant reviews his or her diary entries using the agreed-upon criteria. Each day should be summarized according to how much of the day is spent in each of the following main categories:

(a) leisure/recreation,
(b) work and other forms of obligatory activity, and
(c) self-development/self-care, such as education or personal maintenance.

Further, each category of activity can be evaluated regarding how much of the time was spent with others or alone, was sedentary or active, etc. Through this self-evaluation process, it is anticipated that participants will identify at least one or more areas in which they might like to make some change. Participants should be encouraged to discuss with each other how satisfied they are with the way they are spending their daily lives.

At the close of the second session, participants will determine what criteria they will continue to use in evaluating their daily activities, as well as in what areas they might like to experiment with making changes. Based on the results of this evaluation process, an additional session is scheduled to follow-up on another 10–14 days of diary keeping in which the participants will have decided to consciously change the configuration of daily activities and life patterns.

Session 3 (optional)

The third session will follow-up on the additional days of diary keeping in which participants consciously tried to alter the balance in daily activity choices and are now reflecting on the outcome of this activity. The same evaluation process can be used as was outlined in the second session. The objective at the end of this session and this activity is to continue to empower participants to make changes in their personal daily schedules to reflect a conscious choice for rebalancing the pattern of daily activities.

The outcome of this activity will be to assist the participant in clarifying the role of work, leisure, and personal responsibilities in his or her life by examining the balance among these activity categories in his or her present life. A follow-up activity to this one is to plan the ideal daily diary for future retirement years.

Content Area IV: *Knowledge of Leisure Opportunities and Resources*

Target Goal

The participant will have knowledge about the full range of leisure opportunities that are available in his or her home and community.

Enabling Objectives

- To identify varied forms of leisure that are available at home and in the community.
- To identify factors that influence participation in the leisure services that are available in one's personal life and community.
- To distinguish between factors that can and cannot be changed which influence leisure participation, as well as to identify strategies for overcoming barriers to participation.

Activity Suggestion: *Leisure Resource Catalog for Seniors*

This activity is intended to assist participants in identifying local resources and generating a reference file for their future use. The activity will encompass three to six sessions depending upon the size of the community and the detail that participants seek in their final report. Participants will work in teams, as well as on an individual basis, to gather information, evaluate their findings, and compile the results in a usable format.

Implementation and Materials Suggestions

The final product, "Leisure Resource Catalog for Seniors," will take three to six sessions to complete with each session encompassing one to two hours of meeting time. The leader will need to provide participants with local publications from a variety of sources including: the local visitors and convention office, city and county parks and recreation departments, the local area agency on aging, private and quasipublic recreation organizations (e.g., YMCA), newspaper and other printed media, etc. The group will need to determine the final format and contents for the "Leisure Resource Catalog for Seniors." Additional resources or contacts that are needed by the group as they complete the activity will need to be coordinated by the program leader. Finally, the program leader should have a plan for duplication and distribution to the program participants of the final product including cost estimates and potential underwriters.

Session 1

The first session will introduce the project, outline possible content and format approaches for the final product, determine the scope and depth of detail that will be included in the catalog, and generate a project completion time line. The participants will be guided through a group discussion that determines each of these aspects of the project. For example, it could be decided that only local leisure resources will be included in the catalog rather than including state or regional level resources. Participants may decide to organize resources by categories: programs, services, facilities, and other leisure resources. For all resources included in the catalog, the following kinds of information could be collected: cost, design features, leadership, hours of operation, transportation availability, equipment needed or provided, special clothing, special skills, availability and design of restrooms, food services, membership requirements, barriers to participation by seniors, contact information including phone number(s), and potential interest to older adults. Participants will make all decisions about what will be included and they will be encouraged to work in pairs, if possible.

Sessions 2–5

The first organizational session will be followed by several working sessions where participants will meet to review findings, make changes or adjustments to their project plan, amend decisions regarding content and format, and keep a working compilation of their project. The program leader is to serve as a consultant and facilitator of the group's work. One to two hours should be planned for each of these sessions.

Session 6

The last session will review and evaluate the product in its final draft form. The group will work with the program leader to make plans for the final production, duplication, and distribution of the "Leisure Resource Catalog for Seniors" to members of the program. The leader also should plan an evaluation step to determine if participation in this activity helped to expand the participants' knowledge about leisure resources that are available in their community.

Content Area V: *Decision-Making and Activity Skills*

Target Goal

The participant will create an ideal leisure lifestyle plan for attaining self-fulfillment in retirement.

Enabling Objectives

- To reevaluate one's personal leisure lifestyle and identify areas for modification or development.
- To identify new leisure activity interests.
- To select and practice the use of at least one new leisure activity.

Activity Suggestions: *Planning my Future Leisure Lifestyle and Planning and Implementing a Culminating Leisure Event*

This content area is the highest level in the process of education for leisure-centered living. It is designed to bring together all previous knowledge, values, skills, and attitudes in the development of a leisure lifestyle plan for retirement living. Two suggested activities are provided under this content area: planning a preferred leisure future, and planning/implementing a culminating leisure event for the leisure education program.

The first suggested activity in this area involves making a plan for personal leisure. This activity entails four steps:

1. identifying one to four goals for personal leisure future including the reasons for the goals;
2. identifying one to four activities for attaining each goal, as well as listing the expected benefits for each activity;
3. evaluating the identified activities in terms of time, money, skills, equipment, companionship, transportation, and availability; and
4. making a commitment to pursue at least three of the identified activities including a target date for participation.

This activity is facilitated by the program leader in a single one- to two-hour session.

The second suggested activity can be used as a means for ending the leisure education program. Participants can share their leisure goals and activities from their personal leisure plan. The group leader can facilitate a discussion as to whether the group can brainstorm an activity that the members could do together that would meet at least one goal from each member's personal plan. The outcome from this process would be a culminating leisure event planned and implemented by the group as the finale of the leisure education program. The number of sessions that it would take to complete this second activity will be totally dependent on the group's decision making at this point in the program. It is hoped that independent, self-serving leisure skills are well in place at this point so that the group's next steps are easily identified and completed under the group's direction. The program leader should be merely a facilitator and helper at this point in the process.

If, for some reason, the group is unable to arrive at a decision regarding a culminating event, the leader may want to suggest a social event in order to bring closure to the program and can ask for volunteers to help him or her in planning and implementing the event.

Implementation and Materials Suggestions

The suggested activity, "Planning my Future Leisure Lifestyle," will involve group process skills on the part of the program leader. He or she will organize the session to guide participants through a process of writing their plans. Participants will need paper, writing implements, and a comfortable place to sit and write. The leader will need either a flip chart, blackboard, or overhead projector to use in guiding each step in the process. The session will last from one to two hours with adequate time for debriefing and discussion at the end of the session.

Four process steps will be led by the program facilitator. Participants will first identify one to four goals for their personal leisure future including the reasons for the goals. These will be listed on four separate sheets of paper at the top. Next, participants will identify one to four activities that they would be interested in pursuing for attaining each goal which they will then list down the left hand side of the page. Four activities should be listed under each goal along with the expected benefits from participating in each activity summarized next to each activity and in the middle of the page. On the far right hand side of the page and next to each activity, participants will evaluate the activities in terms of resources that are needed to pursue the activity (Figure 11.3, page 222). The needed resource factors can include: time, money, skills, equipment, companionship, transportation, and availability. Finally, and on a fifth sheet of paper, participants will select three activities from all those listed; the three selected should be ones that they are willing to make a commitment to pursue. For each of these activities, participants will state a target date for participation and any other details that they need to address in order to ensure that participation takes place.

After completing the above process, the program leader provides a forum for participants to voluntarily share their final plan as written on the fifth piece of paper. They should be encouraged to provide constructive feedback to each other, including suggestions for additional activities or ideas on how to negotiate constraints. At the end of this activity, the leader can determine if the group is positioned to consider planning a closing program event. Based on group dynamics, progress throughout the program, and the demonstration of positive attitudes toward leisure along with strong independent leisure skills, the leader may suggest to the group members the idea for a closing event of their choosing.

Figure 11.3

Sample Plan for Future Leisure Lifestyle

Potential Goals:
1. Improve overall health status—mentally, physically, and socially.
2. Expand social and friendship network, improve social well-being.
3. Increase number of pleasure-based recreation activities that are outside my home.
4. Exercise my mind through enrolling in an adult learning class.

Selected Goal: Improve overall health status—mentally, physically, and socially.

Potential activities: Swim aerobics, bicycling, yoga, healthy cooking class.

Goal Planner:

Activity	Benefits	Needed Resources
Swim Aerobics	Socialization, improved flexibility, improved muscle strength, better circulation throughout body	Community program availability and access, transportation, money for fees and special equipment, time
Bicycling	Spend time outside, enjoy nature and feel mentally "clear," increase cardiovascular fitness, find a bicycling companion to develop new friendship	Equipment, locate potential biker friends, time, energy, personal motivation
Yoga	Find inner peace, body and mind integration, discover control	Videotape on yoga, motivation, energy
Healthy Cooking Class	Improve meal planning and preparation, learn new alternatives for improving overall diet, socialization, better physical health	Locate available program in community or on television, plan time, transfer program activities to everyday cooking via personal motivation

Summary

The sample program for preretirement leisure education outlined in this chapter is intended only as an illustration of the content and processes of leisure education with older adults. Any leisure education program that is planned and implemented for a target audience or purpose (retirement preparation, rehabilitation, etc.) will need to be developed in far greater detail than is provided here. It is highly recommended that the reader consult one or more of the resources provided in this chapter to assist in planning and implementing leisure education programs (see Figure 11.4, page 224, and References and Resources, page 226).

Using educational tools and strategies to develop knowledge, values, attitudes, and skills for leisure-centered living is one approach to meeting the needs of older adults as they move through later life events and stages. Leisure education is appropriate for the full range of older adult concerns; that is, from the development of positive retirement lifestyles to the rehabilitation process following a major health event to adapting one's lifestyle when moving into a nursing home. By using the educational process, the activity specialist works in collaboration with the older adult to cultivate independence and control over personal lifestyle. In this regard, leisure education is a highly desired approach with older persons who cherish their autonomy and self-direction.

Figure 11.4

Resources for Developing Leisure Education Programs

Dattilo and Murphy provide the most comprehensive and up-to-date textbook on leisure education available today (*Leisure Education Program Planning: A Systematic Approach,* 1991). These authors give a thorough review of related conceptual literature, as well as provide complete guidelines for developing leisure education programs. This text is a must for the activity specialist who intends to develop leisure education programs at senior centers, adult daycare centers, or skilled nursing facilities.

The curriculum in *The Wake Leisure Education Program: An Integral Part of Special Education* (Bullock, Bedini, and Driscoll, 1991) was initially designed for use in public schools in conjunction with special education curricula for school children with disabilities. Its usefulness to the activity programmer for older adults is twofold: (a) it is an excellent model from which to build an age-appropriate leisure education program for older adults, and (b) it focuses on the concept of *transition* which is also an important aspect of late life development. Leisure education can be instrumental in helping older adults more positively adapt to critical late life transitions (e.g., from work to retirement, from high-level health to impairment), and in coping with changes in their social networks due to death of family members and friends.

Leisure Education: Theory and Practice (Mundy and Odum, 1979) remains an essential resource to professionals who desire to build their expertise in the area of leisure education. Mundy and Odum not only provide a review of the historical roots of leisure education, but they also outline a model for implementation that can be adapted to learners of all ages.

Leisure Education: Program Materials for Persons with Developmental Disabilities (Joswiak, 1989) thoroughly covers the design and implementation of leisure education for people with mental impairment. The concepts and lesson plans in this text can be easily adapted to a wider audience than that of people with mental retardation. The book is very complete and is a valuable resource for any activity professional who may be serving older clients who have cognitive impairments.

Additional useful resources are listed in the References and Resources section at the end of this chapter.

Comprehension Questions

1. Describe the content and processes of leisure education.
2. Explain why leisure education is important in later maturity.
3. Identify the goals of leisure education in older adulthood.
4. Briefly outline a leisure education program to prepare older adults for retirement.

References and Resources

Backman, S. J., & Mannell, R. C. (1986). Removing attitudinal barriers to leisure
   behavior and satisfaction: A field experiment among the institutionalized
   elderly. *Therapeutic Recreation Journal, 20*(3), 46-53.

Bedini, L. A. (1990). The status of leisure education: Implications for instruction
   and practice. *Therapeutic Recreation Journal, 24*(1), 40-49.

Bender, M., Brannan, S. A., & Verhoven, P. J. (1984). *Leisure education for the
   handicapped: Curriculum goals, activities, and resources.* San Diego, CA:
   College Hill Press.

Birren, J. E., & Deutchmann, D. E. (1991). *Guiding autobiography groups for
   older adults: Exploring the fabric of life.* Baltimore, MD: The Johns Hopkins
   University Press.

Boyd, R. (1990). Participation in day programs and leisure activities by elderly
   persons with mental retardation: A necessary component of normalization.
   Research into Action, 7, 12-21.

Brightbill, C. K., & Mobley, T. A. (1977). *Educating for leisure-centered living*
   (2nd ed.). New York, NY: John Wiley & Sons, Inc.

Bullock, C. C., Bedini, L. A., & Driscoll, L. B. (1991). *The Wake leisure education
   program: An integral part of special education.* Chapel Hill, NC: University of
   North Carolina–Chapel Hill, Center for Recreation and Disability Studies.

Dattilo, J., & Murphy, W. D. (1991) *Leisure education program planning: A
   systematic approach.* State College, PA: Venture Publishing, Inc.

Elliott, J. E., & Sorg-Elliott, J. A. (1991). *Recreation programming and activities
   for older adults.* State College, PA: Venture Publishing, Inc.

Gushiken, T. T., Treftz, J. L., Porter, G. H., & Snowberg, R. L. (1986). The development of a leisure education for cardiac patients. *Journal of Expanding Hori-
   zons in Therapeutic Recreation, 1,* 67-72.

Herrera, P. M. (1983). *Innovative programming for the aging and aged mentally
   retarded/developmentally disabled adult.* Akron, OH: Exploration Series Press.

Howe-Murphy, R., & Charboneau, B. G. (1987). *Therapeutic recreation intervention: An ecological perspective.* Englewood Cliffs, NJ: Prentice Hall.

Keller, M. J., McCombs, J., Piligrim, V. V., & Booth, S. A. (1987). *Helping older
   adults develop active leisure lifestyles.* Atlanta, GA: Georgia Department of
   Human Resources.

Kelly, J. R. (1993). *Activity and aging: Staying involved in later life.* Newbury
   Park, CA: Sage Publications, Inc.

Kelly, J. R. (1990). *Leisure* (2nd ed.). Englewood Cliffs, NJ: Prentice Hall.

Kimeldorf, M. (1989). *Pathways to leisure: A workbook for finding leisure opportunities.* Bloomington, IL: Meridian Education Corporation.

Joswiak, K. (1989). *Leisure education: Program materials for persons with
   developmental disabilities.* State College, PA: Venture Publishing, Inc.

Mundy, J., & Odum, L. (1979). *Leisure education: Theory and practice.* New York, NY: John Wiley & Sons, Inc.

Murphy, J. F. (1975). *Recreation and leisure service: A humanistic perspective.* Dubuque, IA: Wm. C. Brown.

Neulinger, J. (1974). *The psychology of leisure: Research approaches to the study of leisure.* Springfield, IL: Charles C. Thomas Publisher.

Overs, R. P., Taylor, S., & Adkins, C. (1974). Avocational counseling for the elderly. *Journal of Physical Education and Recreation, 48*(4), 44-45.

Powers, P. (1991). *The activity gourmet.* State College, PA: Venture Publishing, Inc.

Stumbo, N. J., & Thompson, S. R. (1986). *Leisure education: A manual of activities and resources.* State College, PA: Venture Publishing, Inc.

Thews, V., Reaves, A. M., & Henry, R. S. (1993). *Now what? A handbook of activities for adult day programs.* Winston-Salem, NC: Bowman Gray School of Medicine, Wake Forest University.

Wuerch, B. B., & Voeltz, L. M. (1982). *Longitudinal leisure skills for severely handicapped learners: The Ho'onanea curriculum component.* Baltimore, MD: Paul H. Brookes Publishing Co.

Key Terms

Aerobic Activity

Anaerobic Activity

Biomedical Model of Aging

Flexibility

Maximal Oxygen Consumption

Metabolism

Muscular Endurance

Range of Motion

Strength

Stress Test

Weight Bearing

Wellness

Learning Objectives

1. Identify the activity types that may be utilized in physical activity intervention and health promotion with older adults.
2. Compare and contrast the biomedical model of aging with a wellness model.
3. Discuss the following components of an exercise program: strength training, aerobic training, and flexibility training.
4. Explain the benefits of an exercise program.
5. Discuss concerns and considerations for implementing a fitness program.

Chapter 12

Physical Activity and Health Promotion

Introduction

Historically, aging has been viewed from a biomedical model. According to Estes and Binney (1989), there are two closely related aspects of this model: "(1) the social construction of aging as a medical problem and (2) the praxis (or practice) of aging as a medical problem" (p. 587). The dominance of this model has lead to a society which believes understanding the etiology, treatment, and management of diseases is the needed approach to solving the problems of aging (Estes and Binney, 1989). From the perspective of a biomedical model of aging, decline in physical performance is a normative experience in later life. This situation may be true for many older adults. According to Ferrini and Ferrini (1993), nearly every system of the body deteriorates with inactivity. Consequently, the majority of older adults who do not exercise on a regular basis experience pronounced changes in their physical abilities.

Critics of the biomedical model argue that it has created a mentality that supports the extension of life at all costs and does not consider quality of life (Estes and Binney, 1989). Some gerontologists (Hooyman and Kiyak, 1993) have advocated a shift from a biomedical model of aging which emphasizes treatment of disease to a health promotion model which requires older adults to take responsibility for their own health. According to Hooyman and Kiyak, the goal of health promotion is to reduce the incidence of disabling chronic diseases, and thereby to enhance the elderly's functional independence and overall quality of life, not merely to prolong life. Health promotion, however, does not only focus on the absence of disease. The goal of a health promotion program is high-level wellness. Individuals who have achieved this level of wellness undertake an aggressive program to achieve the highest levels of vitality and quality of life.

A crucial part of a health promotion model is physical fitness. Unfortunately, only about 5% of older adults get a sufficient amount of exercise (Dishman, 1990). Physical fitness is an important factor in the quality of life of many older adults. Ferrini and Ferrini (1993) suggested that fitness is linked to the ability to live independently, to maintain one's home, to engage in leisure activities, and to withstand illness and injury. Other research has shown that participation in physical fitness activities is linked with improved mental health. Mactavish and Searle (1992) found that a five-week, self-selected, physical activity program had a positive impact on perceived competence, locus of control, and self-esteem in a group of older adults with mental retardation.

In addition to maintaining physical fitness, older adults should take the following steps to improve health status:

(a) stop smoking,
(b) limit alcohol consumption,
(c) control one's weight and maintain proper nutrition, and
(d) sleep seven to eight hours a day (Hooyman and Kiyak, 1993).

Keller (1994) recommended the following additional factors as part of an approach to wellness: stress management, safety, and leisure activities.

Developing a Health Promotion Program

The challenge of facilitating a high quality of life for older adults is an ongoing concern for healthcare and recreation professionals. Presently, many older adults are at risk for experiencing significant functional loss in the next 10 to 20 years. There are a number of factors that contribute to this including:

• lack of physical fitness, poor quality lifestyles, and participation in high risk health behaviors;
• increasing levels of individual and societal stress;
• lack of recognition, preparation, and education for qualitative use of leisure;
• absence of or poor affiliation and community life;
• lack of humanistic, high quality structures, environments, and supports at the work place including job requirements and job expectations;
• inadequate quality and safety in personal communities and residences;
• lack of access or availability of health-oriented services; and
• detrimental sociocultural norms and values (Hawkins, 1988).

Comprehensive health promotion programs are designed with all of these factors in mind. According to Butler (1986), health promotion programs encourage three types of fitness: personal, social, and physical. The minimum components of a health promotion program which meet these needs are nutrition, stress management, recreation, and exercise. The first three components are briefly described in the following sections.

Nutrition

There are a number of reasons why older adults often are at risk for problems related to nutrition and a number of factors contribute to malnutrition. These include social isolation, problems with dentures or missing teeth, loss of sense of smell or taste, and the inability to chew or swallow (Hooyman and Kiyak, 1993). Other older adults may be at risk for unneeded weight gain because of the reduced caloric need that accompanies aging (Ferrini and Ferrini, 1993). Obesity is the most common nutrition related problem among older adults. According to the National Center for Health Statistics (1990), 25% of older black and white males, 37% of older white females, and 61% of older black females are obese.

A comprehensive discussion of the nutrition requirements for older adults is beyond the scope of this chapter. However, there are some basic guidelines that can be followed. The following recommendations for older adults are offered:

- consume a wide variety of foods;
- increase consumption of unprocessed foods containing complex carbohydrates (starch and fiber), such as whole grains and legumes; and
- restrict intake of sugar, fat, and cholesterol. Less than 10% of the total calories consumed should be derived from saturated fat (Hooyman and Kiyak, 1993, p. 151).

A number of federal, state, and local programs have been designed to meet the nutritional needs of the older population. The Older Americans Act allocates federal funds to each state to provide congregate and home delivered meal programs. Often senior centers operated by parks and recreation departments are utilized as congregate meal sites. The federal government also finances the Food Stamp Program which is used by approximately 2 million older adults (Hooyman and Kiyak, 1993).

Service providers can impact nutrition in a variety of ways. Nutrition education, cooking classes, and other programs may be offered at senior centers, as part of nursing home activity programs in adult daycare facilities, and as part of rehabilitation activity services. Fitness programs also offer an excellent opportunity to teach nutrition and health. Each class can be followed by a brief discussion or lecture on healthy lifestyles and nutrition. Serving healthy food at programs is another important step to take.

Stress Management

A number of events in older adulthood can contribute to increased stress including death of a spouse, friends, and siblings; relocation to a new residence; change in functional status; and retirement. Regulating stress can contribute to overall health status and to the prevention of specific health problems including hypertension and insomnia (Girdano, Everly, and Dusek, 1990). A number of interventions can be used to manage stress including a variety of types of physical exercise and relaxation techniques.

Recreation

Participation in recreational activity on a regular basis is necessary for a healthy lifestyle. Regular involvement in recreational activity provides opportunities for older adults to meet a variety of needs. These needs include:

(a) strengthening self-concept and self-esteem,
(b) providing for spiritual satisfaction,
(c) promoting a sense of belonging,
(d) supporting companionship and socialization,
(e) improving mental stimulation,
(f) supporting a feeling of social usefulness,
(g) promoting the occupation of time, and
(h) gaining recognition from others in the community (Kaplan, 1960).

Health promotion programs reflect a more comprehensive approach if they also include recreational activity and leisure education as an important component.

Developing an Exercise Program

Successful health promotion and wellness programs just address physical fitness. Participation in regular exercise by older adults is linked to improved health outcomes, including greater independence (Wolinsky, Stump, and Clark, 1995).

An exercise program that is designed to produce optimal results will include a variety of types of exercise which affect different aspects of physical functioning. Exercise may be aerobic (with oxygen) or anaerobic (without oxygen). Aerobic exercises, such as walking, running, and swimming, elevate the heart rate by increasing the participant's oxygen uptake. As the individual uses more oxygen, the harder the heart has to work to distribute that oxygen to the working muscles. Aerobic exercises strengthen the heart and lungs. Anaerobic exercises, such as weightlifting, do not increase oxygen uptake. During anaerobic exercise, the flow of oxygen in the bloodstream cannot keep pace with the intense muscle exertion. A combination of both types of exercise is recommended. The remainder of this section will describe the primary elements of any exercise program: cardiovascular endurance training, strength training, and flexibility training.

Strength Training

Strength training programs should be designed to increase muscular endurance and strength. Muscular endurance refers to the ability of a muscle to sustain work over a period of time. Strength is the ability of an individual to apply force by muscle contraction. Increased muscle strength can improve older adults' speed of walking and enhance their ability to climb stairs, rise from a chair, get in and out of the bathtub, and other important daily activities (Ferrini and Ferrini, 1993).

Approximately one-third of people over the age of 65 experience one or more falls during a year due to balance problems (Lewis and Campanelli, 1990). For many older adults, the results can be devastating, including disability that leads to loss of independence and death. Older adults with chronic illnesses or disabilities that affect balance can benefit greatly from strength training. Strengthened muscles and ligaments aid in maintaining balance (Hooke, 1992). Further, strength training helps reduce muscle tremors which are particularly a problem for individuals with Parkinson's disease and other neuromuscular diseases.

Weight bearing exercise is crucial for women with or at risk for osteoporosis. Exercises such as walking, aerobic dancing, or weightlifting increase bone mineral content and bone strength while reducing the incidence of broken bones (Smith, Raab, Zook, and Gilligan, 1989). Special attention should be given to exercises that prevent bone mass loss in the hips, spine, and wrists since these are the bones most likely to fracture. In addition to reducing risk of injury, weight bearing exercise helps facilitate healing if orthopedic injury occurs (Hooke, 1992).

Cardiovascular Endurance

Any exercise which elevates the heart rate over a sustained period of time is considered aerobic. Common aerobic exercises include walking, swimming, jogging, bicycling, and aerobic dance. Aerobic exercise increases maximal oxygen consumption and strengthens the heart muscle and increases pumping efficiency. Consequently, the individual who exercises regularly can perform activities with less strain.

Maximal oxygen consumption or uptake refers to the amount of oxygen taken in and distributed to working muscles during exercise at maximum rate (Ferrini and Ferrini, 1993). As people age, their maximal oxygen uptake generally decreases (Piscopo, 1985). Adults who have led a sedentary lifestyle may experience a 50% decrease by age 60 which leads to decreased function of the lungs and heart (Clark, 1977). However, older adults who engage in regular vigorous aerobic activity may maintain relatively high maximal oxygen uptake levels.

Aerobic exercise reduces the risk of heart disease in a number of ways. A regular aerobic program will result in a lowered level of LDL cholesterol and an increase in HDL cholesterol. This change in cholesterol levels may lower the risk of heart disease. The progression of atherosclerosis also may be slowed with regular exercise by a change in the proportion of blood lipids (Ferrini and Ferrini, 1993).

Basal metabolism, or the minimum amount of energy needed to maintain the body while at rest, declines over the course of the life span (Piscopo, 1985). As a result, people should decrease caloric intake or maintain or increase levels of physical activity to prevent weight gain. In addition to improving cardiovascular function, aerobic exercise causes a temporary increase in metabolism (the rate at which the body burns calories) that persists for a few hours after exercise.

Persons who maintained a sedentary lifestyle for most of their lives should start an aerobic exercise program with a schedule of 20 minutes of aerobic exercise three times a week and progress to 30 to 50 minutes three to four times a week. Some older adults who walk to the store or do light housework on a regular basis may mistakenly believe that they are engaging in sufficient exercise. For any activity to be effective, it must elevate the heart rate for a sustained period of time and be repeated on a regular basis (Ferrini and Ferrini, 1993).

A treadmill stress test or some other method of assessing baseline fitness should be conducted before an older adult begins a fitness program. This assessment makes it possible for an individualized exercise program to be prescribed which will provide maximum results. In addition to a stress test before initiating an exercise program, participants should be taught to monitor their own heart rate so they can report any irregularities to their fitness instructor (Penner, 1989). A common method of monitoring whether or not one is exercising at the appropriate level is the talk test. If one cannot carry on a conversation without becoming breathless, one is working too hard (Cheney, Diehm, and Seeley, 1992).

Flexibility

Flexibility refers to the ability to move joints through the entire range of motion (Ferrini and Ferrini, 1993). When full range of motion cannot be achieved, it may be difficult to accomplish normal tasks such as reaching, grasping, pinching, stooping, and walking. Adults typically lose muscle elasticity and experience thickening of tissue around the joints as they age. Exercise can counteract this deterioration by stretching the muscles to prevent them from becoming short and tight. Regular flexibility training also may help retard the development of arthritis (AARP, n.d.).

Starting an Exercise Program

There are some risks associated with exercise. These include: muscle soreness, shin splints, tension strains, stress fractures, bone bruises, joint pain, and low back pain. Many injuries can be avoided by designing programs that minimize the risk of falls and teach participants the appropriate posture to use while exercising. Older adults with some health conditions should not engage in vigorous aerobic activity. These conditions include: angina, irregular heartbeat, congestive heart failure, severe hypertension, anemia, and obesity (Ferrini and Ferrini, 1993). In some cases, patients with these conditions may participate in an exercise program, but only under strict medical supervision.

An exercise program should be initiated only after a medical assessment has been completed (Ferrini and Ferrini, 1993). The medical assessment should include a treadmill or similar test to determine the older adult's baseline for a physical fitness program (Hooyman and Kiyak, 1993). Following the assessment, an exercise prescription should be developed by the client and a trained professional. The exercise program should be prescribed according to the individual's abilities. Exercise programs may vary from person to person in terms of type, intensity, duration, frequency, and progression of exercise (Beal and Berryman-Miller, 1988). The program should be monitored by the client and professional on a regular basis. If improvement is not evident after a few months, the rigor of the program may need to be increased.

Individual preferences will vary regarding what time of day is best to conduct an exercise program. Popular times are early morning and late afternoon before dinner. The preferences of participants can be used as the primary determinant of when a program is held. However, it is important to remember that many older adults may experience stiffness in the morning and should wait until at least a half hour after they get up to exercise in order to avoid injury (Cheney, Diehm, and Seeley, 1992). Programs should not be held until two hours after eating, since digestion makes heavy demands on the circulatory system (Cheney, Diehm, and Seeley, 1992). Other considerations regarding the time of day a program is held include facility availability, weather, and program schedules. Exercise programs should not be conducted in extremely hot or humid weather. In warm climates, air-conditioned facilities should be used.

Exercise programs should always have a defined emergency plan that is familiar to all staff and participants. The leader of any exercise program should maintain current cardiopulmonary resuscitation (CPR) certification (Beal and Berryman-Miller, 1988; Penner, 1989).

A Sample Program

Exercise and Wellness

The following program is representative of the types of activities that can be used in a physical fitness program. The program, which covers aerobic activities, strength training, flexibility programs, and stress management, is appropriate for a nursing home, adult daycare, retirement community, senior center, or fitness center. Adaptations can be made easily to each recommended activity to accommodate a variety of skill levels.

Program Purpose

The purpose of this program is to provide older adults with an opportunity to participate in a variety of activities designed to facilitate high-level wellness through the improvement of the physical, mental, and spiritual self. The program is based on the following principles:

1. Older adults have the ability to assume responsibility for their quality of life through an aggressive wellness program.
2. The utilization of a variety of local agencies with expertise in recreation, nutrition, exercise, and stress management will contribute to the success of a holistic wellness program.
3. Older adults prefer to be involved in the planning, implementation, and evaluation of activities and programs, policies, and procedures that are designed to meet their wellness needs.

Activity Area I: *Aerobic Activities*

Target Goal

Participants will be able to walk or engage in aerobic activity continuously for a minimum of 20 minutes three times a week, or the length and frequency specified in their individual treatment plans.

Enabling Objectives

- To plan and implement a varied program of aerobic exercise activities.
- To determine a baseline level of aerobic fitness for each participant through a treadmill or other exercise tolerance test.
- To develop an individual fitness plan for each participant based on his or her fitness assessment.

- To train staff in facilitating and/or leading a variety of aerobic exercise programs.
- To identify and modify a variety of aerobic exercise programs appropriate for a diverse older population.
- To regularly monitor changes in aerobic fitness level of program participants.

Activity Suggestions: *Walking and Dancing*

An ideal aerobic exercise program is one that is flexible enough to accommodate participants with a wide range of fitness levels and functional abilities. Older adults are least likely to have a history of regular participation in exercise programs and may feel uncertain about their ability to be successful in an exercise program. Consequently, programs should be designed to let the participants feel an immediate sense of accomplishment. It is also important to start participants at a level where they will feel challenged, but not discouraged.

Walking is an excellent exercise choice for many older adults. Strain on joints is minimal in walking since it is low impact. Swimming is another activity that is good for people with injured joints or people who are obese. Swimming is not satisfactory, however, for older adults with osteoporosis who need to engage in weight bearing activity. In addition to the physical benefits of walking, there is the opportunity for socialization. Beginning exercisers are more likely to continue if someone participates with them.

An effective strategy for promoting exercise is to organize a walking program that involves staff, clients, and volunteers at the facility. A "Walk around the Country" program has been suggested by Elliott and Sorg-Elliott (1991). In this program, staff and clients work together to build up mileage that is needed to walk across the country to major national attractions. Participants select places of interest and map a route prior to starting the program. Once a route has been established, a chart which indicates progress is located in a prominent area of the facility. Any mileage accumulated while walking, running, or biking for exercise by staff or participants is recorded on the chart. When the "travelers" reach the first "destination" a theme party including slides or videos of the destination, local cuisine, and decorations can be held for all participants. This destination event provides a goal for the exercise participants as well as an opportunity for staff and participants to socialize.

Dance is another type of aerobic exercise program that provides participants with multiple benefits. According to McAdam (1988), dance produces the following benefits: the opportunity to artistically express thoughts, socialization, the opportunity to be creative, and the physical benefits of an aerobic exercise program.

The ideal dance class lasts for 50 minutes to an hour (McAdam, 1988). This time frame includes: 10–15 minutes of warm-up, 10–30 minutes of aerobics, five minutes of cool down, and 10–30 minutes of strength and flexibility training. The purpose of the warm-up period is to gradually elevate the heart level to the desired training level. Walking in time to music or learning new dance steps for the aerobic training are good warm-up activities. The aerobic period consists of rhythmic steps which allow people to keep the heart rate at a fitness training level. The steps should be simple, of moderate tempo, and have long repetitive phrases. In addition, dances are choreographed in a sequence that minimizes stress to any one joint, avoiding hops and jumps, and provides a low-impact option that does not require elevation for people with painful joints. A simple walk with large arm movements is recommended for the cool down period. The cool down period which is essential helps keep blood from pooling. Suggestions for the strength training and flexibility periods are discussed later in this sample program.

Implementation and Materials Suggestions

Good form and posture for participants are necessary in order to avoid injuries. The proper form for walking involves a heel-to-toe movement. The weight of the body should be transferred smoothly from one foot to the other, with one foot always on the ground. The heel should be centered with the foot pointing slightly out. The body should be kept erect by leaning slightly from the ankles. Arms should be loose at the sides and moving in opposition to the legs (Hooke, 1992).

Dance participants should hold their shoulders slightly back and down. To prevent back injury the pelvis should be tilted in and the abdominal muscles held in. Knees should be slightly bent throughout the routine to avoid hyperextension. Elevation of feet off the floor should be minimized. High-impact moves which are popular in many aerobic dance routines can cause excessive stress to the joints and result in injury (Beal and Berryman-Miller, 1988).

Little equipment is needed for most aerobic exercise programs. Participants in the walking program should have comfortable shoes that provide ample support. If participants will be walking outside, they should dress in layers that can be easily removed if needed. The dance program requires a cassette or CD player, straight chairs without arms for participants that exercise from a sitting position, mats for participants who will be doing stretching exercises on the floor, and a microphone for the instructor, if needed. Optional equipment includes balls, hoops, and ribbons that can be incorporated into the dance sequence. Dance program participants should wear comfortable shoes that provide ample support and comfortable clothes which do not restrict movement. The primary problem with this attire is that it prevents the instructor from monitoring posture and form during the program which could lead to potential injury.

Due to the possibility of impact injuries, the preferred location of aerobic programs is a space which does not have a concrete floor. (If a concrete floor is unavoidable, only low-impact activities should be employed and proper shoes must be worn.) The space should have good lighting, proper ventilation, and an open space large enough to allow the participants to move freely. Indoor walking programs require a circular route which is level and contains benches for resting. If an outdoor walking space is available, it should be secured by a fence to prevent confused clients from wandering away from the path. Use of a variety of plantings along the walkway will add interest to the area.

Activity Area II: *Strength Training*

Target Goal

Participants will be able to complete 20 repetitions of strength exercises specified in their individual care plans.

Enabling Objectives

- To plan and implement a varied program of strength training exercise activities.
- To determine target muscle groups for each individual based on the assessment of muscular strength and endurance.
- To train staff in facilitating and/or leading a variety of strength training programs.
- To identify and modify a variety of strength training programs appropriate for a diverse older population, including older adults who use wheelchairs and those who must remain in bed due to a disabling or medical condition.
- To regularly monitor changes in strength level of program participants.

Activity Suggestions: *Resistive Exercises*

Strength training programs consist of resistive exercises. Participants may participate in isotonic exercise in which resistance is provided by a weight or isometric exercise in which resistance is created by contracting a muscle group statically (Lasko and Knopf, 1988). The advantage of isometric exercise is that it does not require equipment or space to perform. However, it is generally not as effective as isotonic exercise so the transfer to functional activities may not be as great.

Greninger and Kinney (1988) recommended the three *I's* for localized strength training:

- Identify the muscle or muscle groups to be exercised.
- Isolate the muscle group by placing the body in the appropriate position. This step is key to preventing injuries and gaining maximum benefits.
- Intensify the muscle group by using weight or resistance to gravity.

In addition, localized strength exercises should only involve one joint at a time. All strength exercises should be done slowly and movements should be made through the full range of motion.

Implementation and Materials Suggestions

It is recommended that one set (eight to 12 repetitions) of eight to 10 resistance exercises be completed by healthy older adults at least two days a week (American College of Sports Medicine, 1990). Localized exercises may be performed standing, sitting, or lying down. According to Hooke (1992), the following posture tips should be followed to reduce the risk of injury and decrease muscle fatigue:

- Standing Position—The body should be erect and relaxed with the head held over the spine. The shoulders should be down, level, and back and the chest should be lifted. The abdominal muscles should be drawn in and the pelvis tucked forward. Knees should not be locked or hyperextended and feet should be shoulder width apart, with body weight slightly forward of the ankles.
- Sitting Position in a Chair—The body should be erect and relaxed with a 90° angle at the hips. The hips should be tilted forward to prevent back injury. The head should be held directly over the spine. The shoulders should be held level and back, the abdominal area drawn in, and the thighs supported by the seat of the chair. Feet should be flat on the floor and placed shoulder width apart.
- Sitting Position on the Floor—The upper body should be erect and relaxed with a 90° angle at the hips. Head, shoulder, and abdomen positions should be similar to the chair position. Feet should be slightly apart and knees may be straight or bent.
- Lying on the Floor or Other Flat Surface—The knees should be bent with feet shoulder width apart and flat on the floor. A small pillow should be placed under the head to support the head and neck.

A variety of equipment has been developed for strength training programs. Small hand-held weights are available in a variety of sizes. Weights of one, three, five, and 10 pounds are sufficient for most programs. Ankle weights also are useful; however, sandbags may be draped over the ankle and used for leg exercises. If cost is a concern to participants, especially those who are exercising at home, program leaders may use soup cans, books, water-filled jugs, or other household goods instead of weights. Many programs use resistance bands for strength training. These bands are fairly inexpensive and are particularly useful for strengthening the arms and legs.

Activity Area III: *Flexibility Programs*

Target Goal

Participants will be able to move targeted joints through the full range of motion or appropriate level as determined at assessment.

Enabling Objectives

- To plan and implement a varied program of flexibility exercises.
- To develop an individual plan for each participant based on the fitness assessment.
- To train staff in facilitating and/or leading a flexibility program.
- To identify and modify a variety of flexibility exercises.
- To regularly monitor changes in level of flexibility of program participants.

Activity Suggestions: *Yoga*

A flexibility program is a necessary element of any well-rounded fitness program. Flexibility exercises may be done on their own or in conjunction with aerobic exercise and/or strength training.

Stretching to music adds interest to a flexibility program. New age music or tapes of nature are soothing and conducive to the slow movements that are part of a flexibility program. Ribbons or brightly colored scarves may be incorporated into the routine for additional interest.

Yoga is an ancient form of exercise that encourages physical, mental, and spiritual development and also increases flexibility (Girdano, Everly, and Dusek, 1990). Hatha yoga is the most popular type of yoga in the Western cultures. This type of yoga utilizes positions and exercises to promote harmony between the physical self and the mental self. Although some yoga positions and exercises may be too advanced for older adults, many are adaptable. Local parks and recreation departments or college physical education departments may be able to recommend an instructor for the yoga program. Yoga programs also may include an educational element wherein participants learn about the various levels of yoga and the culture from which it originated.

Implementation and Materials Suggestions

Prior to beginning stretching, participants should take a walk for three to five minutes or do some other type of warm-up activity (Hooke, 1992). Following the warm-up, general stretches such as long stretches from the toes to fingertips, side stretches, and relaxing shoulder movements are implemented. Stretches for specific muscles may then be done. All major muscle groups should be stretched individually (Clements, 1994).

A number of safety concerns should be addressed when doing stretching exercises. The body should be positioned within its normal range of motion (Clements, 1994). Smooth, gentle movements or static stretching are recommended for older adults (Hooke, 1992). The participant should move very slowly into the stretch and hold it for a period of 10 to 20 seconds before slowly returning to the starting position (Clements, 1994). Participants may try to "bounce" while they are stretching in order to reach further but this should be discouraged. It is important to emphasize that everyone has a different level of flexibility, so progress in this area must be measured on an individual level. All participants should understand that stretching exercises should feel good. Participants should feel "pull, but not pain" (Hooke, 1992, p. 263).

Activity Area IV: *Stress Management*

Target Goal

Participants will develop the skills to incorporate stress management techniques into their lives on a daily basis or as needed.

Enabling Objectives

- To plan and implement a varied program of stress management activities.
- To determine an individual stress management plan that is appropriate for the needs of each participant.
- To train staff in facilitating and/or leading a variety of stress management programs.
- To identify a number of stress management programs appropriate for a diverse older population.
- To regularly monitor perceived changes in level of stress, as well as the reduction of physical manifestations of stress (ulcers, high blood pressure, etc.).

Activity Suggestions: *Relaxation Exercises*

An ideal stress management program is one that contains a variety of techniques. Individual preferences for techniques will vary. It is the task of the instructor or facilitator to introduce these techniques and let the participants decide which are most effective for them.

Yoga or stretch-relaxation exercises help to reduce stress through the reduction of muscle tension. A general lack of physical activity contributes to shortened muscles, tendons, and ligaments and muscle tension. Older adults that experience chronic back or neck pain, or headaches may be feeling the effects of a lifetime of sedentary living or poor posture. Stretching is a natural reflex after the muscles have been tightened or experienced tension and can be used to prevent tension pain in the body (Girdano, Everly, and Dusek, 1990).

Aerobic activity is an excellent stress reducer. All humans have an innate need to respond to stress with physical activity. During stressful situations, the human body produces adrenal hormones which ready the body to "fight or flight" (Girdano, Everly, and Dusek, 1990). In modern times, the fight-or-flight response is typically not an appropriate response to a stressful situation. As a result, the increased hormones are not metabolized and can contribute to ulcers, cardiovascular disease, and a number of other physical illnesses. These resulting health conditions can be prevented with the regular exercise that promotes a healthy and appropriate outlet for stress.

There are many other techniques in addition to exercise that can be used to manage stress. Many of the techniques are simple to teach and can be easily incorporated into daily life as needed. The following is a brief description of three techniques that are described in *The Relaxation and Stress Reduction Workbook* (Davis, Eshelman, and McKay, 1988):

- Progressive Relaxation—Progressive relaxation is used to identify tension in particular muscle groups. While using this technique, participants focus on specific muscle groups, contract those muscles, visualize the tension in the muscles, and then relax the muscles. This sequence is repeated for the following muscle groups:

  (a) hands, forearms, and biceps;
  (b) head, face, throat, and shoulders;
  (c) chest, stomach, and lower back; and
  (d) thighs, buttocks, calves, and feet.

- Breathing—Although breathing is an automatic, natural action, it is not always done correctly. Breathing may be altered by poor posture, tight clothing, disease, or stress. Taking the time to learn proper breathing techniques can contribute to overall health status and reduce the effects of stress. It is difficult to remain stressed or anxious when taking slow, deep breaths. There are many breathing techniques that can be used for stress management. They all involve good posture, deep full breaths, and appropriate use of the diaphragm.

- Meditation—Meditation involves focusing attention on one thing at time. The goal is to become so focused on one object that the participant "lets go" of worries, fears, hate, and other negative emotions. Meditation has long been used by Eastern cultures as a method of strengthening the spirit and the mind. There are three basic types of meditation that can be easily learned. Mantra meditation involves focusing on a word or syllable that one likes or finds pleasing. Breath counting meditation utilizes the counting of slow, relaxed, and unforced breaths. Gazing meditation utilizes an object as the center of attention, rather than a word or syllable.

Summary

In this chapter basic elements of activity programs that are designed to meet the fitness and health promotion needs of older adults are outlined. These activities can be implemented in a variety of settings and can be adapted to multiple fitness levels. A variety of resources are available to help in the development and implementation of an exercise and wellness program (Figure 12.1). Additional texts are listed in the References and Resources section at the end of this chapter.

Figure 12.1

Resources for Developing Physical Fitness Programs

Activities, Adaptation, & Aging is published monthly by The Haworth Press Inc., 10 Alice Street, Binghamton, NY, 13904-1580, telephone 1-800-342-9678. This publication contains valuable articles and other resource materials.

Aerobics and Fitness Foundation, 15250 Ventura Boulevard, Sherman Oaks, CA, 91403, telephone 1-800-233-4886.

American Association of Retired Persons, 1909 K Street, N.W., Washington, DC, 20049 (brochures and audiovisual materials available).

American Diabetes Association, 505 8th Avenue, New York, NY, 10017.

American Heart Association, National Center, 7320 Greenville Avenue, Dallas, TX, 75231.

Arthritis Foundation, 1314 Spring Street N.W., Atlanta, GA, 30309.

Easy Yoga for Seniors. Videotape by Video Vacation, 306 West Avenue, Lockport, NY, 14094, telephone 1-800-441-3006.

Fitness for the Good Years. Videotape by Parade Video, Newark, NJ.

National Resource Center on Health Promotion and Aging, American Association of Retired Persons, 601 E Street, N.W., Washington, DC, 20049.

President's Council on Physical Fitness and Sports, 450 5th Street, N.W., Suite 7103, Washington, DC., 20001, telephone 1-202-272-3430.

Additional useful resources are listed in the References and Resources section at the end of this chapter.

Comprehension Questions

1. Describe the components of a health promotion/wellness program for older adults.
2. Discuss the three basic components of a fitness program for older adults. Why are each of these components necessary?
3. Discuss the influence of physical exercise on health status.
4. Define high level wellness.
5. Discuss considerations for implementing a fitness program.

References and Resources

Administration on Aging. (n.d.). *The fitness challenge . . . in the later years: An exercise program for older adults* (DHHS Publication No. OHD 75-20802). Washington, DC: U.S. Government Printing Office.

American Association of Retired Persons (AARP). (n.d.). *Pep up your life: A fitness guide for seniors* [Brochure]. Washington, DC: Author.

American College of Sports Medicine. (1991). *Guidelines for exercise testing and prescription* (4th ed.). Philadelphia, PA: Lea & Febiger.

American College of Sports Medicine. (1990). The recommended quantity and quality of exercise for developing and maintaining cardiorespiratory and muscular fitness in healthy older adults. *Medicine and Science in Sports and Exercise, 22*(2), 265-274.

Beal, R. K., & Berryman-Miller, S. (1988). *Dance for the older adult.* Reston, VA: The American Alliance for Health, Physical Education, Recreation, and Dance.

Butler, R. N. (1986). Wellness and health promotion for the elderly: An overview. In K. Dychtwald (Ed.), *Wellness and health promotion for the elderly.* Rockville, MD: Aspen Publishers Inc.

Cheney, W. J., Diehm, W. J., & Seeley, F. E. (1992). *The second fifty years: A reference manual for senior citizens.* New York, NY: Paragon House.

Clark, H. H. (1977). Exercise and aging. *Physical Fitness Research Digest, 7*(2). Washington, DC: President's Council on Physical Fitness and Sport.

Clements, C. B. (1994). *The Arts/Fitness Quality of Life Program: Creative ideas for working with older adults.* Baltimore, MD: Health Professions Press.

Corbin, D. E., & Metal-Corbin, J. (1990). *Reach for it: Handbook of health, exercise and dance for older adults* (2nd ed.). Dubuque, IA: Eddie Bowers Publishing Inc.

Davis, M., Eshelman, E. R., & McKay, M. (1988). *The relaxation and stress reduction workbook.* Oakland, CA: New Harbinger Publications, Inc.

Dishman, R. K. (1990). Determinants of physical activity and exercise for persons 65 years of age and older. In W. W. Spirduso and H. M. Eckert (Eds.), *The Academy Papers: Physical activity and aging.* Champaign, IL: Human Kinetics Inc.

Elliott, J. E., & Sorg-Elliott, J. A. (1991). *Recreation programming and activities for older adults.* State College, PA: Venture Publishing, Inc.

Estes, C. L., & Binney, E. A. (1989). The biomedicalization of aging: Dangers and dilemmas. *The Gerontologist, 29*(5), 587-596.

Ferrini, A. F., & Ferrini, R. L. (1993). *Health in the later years* (2nd ed.). Madison, WI: Brown & Benchmark.

Girdano, D. A., Everly, G. S., Jr., & Dusek, D. E. (1990). *Controlling stress and tension: A holistic approach.* Englewood Cliffs, NJ: Prentice Hall.

Greninger, L. O., & Kinney, M. B. (1988). *Therapeutic exercises for older adults.* Dubuque, IA: Eddie Bowers Publishing Inc.

Hawkins, B. (1988). *Health promotion and high level wellness in health, physical education, and recreation.* Bloomington, IN: Indiana University School of Health, Physical Education, and Recreation.

Hooke, A. P. (1992). *Active older adults in the YMCA: A resource manual.* Champaign, IL: YMCA of the USA.

Hooyman, N. R., & Kiyak, H. A. (1993). *Social gerontology: A multidisciplinary perspective* (2nd ed.). Needham Heights, MA: Allyn & Bacon.

Kaplan, M. (1960). *Leisure in America: A social inquiry.* New York, NY: John Wiley & Sons, Inc.

Keller, M. J. (1994). Wellness programs with older adults residing in retirement communities. In M. J. Keller & N. J. Osgood (Eds.), *Dynamic leisure programming with older adults.* Arlington, VA: National Recreation and Park Association.

Lasko, P. M., & Knopf, K. G. (1988). *Adapted exercises for the disabled adult: A training manual* (2nd ed.). Dubuque, IA: Eddie Bowers Publishing Inc.

Lewis, C. B., & Campanelli, L.C. (1990). *Health promotion and exercise for older adults.* Rockville, MD: Aspen Publishers Inc.

Mactavish, J. B., & Searle, M. (1992). Older individuals with mental retardation and the effects of physical activity intervention on selected social psychological variables. *Therapeutic Recreation Journal, 26*(1), 38-42.

McAdam, M. (1988). Dance as a vehicle to fitness for the healthy older adult. In R. K. Beak & S. Berryman-Miller (Eds.), *Dance for the older adults* (pp. 16-27). Reston, VA: American Alliance for Health, Physical Education, Recreation, and Dance.

National Center for Health Statistics. (1990, October). Current estimates from the National Health Interview Survey, 1989. *Vital and Health Statistics, 10*(176).

Penner, D. (1989). *Eldercise: A health and fitness guide for older adults.* Reston, VA: American Alliance for Health, Physical Education, Recreation, and Dance.

Piscopo, J. (1985). *Fitness and aging.* New York, NY: John Wiley & Sons, Inc.

Rejeski, W. J., & Kenney, E. A. (1988). *Fitness motivation: Preventing participant dropout.* Champaign, IL: Life Enhancement Publications.

Smith, E. L., Raab, D. M., Zook, S. K., & Gilligan, C. (1989). Bone changes with aging and exercise. In R. Harris & S. Harris (Eds.), *Physical activity, aging and sports: Volume 1 Scientific & Medical Research.* Albany, NY: Center for the Study of Aging.

Teaff, J. D. (1990). *Leisure services with the elderly.* Prospect Heights, IL: Waveland Press, Inc.

Wolinsky, F. D., Stump, T. E., & Clark, D. O. (1995). Antecedents and consequences of physical activity and exercise among older adults. *The Gerontologist, 35*(4), 451-462.

Key Terms

Life Review
Motivation
Reality Orientation
Reminiscence
Remotivation
Resocialization

Sensory Stimulation
Spirituality
Therapeutic Humor
Triggers
Validation Therapy

Learning Objectives

1. Identify the activity types that may be utilized in cognitive therapeutic activity intervention with older adults.
2. Describe common treatment modalities that are used with older adults who have cognitive impairment, as well as with unimpaired persons.
3. Discuss therapeutic activity intervention in the following areas: reminiscence and life review, validation therapy, reality orientation, sensory training, spiritual activities, therapeutic humor, remotivation, and resocialization.
4. Describe a sample cognitive activity intervention program for elderly clients.
5. Explain common motivational and leadership techniques that can be used to enhance participation by older adults in therapeutic cognitive activities.

Chapter 13

Cognitive Activity Intervention

Introduction

Outreach programs for the elderly are seriously limited. Persons over the age of 65 tend to receive much less therapy or skilled outpatient treatment than is recommended for depression, anxiety, alcohol problems, and other mental disorders that are prevalent among this segment of the population (Kane and Kane, 1989). Some elderly clients in nursing facilities suffer from Alzheimer's disease. However, geriatric assessments in nursing homes tend to ignore psychiatric diagnoses, and, similarly, physicians in geriatric practice often fail to deal with mental health problems (Waxman, Carner, and Berkenstock, 1984). As a consequence, activity specialists in nursing homes, senior centers, adult daycare centers, and rehabilitation facilities may encounter elderly persons who are in need of programs, whether or not they have been formally diagnosed with a cognitive disorder (e.g., Alzheimer's disease or other forms of dementia) or are experiencing symptoms related to depression.

This chapter discusses the rationale for therapeutic activity intervention that is aimed at cognition and related aspects of mental health. Various therapeutic cognitive activities that are commonly utilized with older persons, especially those residing in nursing or rehabilitation facilities, are discussed. The following therapeutic activities are included: reality orientation, sensory stimulation, spiritual activities, therapeutic humor, remotivation, and resocialization. A sample treatment program is described for the purpose of assisting activity specialists in understanding and supporting individual cognitive needs and abilities. Common motivational and leadership techniques that can be used to enhance participation in cognitive activities also are considered.

Rationale for Therapeutic Cognitive Activity Intervention

Therapeutic activity intervention is comparable to generic rehabilitation programming because positive behavioral change is promoted in the older person in the cognitive, sensorimotor, and affective domains. Specifically designed programs based upon individual need can assist in the facilitation of positive behavioral change. The older adult who is able to adapt to changes may be more likely to function as a complete human being through the integration of these changes into all areas of his or her environment (Greenblatt, 1988). In this chapter, therapeutic activities that target behavioral change in cognitive functioning and those activities which are aimed at promoting optimal mental health are addressed.

Chapter 6 of this text presents several psychological illnesses and psychiatric disorders commonly experienced by older persons. Typical disruptions in the functional mental health of older adults include depression, anxiety disorders, psychotic illnesses, alcoholism, and drug abuse/misuse. Organic diseases, on the other hand, encompass dementia-related syndromes including Alzheimer's disease. Whether the older individual suffers from a cognitive disease or temporary loss in mental functioning due to depression, cognitive therapeutic activity intervention will focus on enhancing overall mental health in areas of judgment and decision making, memory (long and short term), affect and emotional stability, reasoning, orientation, and self-identity. Because an estimated 20% of the older population suffer from depression and 15% to 20% experience some form of mental illness, therapeutic cognitive activities are recognized as an important aspect of any activity program for seniors.

Meeting Cognitive Needs through Activity Intervention

Cognitive impairment in older persons may be caused by either organic brain disease (e.g., Alzheimer's disease or multi-infarct dementia) or difficulties in mental functioning associated with depression, drug misuse/abuse, and alcoholism. In either case, the older person displays the need for cognitive support and therapy. A variety of approaches are used to enhance the mental functioning and health of older persons who are experiencing mental health problems. Reminiscence, life review, validation therapy, reality orientation, sensory stimulation, spirituality, therapeutic humor, remotivation, and resocialization are common approaches that are covered in this chapter.

Reminiscence and Life Review

Reminiscence refers to the vocal or silent recall of events in a person's life either alone or with other persons. The term *life review* is usually applied to the process of reviewing, organizing, and evaluating one's life as a whole in order for the individual to consider one's life as unique. The themes of life review generally are a person's own hopes and expectations (Woods, Portnoy, Head, and Jones, 1992).

Reminiscence involves certain positive qualities such as fantasy, simplicity, fun, comfort, empathy, affiliation, history, heritage, legacy, and self-preservation. Reminiscence also is intellectual, rational, emotional, therapeutic, and cultural and involves both passive and active components (Ebersole, 1988). Life review, as a task to be completed in the final phase of life, embraces the positive functions of reminiscence. Both life review and reminiscence are aspects of the personal adaptation process, and both produce social benefits. Therefore, life review may be thought of as a form of structured reminiscence (Butler, 1963).

Assisting older persons with life review promotes self-acceptance, but it is likely that the nature of life review will evoke a sense of regret and sadness at the brevity of life. However, most persons have the capacity to reconcile their lives and to find meaning, especially with the support of others. The success of life review is difficult to determine because much of the process often occurs within an individual and overt indications of change are not always apparent. For the most part, it's best to encourage achievements within the reminiscence session rather than to analyze changes and positive results that may occur outside of the group (Butler, 1963; Woods, Portnoy, Head, and Jones, 1992).

Reminiscence and life review have not always been recognized as valuable experiences for elderly persons and staff members. In the past, reminiscence was viewed as a negative attribute of older persons. Dwelling in the past and repeating stories about the old days were seen as indicators of regression. In more recent years, reminiscence and life review have been recognized as valuable at any life stage and, most particularly, during periods of transition (Woods, Portnoy, Head, and Jones, 1992).

Group reminiscence can be used to meet many levels of human need. As older persons socialize, they express themselves, share, and mutually value each other for their contributions. In group reminiscence, participants can develop the strength and self-esteem required to actualize their potentials (Ebersole, 1988). In order to accomplish predetermined treatment goals and objectives, it is helpful to begin with each individual and to ascertain what the person can do; that is, to focus upon abilities rather than disabilities.

The overall aims of a reminiscence group include: (a) improved affect, (b) increased socialization, and (c) increased opportunities for others to listen to excerpts from the participant's life. Reminiscence stimulates interest, attention, and interaction and can be enjoyed by both clients and activity staff. There also is hope that staff members will retain the knowledge learned about clients during reminiscence and utilize this information during other caregiving activities (Woods, Portnoy, Head, and Jones, 1992).

Reminiscence groups provide a supportive setting for the discussion of problems and the expression of feelings. They promote elevation of mood through enjoyable, entertaining activity. Reminiscence also facilitates supplementary description of self to others, offers opportunities for continuity, and contributes to autonomy and control. The activity specialist can utilize reminiscence periods for the evaluation of treatment efficacy by monitoring client confusion, depression, social interaction, and self-esteem prior to intervention during therapy, and after termination of the group. Older adults who exhibit impaired memory processes often have the ability to discuss events from the past because of the richness of the association with strong affective memories, repetition, and possibly, memory storage in different areas of the brain other than those that have been damaged by dementia or other illnesses (Burnside and Schmidt, 1994; Harrison, 1980; Holland, 1987; Morris and Koppelman, 1986).

In the course of reminiscence, triggers are employed which may be specific, as well as implied. *Triggers* are any type of stimuli that prompt recall. Music, photographs, food, poetry, faces, colors, objects, and odors all may act as triggers. These triggers can be used intentionally to facilitate or access particular memories or spontaneously during ongoing conversation. Random environmental events also can function as triggers, and questions alone may be appropriate to inspire and focus recall (Woods, Portnoy, Head, and Jones, 1992).

Validation Therapy

Validation therapy is a means of categorizing the behaviors exhibited by disoriented elderly persons. It is also a method of communication, as well as a theory of late-onset disorientation. The process of validation cannot restore damaged brain tissue, but it can assist in the stimulation of dormant yet intact capacities by acknowledging basic human needs. Validation therapy does not judge, analyze, or intend to change the disoriented person. The goals of becoming and remaining oriented are not emphasized. The activity specialist understands that validation therapy is used to assist the elderly individual in attaining his or her own goals. A validation approach suggests the acceptance of the feelings of the older person with dementia.

Validation is a humanistic approach for providing disoriented older persons with the opportunity to resolve their unfinished conflicts through (a) the expression of their feelings, (b) acknowledgment of their lives through reminiscence, and (c) coming to peace with their losses (Babins, 1988; Feil, 1989). Validation includes reflection of a person's feelings, assistance in the expression of unmet human needs, restoration of well-established social roles, facilitation of perceptions of well-being, and stimulation of interactions with others (Feil, 1989).

Reality Orientation

Reality orientation is a psychological treatment approach for attending to the problems of confused older adults (Folsom, 1986). The specific procedures for reality orientation are pragmatic, focused upon daily routines, behavior, and principles of reinforcement to assist clients in maintaining a sense of self, time, and place. Reality orientation concentrates on supporting clients at their highest level of current functioning while actively presenting them with reality through environmental management, teaching/training, and consistent attitudes of family and staff members (Bowlby, 1993; Edinberg, 1985).

Sensory Stimulation

Sensory stimulation is an individual or group activity for cognitively impaired older adults who have difficulty in relating and responding to their environments. Meaningful and familiar smells, movements, sights, sounds, tastes, and tactile sensations from the immediate and larger surroundings are systematically presented in a format that can be understood by the individual. By focusing attention on specific, concrete, sensory cues, individuals can explore and relate "sensory props" to familiar life experiences. From this process they are enabled to make appropriate responses to the world. Sensory stimulation is designed to compensate for the sensory deprivation that elderly persons often suffer as a result of dementia. It has been suggested that individuals who have the ability to participate in the social and self-care aspects of their lives function at a higher level, have higher self-esteem, are calmer, and tend to be more alert (Bowlby, 1993).

Spirituality

Spirituality or religious activity may not necessarily be a part of the daily life experiences of all older adults. However, for those persons to whom religion has played a continuing and significant role, maintaining their involvement may be a major contributor to self-respect and perceived well-being. Religious behavior is reported to be an effective means of coping and is common among older adults regardless of sex, race, socioeconomic status, or place of residence. There is a significant correlation between positive morale and involvement in religious activities (Bowlby, 1993).

As a lifelong means of coping with stress, personal religious practices are negatively affected by the progression of dementia. Individuals afflicted by dementia will require additional support and assistance in order to adapt their means of coping through participation in religious activities. Religious activities can be modified to be compatible with the individual's present abilities. Inclusion in religious activities must be based on ongoing experiences and practices (weekly devotions, celebration of religious holidays, etc.), and may be supported by the use of a peer companion system. Spiritual and religious activities should continue to be purposeful and adult-oriented. Religious activities represent a unique method of communication to provide opportunities for reminiscence and to offer meaning even when standard communication has regressed (Bowlby, 1993).

Therapeutic Humor

There is a complex system of mutual functioning between the human psychological and physiological processes. Laughter is an observable reaction to humorous situations in which muscles are stimulated, heart rate is intensified, and respiration is increased, thereby expanding the exchange of oxygen (Fry, 1971). However, the natural healing powers of the body are often ignored. It is important to recognize that positive emotions (e.g., the experience of humorous moments or material) may produce chemical changes in the brain that are effective in the obstruction of pain. Laughter also facilitates the reduction of stress and, therefore, the remission of stress-related illnesses and related pain (Adams and McGuire, 1986).

Improvements in quality of life for those elderly persons who view humorous movies, television programs, or live performances are possible and have been documented. Activity interventions that are founded upon the effective use of humor are beneficial in the care and treatment of older persons. The application of *therapeutic humor* activities that promote amusement and laughter are exceedingly valuable, especially in the later stages of life when additional challenges and compromises in health may be present (Adams and McGuire, 1986).

Remotivation and Resocialization

Remotivation activity intervention attempts to make older adults aware of current surroundings while providing opportunities for socialization. Remotivation activities employ the practice of memory and/or cognitive skills, as well as verbal abilities, through which the participant gains a sense of dignity and self-esteem. Remotivation groups consist of structured sessions that are usually held once or twice a week for 12 sessions. Meetings last from 30 minutes to one hour depending upon the attention of the group (Dennis, 1994).

Resocialization activity intervention is a less structured discussion approach used to maintain cognitive functioning and to focus upon relationships and feelings. Resocialization is a method used for the readjustment of confused or withdrawn clients (Edinberg, 1985). Resocialization groups provide the elderly client with opportunities to establish new relationships and to renew long-term friendships (Herrera, 1983). The differences among reality orientation, remotivation, and resocialization are described in Table 13.1.

Motivational and Leadership Techniques

Motivation can be defined as a process that arouses and instigates behavior, provides purpose and direction, permits behavior to continue, and guides behavior preferences (Wlodkowski, 1978). Some factors that may be effective in the motivation of desired behaviors include: explanation of benefits; avoidance of pretense; opportunities for competition; and attractive, supportive environments (Teaff, 1985). Other motivating factors include:

(a) a comfortable, relaxed, nonthreatening environment;
(b) a structure based upon successful experiences;
(c) the promotion of dignity;
(d) the availability of trained, competent leadership; and
(e) the use of persuasive, informative promotion of activities (McGuire, 1987).

A responsibility of the activity specialist is to enhance motivation for participation, and this may require considerable leadership creativity. Activities generally are not longer than two hours, with 45 minutes to an hour being the most appropriate duration. The length of an activity depends upon its nature, number of rest periods provided, and interest and endurance of the participants. The physical setting where activities are conducted also is an important consideration. It is difficult to conduct discussion groups in a large room where other activities are being accommodated

Table 13.1

Differences between Reality Orientation, Remotivation, and Resocialization

Reality Orientation	Remotivation	Resocialization
Structured	Structured	Unstructured
Refreshments may be served	Refreshments not served	Refreshments served
Reminds of who, where, why, and what	Stimulates desire to function in society	Encourages participation
Group size: 3 to 5	Group size: 5 to 12	Group size: 5 to 17
Meeting one-half hour daily	Meeting one to two times per week for one-half to one hour	Meeting three times per week for one-half to one hour
Planned procedures; reality-centered objects	Preselected and reality-centered objects	No planned topic; group-centered feelings
Periodic reality orientation	Progress ratings	Periodic progress notes
Emphasis on time, place, person	No discussion of religion, politics, or death	Any topic freely discussed
Use of part of the mind still intact	Untouched area of mind	Store of memories and experiences
Greeting, handshake and/or physical contact upon leaving	No physical contact	Greeting, handshake upon leaving
Conducted by trained aides and activity assistants	Conducted by trained psychiatric aides	Conducted by RN/LPN, aides, and program assistants

Note: Adapted from Barnes, Stack, & Shore, 1973.

simultaneously. If a small, quiet room is not available, moving furniture to provide a secluded corner for discussion may be an acceptable alternative (Salamon, 1986).

If there is only one group leader, it is better to keep group size small—six to eight members. The intensity of a group experience is likely to diminish proportionately as membership increases. It is best not to mix participants who have high-levels of cognitive impairment with alert individuals in the same group which may create additional problems. The group is placed in a circle to maximize vision and hearing. Individual attention is provided at the beginning and end of a group session. Personal names are used often. The number of rules usually are few and simple. The purposes and goals of the group are developed in collaboration between the leader and the group members. Touching and closeness are of critical importance. The group leader will share things about herself or himself; group members often will not allow the leader to escape being an active member of the group. Dealing with sad themes also is a part of the group leader's role (Burnside, 1978).

Leadership involves human behavior and social interactions. Because elderly participants are unique, optimizing their performance in learning, problem-solving, and memory tasks may require special methods during certain activities. In various learning tasks, the activity specialist enhances participation through the use of:

- slow, preferably self-paced, instruction;
- concrete, directly relevant material;
- repeated exposure to the material to be learned;
- a narrow focus to avoid diffusion of interest;
- generalization;
- a structured learning process; and
- multiple opportunities for feedback (Patrick, 1987).

The "here and now" can be effectively used to initiate a group. The use of common topics such as the weather or the seasons is acceptable for beginning a group session. Through the use of praise and compliments that are sincere and free-flowing, self-esteem is nurtured. The group leader also must be willing to express his or her own feelings (Burnside, 1978).

Activity programs emphasize the dignity of the individual. Depersonalization occurs when programming details and rules take precedence over the specific needs of the participants. Choice, independence, and control in activity programs is encouraged for all persons who are involved in the program. Those individuals who take part in activity programs prefer to have input into all aspects of the program including activities, leadership, scheduling, and accessible locations. Strong activity programs reflect flexibility in order to address the needs of the participants rather than to force individuals to meet fixed requirements. Individuals need challenges and excitement in their lives. Stimulation is vitally important for persons who reside in nonstimulating institutions or who live fairly passive lives. Activity programs can incorporate stimulation into the daily routines of elders through incorporating variety and progression (McGuire, 1987).

Additional motivational techniques may include:

(a) praise after successful completion of a task,
(b) opportunities for participants to feel useful,
(c) the use of frequent reminders,
(d) being careful to speak directly to the individual,
(e) providing continual reinforcement of reality, and
(f) by extending personal invitations.

Other areas to consider when attempting to motivate and encourage participation are promoting self-esteem and status, relating to lifelong interests, overcoming boredom, socializing, building legitimacy and relevancy of the activity tasks, and providing refreshments (Cunninghis, 1989).

A Sample Program

Cognitive Remediation

The following program is suggested as representative of the types of thera-peutic activities—reminiscence and life review, validation therapy, reality orientation, sensory stimulation, spirituality, therapeutic humor, and remo-tivation and resocialization—that can be used to remediate the cognitive abilities of older adults when impairment is present. The program is adapt-able to a variety of surroundings, public recreation facilities, senior centers, adult daycare centers, retirement communities, rehabilitation centers, and nursing homes to name a few. The activity specialist will develop additional program components such as facility preparations, equipment and supplies, expenses, staffing, and publicity in order to effectively utilize the proposed framework.

Program Purpose

The purpose of this program is to provide older adults with an opportunity to experience a diversity of cognitive activities that influence awareness, promote self-esteem, reduce feelings of isolation, encourage interaction with others, reinforce desired behaviors, challenge and stimulate the client, and provide an environment where achievement and recognition are possible. The program is based upon the following principles:

1. Older persons prefer a variety of unique program activities in order to address individual cognitive abilities, interests, and requirements. The following objectives are relevant for enhanced activity involvement:

    (a) to support recognition of surroundings,
    (b) to foster appreciation of self,
    (c) to maintain supportive environments,
    (d) to cultivate and nurture supportive relationships,
    (e) to arouse the senses,
    (f) to provide opportunities for mastery,
    (g) to enhance possibilities for acknowledgment, and
    (h) to inspire pertinent emotion and behavior.

2. The utilization of local community resources, associations, and agencies to assist in meeting the mental health needs of older adults will contribute to the success of a therapeutic cognitive activity program.
3. Older individuals prefer activities that encourage self-renewal.
4. Older persons prefer to be involved in the planning, implementation, and evaluation of activities and programs, policies, and procedures that are designed to meet their mental health needs.

Activity Area I: *Reminiscence and Life Review*

Target Goal

Reminiscence and life review activities are planned and implemented in order to provide the following benefits to older adult participants:

(a) reduce apathy and confusion,
(b) relieve depression,
(c) increase social interaction,
(d) increase life satisfaction,
(e) improve morale,
(f) enhance self-esteem,
(g) evoke creativity,
(h) increase control over the environment, and
(i) evaluate ego integrity (Burnside and Schmidt, 1994).

Enabling Objectives

*   To assess the interests of potential group members and to provide a variety of program formats that correspond to these interests.
*   To determine resources that are required for successful reminiscence group activities.
*   To devise an agenda of prospective reminiscence topics or themes, and to gather provoking reinforcements.
*   To evaluate reminiscence activities and group participants for progress and changes, as needed.

Activity Suggestions: *Memory Stimulation*

A number of topics can be effectively used to stimulate reminiscence and life review in group or individual discussion sessions (Jones and Miesen, 1992). Suggested topics are organized in Figure 13.1 (page 262).

In addition to using a topical approach, lead questions also produce quality reminiscence or life review sessions. Haight (1992) recommended the use of the following lead questions:

Figure 13.1

Examples of Stimulus Topics for Reminiscence and Life Review

Childhood:
    Games played, hobbies
    Favorite toy
    Favorite food
    Where did you grow up?
    What did you want to be?
    Family stories, traditions
    Celebrations, holidays, movies
    Schooling, clubs
    Religious beliefs and practices

Adolescence:
    Entering high school
    Graduation
    Clubs, activities, music
    Favorite books
    Best friends
    Hobbies
    Part-time jobs
    Clothing, cars, dating
    Radio programs, television
        programs

Early Adult Years:
    Dating
    First pay check, salary
    When did you move from
        parents' home?
    Entertainment
    Furnishing own home
    Things done alone
    Where did you meet spouse?

Marriage:
    How long did you know spouse
        before marriage?
    Age at marriage
    Wedding—best man, maid of
        honor
    Planning for marriage
    First home as married couple
    Adjusting to marriage
    Were you surprised to marry
        person that you did?

Childbearing/Family Building:
    How many children?
    Special events in their lives
    Help from spouse in rearing
        children
    Positive and negative aspects
        of being a parent
    Child's first words
    Children moving from home

Work and Avocations:
    Clubs or organizations
    Church
    Politics
    Type of work
    Changes in work

Health:
    Major illnesses
    General health
    Fitness
    Involvement in activities

Memories of People/Pets:
    Parents, brothers, sisters
    Grandparents
    Relatives
    Friends
    Teachers, actors, heroes
    Pets
    Helping mother and father

Memories of Places:
    Holidays, vacations
    Hideaways
    Bedroom, home
    Where have you lived?

Memories of Events:
    Holidays, vacations
    Celebrations

Other Memories:
    Historical events
    How did you view self?
    Being an American

Figure 13.1 Continued

Favorite Things:	*Hardest Times and Things that*
People	*Might Have Happened*
Places	*Differently:*
Events	Job loss
Seeking Advice:	Parents' death
Getting along with others	Children leaving home
Marriage, rearing children	
Work, handling finances	
Preparation for retirement	

Note: Developed from information contained in Jones & Miesen, 1992.

1. If you could stay the same age all of your life, what age would you choose? Why?
2. What are the best things about the age that you are now?
3. What are the worst things about being the age you are now?
4. What are the most important things to you in your life today?
5. What do you fear will happen to you as you grow older?
6. What do you hope will happen to you as you grow older?
7. Have you enjoyed participating in the review of your life?

With any group process there are certain procedural steps that will enhance a successful outcome for the participants. Orienting the participants to the environment, each other, and the goals of the group is the first step. As discussion is set up by the suggestion of a topic or a lead question, the group leader can facilitate conversation by seeking a response from participants who are known to be more comfortable in group situations. As discussion progresses, the regulation of participation to ensure involvement of all participants will be an important task for the leader. Pointing out important relationships, events, and happenings on an individual basis and linking them across participants helps the group to develop an "identity." Finally, closing the discussion with a summary of the main contributions and any issues that may need to be continued for resolution, is important to the overall success of reminiscence or life review as a group activity. A positive experience for all participants is enhanced by creating an environment of support and acceptance. Two-way communication, a lack of pressure, room for sharing personal mementos, and affirmation of the importance of each participant are just some of the ways to build a supportive environment for reminiscence or life review activities.

Life review and reminiscence need not only be undertaken as a group activity. Individuals can be encouraged to engage in bibliotherapy as a means for completing a life review. For individuals who are not interested in writing, the audiotaped or videotaped life review can provide both therapeutic benefits as well as a documented record for other family members (Dreher, 1987).

Implementation and Materials Suggestions

There are several important factors to consider in selecting the members for reminiscence or life review groups. Potential group members are approached individually. Following an explanation of the purpose of the group, a verbal contract is established. Personal choice and an understanding of the commitment needed for participation in the group significantly add to active involvement in the group process. It also is important to inform each prospective member of the others involved. It is unrealistic to expect people to gather arbitrarily and share important memories without an orientation to the process and to the other members of the group (Ebersole, 1988).

Reminiscence groups meet regularly at the same time and place each week. Group meetings become anticipation, which adds to the structure of the participants' lives. Occasionally, a group member may be unable to get out of bed or to attend the group meeting. Barring restrictive factors, the group can meet at the member's bedside or contact the absent participant. Consideration of the relevance for such an action would include: meaning to other members, adaptability of the group, and the possibility of manipulation (Ebersole, 1988).

The group process includes a beginning, a working phase, and termination. The working phase may present the most difficulty when occasions arise that the reminiscence group leader is facilitating group members with sad subject matter. Termination also can be painful, but if planned early, it can contribute to growth experiences (Ebersole, 1988).

Short-term groups are more effective when there is more structure. For long-term groups, as the group members become more familiar with each other, the group process should flow with a decrease of structured content. In either case, maintaining the flexibility needed to meet the needs of the participants is important. The content areas for reminiscence can be enhanced by the use of music, bright visual aids, and objects or memorabilia that are not fragile or difficult to handle. Various scents and aromas are among the most powerful stimuli for reminiscence (Ebersole, 1988).

Short-term reminiscence groups (10 weeks or less) should be small and focused on particular group needs. Long-term groups can be conducted indefinitely with periodic reassessment and redefinition of goals. Group members should be actively involved in the process and in the admission of new members once the group is well-established. It also is important to consider all personnel affected by group meetings because they will impact the success or failure of the group. Other staff members can assist by reminding group participants of meeting times and by helping them to prepare for and attend the meetings on time (Ebersole, 1988).

Reminiscence may be transformed into a social visit or occasion on an individual basis by conducting the session in a client's room or in other areas in which the client may feel comfortable such as the lounge, cafeteria, or garden. Occasionally, a family member of the client can be present in order to provide triggers that may elicit a response or to confirm factual details in the life review process (Woods, Portnoy, Head, and Jones, 1992). Community outings also are an important adjunct to reminiscence groups. Attending a nostalgic movie, seeing a band concert in the park, viewing a live fireworks display, or eating at a restaurant with a memorable decor are all catalysts for reminiscence (Ebersole, 1988).

Activity Area II: *Validation Therapy*

Target Goal

The use of validation therapy with confused, disoriented, or demented older persons is targeted toward assisting them to be as happy as possible by accepting them as they are and, thereby, reducing anxiety and frustration. It is anticipated that personal well-being will be promoted through the use of validation therapy (Feil, 1989).

Enabling Objectives

- To assess the capacities of potential group members and to supply purposeful activities that satisfy the needs of the individual.
- To ascertain the resources essential for successful implementation of various validation activities.
- To plan a feasible program of topics and themes and to determine positive reinforcements.
- To evaluate validation activities and group members for progress and to make alterations as needed.

Activity Suggestions: *Unresolved Conflicts*

Issues and themes for discussion usually include death, family relations, loneliness, and disappointments. The selection of a topic is based on areas of conflict for the individual. Questions, manipulation of an assortment of items, singing, acting out, and role play are methods that can be used by clients to express themselves (Babins, 1988).

Implementation and Materials Suggestions

Validation therapy can be used in association with other programs without attempting to alter the older person's concept of reality. A group of five or six people can meet to converse about unresolved personal conflicts. The activity specialist facilitates the discussion by posing basic questions such as who, what, where, and when. These questions provide opportunities for individuals to describe relevant events in their lives (Babins, 1988).

Individualized plans will consider the older adult's abilities for attaining desired outcomes. Through the use of tolerance and recognition, activity leaders and other group members will have the ability to validate and affirm the value of each individual. Validation requires that meaningful expressions of the person's inner-self are acknowledged and accommodated (Taft, Delaney, Seman, and Stansell, 1993).

Activity Area III: *Reality Orientation*

Target Goal

According to Herrera (1983), reality orientation activities can be effectively used to reach several treatment goals:

- to promote the awareness of daily living factors in the immediate environment;
- to develop and/or maintain interactions with surroundings, peers, and caregivers;
- to supply information regarding person, time, place, and things;
- to correct disoriented information; and
- to reinforce behaviors that approximate or reflect meaningful interactions with the environment.

Enabling Objectives

- To assess the needs and abilities of potential group members and to provide meaningful reality orientation activities that address these needs and capacities.
- To determine the resources necessary for successful implementation of reality orientation activities.
- To devise a probable agenda of topics and themes and to gather motivating reinforcements.
- To evaluate reality orientation activities and group participants for progress and for changes as required.

Activity Suggestions: *Reinforcement of Person, Time, and Place*

Basic, current, and personal information is presented and reviewed with group members. The group leader should attempt to improve individual members' ability to identify information related to person, time, and place, and to act upon the information in an appropriate manner. The reinforcement of group members for correct responses and the repetition of information are aspects of the treatment process. Discussion is centered on a variety of subjects that are related to the interests of the participants such as holidays, weather, and current events (Herrera, 1983; Williams, 1994).

Implementation and Materials Suggestions

Instructional aids such as large calendars, clocks, telephones, mailboxes, and a reality orientation board are used to stimulate the group of participants. Verbal and nonverbal communication is used to emphasize various concepts. Positive reinforcement is employed within a strategy of active or passive friendliness, depending upon the preferences of the client (Herrera, 1983; Williams, 1994).

Activity Area IV: *Sensory Stimulation*

Target Goal

The target goal of activities in this area is to stimulate the individual senses on a regular basis in order to maintain his or her functional abilities in daily life (Herrera, 1983).

Enabling Objectives

- To assess the needs and abilities of possible group members and to provide beneficial sensory stimulation activities that consider these needs and capacities.
- To determine the resources required for effective implementation of sensory stimulation activities.
- To prepare a reasonable schedule of subjects and themes and to consider potential motivating reinforcements.
- To evaluate sensory stimulation activities and group members for progress and for changes as needed.

Activity Suggestions: *Touch, Vision, Hearing, Taste, and Smell*

Sensory stimulation activities can follow any of the following strategies (Elliott and Sorg-Elliott, 1991):

- the participant's skin can be stroked with various textures;
- hand gestures may be used to act out hello, stop, thin, tall, etc.;
- the participant can clap hands, reach out, make a fist, laugh, smile, frown, etc.;
- a tape recording of people laughing, crying, or clapping may be played in order to determine if the participant can identify the actions;
- different sizes and textures of balls may be passed, squeezed, and kicked;
- the participant can be asked to recognize other persons by name;
- a ball may be bounced and the participant can count the number of times that it is bounced;
- the game "Simon says" may be used to accomplish exercises such as lifting the arms over the head, moving the arms to the side, stepping to the front and stepping to the back, etc.;
- a telephone can be used with the participant being encouraged to answer the phone when it rings; and
- a variety of short songs can be played on a small portable cassette player near the participant.

Implementation and Materials Suggestions

A variety of activities and objects may be used to awaken the senses such as:

(a) flashlights in a darkened room and colorful objects to stimulate vision;
(b) sharp smells contrasted with sweet smelling substances to exercise the sense of smell; and
(c) recordings, musical instruments, and whispering to provide a diversity of sounds that sharpen hearing.

Candy, pickles, and potato chips can demonstrate differing types of taste. Soft, hard, smooth, rough, hot, and cold objects offer stimuli for the sense of touch (Herrera, 1983).

Activity Area V: *Spirituality*

Target Goal

Spiritual activities are used to provide a means of coping with stress, promote self-esteem, and foster a general sense of well-being (Bowlby, 1993).

Enabling Objectives

- To assess the needs of individual participants in regard to spiritual needs.
- To provide meaningful religious activities that address these needs.

- To determine the resources and services that are available in the community for meeting the religious needs of the program participants.
- To maintain a reasonable schedule of spiritual activities as motivation and reinforcement of personal religious beliefs for participants of various faiths.
- To evaluate spiritual activities, group members, and spiritual changes, if any, in individual participants.

Activity Suggestions: *Religious Services*

Spiritual activity groups can serve the purposes of worship, education, support, and introspection. Spiritual gatherings may include regularly scheduled worship services, religious discussions, singing of hymns, world religious education sessions, and intergenerational religious projects (Szekais, 1986).

Implementation and Materials Suggestions

Generally, younger participants are involved in more formal or organized religious activities, and older individuals engage in more private devotional endeavors. The spiritual well-being of older persons is increased by the relationship one has with one's God, self, community, and the environment. Engaging in organized religious activities is a means for affirming, nurturing, and celebrating the wholeness of life (Young and Dowling, 1987).

Spiritual groups can be structured to meet the needs of individuals at the same level of impairment or to include individuals of various functional skill levels. Regular worship, as well as the sharing of spiritual beliefs and values through discussion groups, are activities that are responsive to the innermost needs of many elderly persons (Szekais, 1986).

Activity Area VI: *Therapeutic Humor*

Target Goal

Participants in activities that use therapeutic humor receive many benefits. The goals of therapeutic humor activities are to enhance self-concept, provide a means for coping with stress, and promote positive affect and psychological well-being (Martin, Kuiper, Olinger, and Dance, 1993).

Enabling Objectives

- To assess the interests and abilities of older persons for their involvement in activities and events that involve humor and laughter.
- To provide activities that satisfy these interests and abilities.
- To determine the resources necessary for the beneficial implementation of humorous activities.

- To maintain a feasible schedule of humorous and laughter-provoking activities and to clarify appropriate reinforcements for the perpetuation of humor and laughter.
- To evaluate the use of therapeutic humor with individual group members and to make changes as needed.

Activity Suggestions: *Evoking Laughter*

Reminiscence activities such as humorous anecdotes, favorite stories, and viewing old television comedy shows (e.g., "I Love Lucy" or "The Honeymooners") and humorous movies can reaffirm the pleasures of life. Sing-alongs, topical or thematic parties, humorous readings, and the use of exaggeration and absurdity also are effective for evoking laughter and enjoyment (McGuire and Boyd, 1993).

Implementation and Materials Suggestions

The physical act of laughing, the social act of joke telling, and involvement in movies, other humorous activities, and productions may each result in better physical and emotional health. The ability to see the humor in detrimental situations also is an effective way to alleviate potentially harmful or unhealthy consequences. Humor can be used to transform difficult circumstances into humorous situations. Laughing with others is natural and communicates the themes of community, vitality, and disclosure (McGuire and Boyd, 1993).

Activity Area VII: *Remotivation and Resocialization*

Target Goal

Remotivation and resocialization activity programs are targeted to meet several treatment goals for participants (Burnside, 1978; Dennis, 1994). These treatment goals include:

- to establish a climate of acceptance,
- to create a bridge to reality,
- to share and to appreciate the function of the world,
- to maintain an atmosphere of appreciation,
- to improve communication,
- to decrease withdrawal and isolation, and
- to care for and enjoy the company of other persons.

Enabling Objectives

- To assess the interests and abilities of potential group members.
- To provide beneficial remotivation and resocialization activities that address these interests and capabilities.
- To determine the resources necessary for the successful implementation of remotivation and resocialization activities.
- To maintain a reasonable schedule of remotivation and resocialization activities and to discover acceptable reinforcements.
- To evaluate resocialization and remotivation activities and group members in order to determine progress and to make changes as needed.

Activity Suggestions: *Discussion Groups and Word Games*

Examples of topics for remotivation groups include: vacations, holidays, hobbies, gardening, sports, pets, art, nature, transportation, weather, and animals (Dennis, 1994). Familiar activities such as spelling bees, name the tune, finish the proverb or weather saying, and simple math problems may be used in resocialization groups. Other examples of resocialization activities might include: discussion of well-known topics and objects, open-ended statements, word scrambles, and special dinners (Elliott and Sorg-Elliott, 1991).

Implementation and Materials Suggestions

Each remotivation session is based on a different topic. The topics that are used will represent the diverse backgrounds, experiences, and interests of elderly group members and must directly tempt as many senses as possible. Visual aids and appropriate objects can be used to maintain a high level of attention, interest, and response. Visual aids are passed from one person to another in order to encourage communication among group members. The group is structured to focus discussion on the things that constitute the real world of the participants (Dennis, 1994).

Resocialization groups provide elderly participants with frequent exposure to experiences which promote the feeling that life is worth living. Group members focus upon their relationships with each other. The group leader provides a model of behavior with his or her actions during the group, recognition of group members, and nonevaluative conversation. Resocialization activities should establish an atmosphere of acceptance and freedom of expression where group participants may discuss the concerns of daily living and enjoyable experiences that conceivably might be dismissed as insignificant (Herrera, 1983).

Summary

A variety of therapeutic cognitive activities are introduced in this chapter including reminiscence and life review, reality orientation, sensory training, spiritual activities, the application of therapeutic humor, remotivation, and resocialization. The use of these activities is intended to emphasize abilities rather than to focus on disabilities. The human needs of older persons require that activity staff positively and creatively work to meet the mental health concerns of the aging participant. Interventions and methods are designed to nurture the potentials of elderly individuals as well as to assist in their adjustments and transitions that often accompany the older adult life stages.

Various motivational and leadership skills and techniques are presented along with a listing of additional activity resources (see Figure 13.2 and the References and Resources, page 275). The sample program of therapeutic cognitive activities illustrates programming to meet the cognitive and affective needs of older persons. Supportive, caring environments which actualize control, choice, adaptation, and coping skills can effectively influence the well-being of elderly individuals.

Figure 13.2

Resources for Cognitive Remediation Programs

Activities, Adaptation, & Aging is a practical journal published quarterly and includes articles on activities. Available from the Haworth Press, 10 Alice Street, Binghamton, NY 13904-1580. Telephone: 800-342-9678.

Activity Director's Guide is a newsletter published monthly for activity specialists. Available from Eymann Publications, Inc., 1490 Huntington Circle, Box 3577, Reno, NV 89505.

Activity Ideas for Older Adults is a mail-order company offering a small catalogue of books, pamphlets, games, and other resources for working with older adults. Contact: Elderpress, 731 Treat Avenue, San Francisco, CA 94110.

The American Association of Retired Persons (AARP) offers resources for reminiscence, intergenerational programs, and other books on various topics, as well as audiovisual materials for loan. Contact: American Association of Retired Persons, 1909 K Street, NW, Suite 400, Washington, DC 20036. Telephone: 202-296-5960.

Bifocal offers a selection of resources for reminiscence, including slide-tapes, videos, and resources on particular themes. Contact: Bifocal, 911 Williamson, Madison, WI 53703. Telephone: 608-251-2818.

Eldergames offers a variety of materials for various functional levels such as memory games, trivia questions, and fabric books for stimulation. Contact: Eldergames, 11710 Hunters Lane, Rockville, MD 20852.

Keep in Touch is a practical guide for groups and activities with disabled older adults. Available from M. Judd, 1379 Dudley Circle, Winnipeg, MB, Canada R3M 1P1.

Mental Aerobics is a book of quizzes, holiday theme activities, word games, and memory games designed for older adults. Available from Mental Aerobics, 4417 Torrington Road, Victoria, BC, Canada V8N 4N8.

Nottingham Rehabilitation Equipment offers a selection of adapted adult games, large-piece adult jigsaw puzzles and games, and an assortment of pictures, slides, and music for use in reminiscence. Contact: Nottingham Rehabilitation Equipment, Physio E. R. P., 1170 Burnamthorpe Road West, #32, Mississauga, ON, L5C 4E6. Telephone: 416-566-4092.

Potentials Development is a mail-order company with a catalogue of booklets and small publications that provide practical plans for activities of many types with older adults. Contact: Potentials Development, 775 Main Street, Buffalo, NY 14203.

Sensory Stimulation Products for Alzheimer's Patients is a small selection of self-directed activities for persons with advanced Alzheimer's disease and related disorders. Contact: Geriatric Resources, Inc., 5450 Barton Drive, Orlando, FL 32807. Telephone: 800-359-0390.

Additional useful resources are listed in the References and Resources section at the end of this chapter.

Comprehension Questions

1. Describe four different activity types that can be used in cognitive intervention with older adults.
2. Outline a sample activity program to use with older adults who have cognitive impairment. Include the target goals, enabling objectives, suggested activities, and implementation plan.
3. Discuss motivational and leadership strategies that can be effectively used with older adults who have cognitive impairment to encourage their participation in therapeutic activity programs.

References and Resources

Adams, E. R., & McGuire, F. A. (1986). Is laughter the best medicine? A study of the effects of humor on perceived pain and affect. In P. M. Foster (Ed.), *Therapeutic activities with the impaired elderly* (pp. 157-175). Binghamton, NY: The Haworth Press, Inc.

Babins, L. (1988). Conceptual analysis of validation therapy. *International Journal of Aging and Human Development, 26*(3), 161-168.

Barnes, E., Stack, A., & Shore, H. (1973). Guidelines to treatment modalities and methods for use with the aged. *Gerontologist, 13*(4), 513-527.

Bowlby, C. (1993). *Therapeutic activities with person's disabled by Alzheimer's disease and related disorders.* Gaithersburg, MD: Aspen Publishers Inc.

Burnside, I. M. (1978). *Working with the elderly: Group processes and techniques* (2nd ed.). North Scituate, MA: Duxbury.

Burnside, I. M., & Schmidt, M. G. (1994). *Working with older adults: Group processes and techniques* (3rd ed.). Boston, MA: Jones & Bartlett Publishers, Inc.

Butler, R. N. (1963). The life review: An interpretation of reminiscence in the aged. *Psychiatry, 26,* 65-76.

Cunninghis, R. N. (1989). The purpose and meaning of activities. In E. S. Deichman & R. Kociecki (Eds.), *Working with the elderly* (pp. 151-170). Buffalo, NY: Prometheus Books.

Dennis, H. (1994). Remotivation groups. In I. M. Burnside & M. G. Schmidt, *Working with older adults: Group processes and techniques* (3rd ed.) (pp. 153-162). Boston, MA: Jones & Bartlett Publishers, Inc.

Dreher, B. B. (1987). Communication skills for working with elders. *Springer Series on Adulthood and Aging, 17.* New York, NY: Springer Publishing Co., Inc.

Ebersole, P. P. (1988). Establishing reminiscing groups. In I. M. Burnside (Ed.), *Working with the elderly: Group processes and techniques* (2nd ed.) (pp. 236-254). North Scituate, MA: Duxbury.

Edinberg, M. A. (1985). *Mental health practice with the elderly.* Englewood Cliffs, NJ: Prentice Hall.

Elliott, J. E., & Sorg-Elliott, J. A. (1991). *Recreation programming and activities for older adults.* State College, PA: Venture Publishing, Inc.

Feil, N. (1989). Validation therapy with late-onset dementia populations. In G. M. M. Jones & B. M. L. Miesen (Eds.), *Caregiving in dementia: Research and applications* (pp. 199-218). New York, NY: Routledge.

Folsom, G. S. (1986). "Worth repeating" reality orientation: Full circle. In P. M. Foster (Ed.), *Therapeutic activities with the impaired elderly* (pp. 65-73). Binghamton, NY: The Haworth Press, Inc.

Fry, W. F. (1971). Laughter: Is it the best medicine? *Stanford, M. D., 10,* 16-20.

Greenblatt, F. S. (1988). *Therapeutic recreation for long-term care facilities.* New York, NY: Human Sciences Press.

Haight, B. (1992). The structured life-review process: A community approach to the aging client. In G. M. M. Jones & B. M. L. Miesen (Eds.), *Caregiving in dementia: Research and applications* (pp. 272-292). New York, NY: Routledge.

Harrison, C. L. (1980). Therapeutic art programs around the world—XIII: Creative arts for older people in the community. *American Journal of Art Therapy, 19,* 99-101.

Herrera, P. M. (1983). *Innovative programming for the aging and aged mentally retarded/developmentally disabled adult.* Akron, OH: Exploration Series Press.

Holland, L. (1987). Life review and communication therapy for dementia patients. *Clinical Gerontologist, 6*(3), 62-65.

Jones, G. M. M, & Miesen, B. M. L. (1992). *Caregiving in dementia: Research and applications.* New York, NY: Routledge.

Kane, R. L., & Kane, R. A. (1989). Transitions in long-term care. In M. G. Ory & K. Bond (Eds.), *Aging and health care: Social science and policy perspectives* (pp. 217-243). New York, NY: Routledge.

Martin, R. A., Kuiper, N. A., Olinger, J., & Dance, K. A. (1993). Humor, coping with stress, self-concept, and psychological well-being. *Humor, 6*(1), 89-104.

McGuire, F. A. (1987). Recreation for the frail elderly. In M. J. Keller & N. J. Osgood (Eds.), *Dynamic leisure programming with older adults* (pp. 99-106). Alexandria, VA: National Recreation and Park Association.

McGuire, F. A., & Boyd, R. K. (1993). The role of humor in enhancing the quality of later life. In J. R. Kelly (Ed.), *Activity and aging* (pp. 164-173). Newbury Park, CA: Sage Publications, Inc.

Morris, R., & Koppelman, M. (1986). Memory deficits in Alzheimer-type dementia: A review. *Quarterly Journal of Experimental Psychology, 38,* 575-603.

Patrick, G. D. (1987). The uses of recreation in geropsychiatry. In M. J. Keller & N. J. Osgood (Eds.), *Dynamic leisure programming with older adults* (pp. 85-97). Alexandria, VA: National Recreation and Park Association.

Salamon, M. J. (1986). A protocol for recreation and socialization programs for the aged. In P. M. Foster (Ed.), *Therapeutic activities with the impaired elderly* (pp. 47-56). Binghamton, NY: The Haworth Press, Inc.

Szekais, B. (1986). Therapeutic group activities. *Activities, Adaptation, & Aging, 8*(3-4), 11-20.

Taft, L. B., Delaney, K., Seman, D., & Stansell, J. (1993). Dementia care: Creating a therapeutic milieu. *Journal of Gerontological Nursing, 19,* 30-39.

Teaff, J. D. (1985). *Leisure services with the elderly.* St. Louis, MO: Times Mirror/Mosby.

Waxman, H. M., Carner, E. A., & Berkenstock, G. (1984). Job turnover and job satisfaction among nursing home aides. *Gerontologist, 24*(5), 503-509.

Williams, E. M. (1994). Reality orientation groups. In I. M. Burnside & M. G. Schmidt (Eds.), *Working with older adults: Group processes and techniques* (3rd ed.) (pp. 139-152). Boston, MA: Jones & Bartlett Publishers, Inc.

Wlodkowski, R. J. (1978). *Motivation and teaching: A practical guide.* Washington, DC: National Education Association.

Woods, R. T., Portnoy, S., Head, D., & Jones, G. M. M. (1992). Reminiscence and life review with persons with dementia: Which way forward? In G. M. M. Jones & B. M. L. Miesen (Eds.), *Caregiving in dementia: Research and applications* (pp. 137-161). New York, NY: Routledge.

Young, G., & Dowling, W. (1987). Dimensions of religiosity in old age: Accounting for variation in types of participation. *Journal of Gerontology, 42*(4), 376-380.

Key Words

Adaptation
Adjustment
Creativity
Intergenerational
Psychosocial
Socialization
Social Network

Learning Objectives

1. To become familiar with the use of activities that meet the psychosocial needs of older adults.
2. To identify common activities that are used in psychosocial therapeutic intervention with elderly clients.
3. To describe a sample psychosocial activity plan in therapeutic intervention with elderly clients.
4. To understand and apply therapeutic activity intervention in the following areas: intergenerational activities; socialization activities and special events; hobbies, crafts, and games; travel and outdoor activities; and specific therapies (e.g., pet, horticulture, music, art).

Chapter 14

Psychosocial Activities

Introduction

Socializing plays an important role in most peoples' lives. A broad range of activities may be used to address the psychosocial needs that are common to older adults (Zgola, 1987) such as:

(a) maintaining social relationships,
(b) expressing one's identity through appropriate and valued social roles,
(c) supporting self-esteem,
(d) communicating feelings with others and talking about things that are important,
(e) preserving a sense of autonomy and control over one's life, and
(f) generally maintaining a sense of connection with the social customs and aspects of everyday life in the community.

Previously in this book the importance of activity in adjusting to later life changes in health, physical functioning, mental alertness, and social roles was stressed. In this chapter focus is specifically on changes in the psychosocial domain; that is, the use of activities in meeting psychosocial needs associated with older adulthood.

The first section of this chapter provides a brief review of the major psychosocial needs and adjustments experienced by older adults. Following this review is a discussion of the range of activities that can be used to promote successful aging in the psychosocial domain. Next a sample psychosocial activity plan which blends a variety of activities in this area to illustrate appropriate programming strategies is presented. The sample plan also is intended to show the use of psychosocial activities as therapeutic intervention in the care and treatment of older persons. Completing this chapter is a list of additional references and resources for use in the psychosocial program development process.

Psychosocial Needs in Later Maturity

Individuals are challenged by developmental tasks that accompany the different stages of life across the life course. Old age, as in the other major periods of life, is no exception. The ability to adapt to changes that typically occur in later maturity varies from person to person, with some individuals showing greater capability to handle the major challenges associated with growing older. Three major areas in which older persons experience developmental tasks in older adulthood are:

(a) adjusting to new life circumstances produced by the changes in social roles that often accompany retirement from one's lifelong occupation (e.g., job or childrearing);

(b) the loss of one's spouse, family members, and friends through death; and

(c) the loss of one's own youthful vitality, vigor, and physical reserves including dealing with one's own mortality.

Adapting to changes in these three broad areas can have a dramatic impact on the psychosocial functioning and well-being of older adults.

The ability of older persons to manage adjustments in these major areas is greatly influenced by individual personality and abilities, past experiences, health status, and the existing social network of family members and friends (Hooyman and Kiyak, 1988). While personality is relatively stable across the life span, it can either serve to help or to hinder in the process of handling later life events. Individual abilities in adapting to major change and coping with stress vary greatly from one individual to the next. Awareness of the aging process, personal coping style, and the importance of flexibility, reevaluation, and acceptance in adapting to major change are factors that influence successful aging in the psychosocial domain.

Retirement from lifelong occupation to part-time employment or to full retirement constitutes a major change in the daily life activity patterns, as well as the social roles, of an increasing number of men and women. For many individuals identity is tied closely with both the nature of their work and the people at the workplace with whom they come into daily contact. At retirement, changes in role, social networks, daily rhythms, and social expectations may potentially impact the individual's psychosocial well-being. By taking time to recognize the needs that are fulfilled primarily through involvement in the workplace, the older individual can actively plan new involvements and environments that can satisfy these same needs. For example, many older persons retire from their lifelong occupation and begin new part-time jobs doing things that they always wanted to try; while other individuals put their energies into community leadership, volunteerism, and family-based activities (e.g., caring for grandchildren). Part-time work, volunteerism, and community leadership are some of the important ways in which older adults remain connected with society and their communities. Replacing the work role with other activities that serve to maintain one's involvement in the community represents one avenue for adjusting to the major life changes that accompany retirement. It should also be recognized that many older persons experience little adjustment difficulty at retirement and look forward to increasing their involvement in favorite activities (e.g., travel, sport, social, educational, family caregiving) through which their identity needs are adequately expressed and fulfilled.

Dealing with the loss of one's lifelong partner, other family members, and close friends is another major area in later maturity that challenges older persons to adapt to dramatic changes. The shrinking of one's primary social network is a persistent theme in the daily lives of older people. The loss of persons on whom one has depended for daily social exchange and support is a potent force in the psychosocial adjustment of older persons. Maintaining an active life filled with opportunities to socialize with others, to expand one's social network to persons of all ages (thus buffering the persistent loss of age peers), and to celebrate the cultural heritage that holds together the social fabric of community are some of the ways in which elders can cope with these losses. Leisure activities and recreation centers provide the structure through which social networks can be built and strengthened, especially through a focus on intergenerational programming.

A third major area of psychosocial adjustment in later life is learning to accept and adjust to the loss of one's own physical reserves and the eventuality of one's own death. The accumulated effects of declines in physical functioning affect all older persons. Some older adults continue to lead vigorous and active lifestyles while experiencing few limitations in their physical capabilities. Others, however, experience declines to such an extent that physical independence is impacted, and eventually these individuals may have impaired functioning. Physical functioning and independence are greatly influenced by several factors including: chronological age, physical fitness, health/disease status, and genetic endowment. While probably all older persons will eventually experience some reduction in their physical reserves, it is not until very late in life that many individuals will experience limitations in activity involvement due to declined physical status. Therefore, leisure activities that promote fitness and help to prevent decline are instrumental to the physical well-being of older adults.

The recognition of one's own mortality, coupled with declines in physical functioning, may pose a significant sense of personal loss. The preservation of a social network can greatly help older persons to deal with these losses, as well as to maintain a sense of quality in their lives. Older persons' involvement in travel, group outings, special events, games, hobbies, holidays, celebrations, and low impact physical recreation activities can have direct psychosocial benefits.

The maintenance of identity through meaningful role involvement and environmental supports is important in promoting continuity and activity involvement throughout the life course. Assisting older persons to adapt to the developmental tasks that are typical in later life becomes the focus and purpose of psychosocial activity programs. These programs primarily support the following psychosocial needs: social role and identity, belongingness, self-esteem, adjustment, companionship and meaningful relationships, autonomy and independence, happiness, creativity, socialization, and pleasure. Psychosocial activity programs can be found in a variety of settings that provide care and treatment services to older persons, including senior centers, adult daycare centers, nursing facilities, rehabilitation centers, hospitals, and the home. In the next section just how activities can help older persons manage the major developmental tasks associated with later life is discussed.

Meeting Psychosocial Needs through Activities

Successful aging has been described as the ability to adapt to the major life events and challenges that typically present themselves in later maturity (Hooyman and Kiyak, 1988). In the previous section, three broad areas in which major developmental challenges typically occur in older adulthood were discussed:

(a) social role changes and identity,
(b) loss of one's significant other(s), and
(c) loss of one's own physical independence, as well as confronting one's own eventual death.

This section will briefly discuss factors that influence how individuals cope with changes and challenges in these areas and how activities can be therapeutically used to support personal capabilities and adaptation in later maturity.

The ability of older persons to adapt to the major challenges that typically occur in older adulthood is greatly influenced by individual personality, physical health status, earlier life experiences and history, and the availability of a wide range of social supports (e.g., family, income stability, suitable housing, accessible recreation, valued social roles). As older persons confront late life events that threaten independence/autonomy, instigate emotional instability, remove valued social roles, alter living arrangements and standards, or dramatically affect lifestyle patterns, a series of reactions or defenses may result. Typical reactions include feelings of loneliness, fear, anger, depression, and anxiety. These reactions often produce negative behaviors or defense mechanisms such as repression, denial, withdrawal, projection, regression, fixation, manipulation, and displacement or rationalization. Older persons who are able to recognize their personal strengths and abilities will most likely cope more positively with reactions and show fewer negative defense mechanisms. However, many older people may not deal well with these reactions and may present poor defense mechanisms, thus displaying poor coping skills. Personal coping style in late life typically mirrors the coping behaviors that were characteristic of earlier life adjustments.

Successful coping is related to self-esteem and self-concept, health status, and one's ability to "think through" or cognitively process the events that are impacting one's life, as well as the stability of one's social network of friends and family members (Hooyman and Kiyak, 1988). Having constructive outlets through which to express oneself, a supportive environment, and others who are able to give emotional reassurance are helpful strategies for most persons who are experiencing the stresses associated with major life changes in older adulthood. Activities that build self-esteem (e.g., celebrating birthdays) and promote positive self-concept (e.g., developing a hobby into a special skill such as woodworking) can be useful in providing a supportive, constructive environment through which successful coping may be promoted.

Activities to build self-esteem should address how the person feels about himself or herself. Personal feelings of worth can be promoted through recognition by others. This acknowledgment can be promoted by providing individuals with opportunities to lead activities, honoring them for making contributions to a group or an activity, or appreciating the importance of their existence through celebrating birthdays or other special occasions.

Self-concept, on the other hand, relates to the identity that each person constructs for himself or herself. Identity can be built and reinforced through activities that produce outcomes that the individual values and outcomes that are viewed as instrumental or valued by others. There are many activities that can promote a positive self-concept for individuals, especially when they feel valued and successful while pursuing these activities. Hobbies, sports and physical recreation activities, volunteering, community leadership service, continuing education, and many other activities can be effectively used in strengthening the self-concept of older persons.

Activities that promote fitness, health promotion, and a sense of well-being also can aid older adults in the process of successfully coping with the ongoing stress and challenges of older adulthood. By understanding that physical activities not only impact overall health and fitness but also promote the inner strength needed to manage stress, the activity leader will be proactive in supporting positive coping. Physical recreation activities can include walking, low-impact games, dancing, travel, and outdoor activities, to name just a few examples.

In regard to supporting the individual in cognitively processing his or her personal stresses, socialization and group activities can be useful in setting the environment for sharing his or her experiences and feelings with others. Some activities that can be used to meet these purposes include:

(a) self-help support groups;
(b) club activities;
(c) games, crafts, and hobby groups; and
(d) horticulture, art, and music therapies.

Several objectives associated with assisting older persons with successful coping are:

(a) to maintain social engagement with others,
(b) to promote the pursuit of meaningful activities,
(c) to assist in setting new directions for personal growth and adaptation,
(d) to promote feelings of self-worth, and
(e) to prevent disablement due to deteriorating health.

The attainment of these objectives is aided by the implementation of a well-designed and skillfully led program of activities that meet psychosocial needs associated with later maturity.

In summary, there are several major activity categories that can be used to enhance successful aging in the psychosocial domain. These include but are not limited to: intergenerational activities; socialization activities and special events; hobbies, crafts, and games; travel and outdoor activities; and specific therapies (e.g., pets, horticulture, music, art). A wide range of specific activities are available under each of these main categories, and the reader is encouraged to consult the resources at the end of the chapter for activity ideas. Activities are selected from these categories to build a program that will:

(a) promote dignity and a sense of identity,
(b) provide meaning and connectedness within society and community, and
(c) support personal resolve to one's eventual mortality.

The sample program that follows is intended to demonstrate one approach to blending activities in meeting these psychosocial needs.

A Sample Program

Social Activities

The following program presents five kinds of activities that can be used to meet the psychosocial needs of older adults. The program can be adapted to a wide range of environments including community recreation centers, senior centers, adult daycare centers, church-based organizations, retirement communities, assisted living centers, nursing homes, and rehabilitation centers. The activity specialist will need to provide further program development details, such as facility arrangements, materials, costs, staffing, and advertising, in order to apply the outline as provided.

Program Purpose

The purpose of this program is to provide older adults with a diverse range of psychosocial activities that are instrumental in supporting identity, social roles, social network, positive coping, and optimal health and well-being. The program is developed and implemented based on the following principles:

1. Older persons desire a varied and diverse program of activities to meet their identified psychosocial needs and interests. Of particular interest are the following activity involvement objectives:

   (a) to maintain social relationships with others,
   (b) to promote the pursuit of meaningful activities,
   (c) to set new directions for personal growth and adaptation,
   (d) to promote feelings of self-worth, and
   (e) to prevent social isolation due to deteriorating health.

2. It is desirable to develop partnerships with local, community-based organizations and agencies in meeting the psychosocial needs of the senior members of the community.
3. Older persons prefer activities that promote self-development, independence/autonomy, and positive coping skills.
4. Older persons desire to participate in the planning, implementation, and evaluation of activities and programs that are designed to meet their psychosocial needs.

Activity Area I: *Socialization Activities and Special Events*

Target Goal

Participants will have a regular calendar of social events that provides for a diversity of interests, promotes recognition of special dates both personal and cultural, and integrates activities with community events and happenings.

Enabling Objectives

- To assess the social activity interests of potential participants and select varying program formats to match these such as parties, celebrations, special performances, and special events (e.g., art fairs, white elephant sales).
- To assess community resources and the calendars of other community organizations for the purpose of identifying existing programs and activities in order to avoid duplication and to promote collaboration.
- To develop a calendar of major religious, cultural, and community events, and to publish and disseminate the calendar to prospective participants in the community and in long-term care facilities.

Activity Suggestions: *Developing Social and Activity Calendars*

The activity calendar for the socialization and special events category includes both formal organized events as well as informal activities. For example, a monthly birthday party is scheduled for celebrating all birthdays that occur within each month. The social events calendar also includes the celebration of major holidays as a very popular way to promote social gatherings. In addition, regularly scheduled informal drop-in conversation times that are accompanied by refreshments should be included on the monthly calendar. These informal conversation hours are appreciated by many individuals who are either less inclined to participate in large social gatherings or prefer to socialize informally on a regular basis.

The monthly social calendar also reflects theme parties that include a half-hour special program, and seasonal festivals as they are appropriate. Theme parties are developed around any topic of interest to prospective participants. The following can serve as possible themes for half-hour programs: my favorite book or poem, favorite jokes, sharing Christmas ornament ideas, the oldest thing I own, photograph sharing day, or stories about my children and grandchildren. By building upon themes generated by the participants themselves, half-hour socials are easily initiated and sustained as a regular aspect of the monthly social calendar.

Festivals serve as excellent opportunities to join with other community organizations in planning and conducting a program of annual festivals (e.g., Fall Foliage Festival, Festival of the Winter Solstice, Spring Blossom Festival, and Summer Breezes Festival). Festivals can be developed around cultural events, seasonal happenings, or historically significant dates to the community or state. Festivals often involve socializing, special displays, events, and exhibits. Festivals are excellent social events that serve to connect all generations and members of the community together in celebrating life and the culture that binds them together.

The social calendar is complete when an ample number of additional social events are provided such as dances, special parties (e.g., game parties, progressive lunches or dinners), special events (Health Fairs), and clubs (e.g., creative writing, hobbies, debate, politics, quilting, woodworking) The list is endless regarding ideas for the social calendar; therefore, program staff will be wise to form a social committee of older persons to guide the ongoing development and implementation of the social program.

Implementation and Materials Suggestions

Probably the single most important suggestion for social activity specialists is to remember that what is done *by* (as opposed to *for*) older people is the key to successful programming. Involving the participants in all phases of social program planning, implementation, and evaluation will help to ensure that the program reflects this basic principle and, therefore, that the participants' interests and needs are met. The second principle to ensure success is the importance of using other community resources. All the social needs and interests of older persons as briefly summarized above cannot be met in most communities by a single senior center, one club, or an individual facility. Therefore, a skillful activity specialist will know what other resources, expertise, facilities, programs, organizations, and services are available in the community for meeting the social needs of older adults.

There are other important ingredients to a successful social program. They are:

(a) the use of motivational techniques to attract and maintain the involvement of participants,

(b) the selection and preparation of good leaders,

(c) the skillful utilization of volunteers,

(d) the development of a sound program structure (e.g., selection of activity type, time allotment, materials and facilities, other environmental arrangements and supports),

(e) the consideration of all safety considerations and preparations, and

(f) the need for transportation.

In regard to social events and special programs, the core considerations for program elements and implementation requisites will need to be addressed. These details include a list of materials, costs, adaptations, specified procedures for conducting the program, length of time needed for the activity or program, the goals and objectives of the program, maximum size of group, and any special concerns that will need to be addressed. These considerations are specified as the written program plan is developed by the activity staff in collaboration with older adult advisory members.

Activity Area II: *Intergenerational Activities*

Target Goal

Participants will have access to a variety of activities that are designed to connect them with members from the younger generations in the community.

Enabling Objectives

- To assess the interests of older persons in activities and events that involve younger generations.
- To evaluate community agencies and organizations for opportunities to develop intergenerational activities (e.g., schools, daycare centers, churches, youth organizations, and family organizations).
- To plan and conduct at least four to six intergenerational activities or programs on an annual basis.
- To assess young people's organizations for the interest and willingness of younger people to interact with older people in specific activities and programs.

Activity Suggestions: *Storytelling and After-School Tutoring*

Intergenerational activities and programs are growing in their importance and popularity as members from the different generations in the community continue to lead lifestyles that tend to isolate them from one another. Intergenerational activities and programs are those in which the primary goal is to bring older persons in direct contact with younger persons, and vice versa, while engaging in collaborative activity. A broad range of activity formats can be used to facilitate this goal. For example, older persons can develop a program of regular visits to child daycare centers for the purpose of conducting a storytelling and/or reading hour. In this way, older persons can provide grandparenting to younger children whose natural grandparents may either live far away or may be deceased. In return, the younger children provide opportunities to the older adults to experience memories of when they were younger and rearing their own children. This type of intergenerational program also provides direct benefits to the childcare center in that an expanded availability of adults to give more one-on-one attention to the children is possible.

Another intergenerational activity that can be successfully developed is extending invitations to young people from local schools or youth clubs to visit the senior center for the purpose of providing a special program such as a demonstration of a group project, the reading of short stories or poems written by the youth (or the elders), or a musical or theatrical performance. Inviting young people to participate in senior center activities like board games, cards, hobbies, and crafts, is another strategy that can be used to expand the senior program to include younger people.

Community and civic organizations often join forces with senior center participants to plan special, community-wide programs that target families and the younger generations. For example, after-school tutoring and job-mentoring activities are desperately needed by younger people. The wisdom and time that older persons have at their disposal could be used to help meet this need through specifically developed intergenerational programs.

Also, many families today have two working parents or reflect the single working-parent home. Children in these situations often need someone to talk with and someplace to go. Senior citizens can be effective advocates in meeting some of the needs of these youth. These activities involve taking the initiative to develop the idea for the joint program and then locating other community organizations to join forces in providing these needed services to young people. This approach can reduce the isolation that often develops when senior citizens are viewed as "having their own center and programs." By opening up the senior center at specific times to meet youth needs through directed programs and activities, senior citizens and community agencies may be enabled to join together to strengthen the community as a whole.

Last, intergenerational dance classes and dances can be used effectively to bridge the generations. Young people generally enjoy dancing and, with an effective marketing approach, they may become interested in learning various new and old dance styles from older adults. Dancing is an activity that is of interest to people in all generations, and is an activity through which connections can be built across the generations.

Implementation and Materials Suggestions

The development and implementation of intergenerational activities and programs depends upon several key ingredients:

(a) interested and willing senior citizens,
(b) enthusiastic leaders and facilitators who also understand child development and youth,
(c) community support,
(d) commitment of organizations and facility managers to provide the needed space and resources to support intergenerational events, and
(e) young people of all ages who are interested in spending time with older adults.

Beyond these basics, standard program development steps are pursued to establish and carry on intergenerational programs. These steps include assessing needs and interests, identifying program resources and leadership, planning the details of the program, conducting the program, and providing evaluation feedback about the program. Throughout the program planning process, consideration is given to materials, program costs, time and space requirements, transportation, and other environmental supports (e.g., adequate lighting, heating and cooling, refreshments, safety). The success of intergenerational programs, however, rests largely on the motivation, involvement, and commitment of the participants to the overall program goals.

Consideration is given to the interaction skills that will be needed by participants in order to insure a successful program. Some aspects of social interaction that are addressed when planning an intergenerational activity or program include the following:

1. Does the program or activity emphasize cooperation or competition?
2. What size group is the activity or program best suited for?
3. Does the activity and environment serve to promote a high degree of interaction?
4. What degree of physical proximity does the activity entail and will it fit within a "comfort zone" for all participants?
5. How much initiative is required by both older and younger participants?
6. Is the activity structured so that it is appropriate for participants of all ages?

Group leadership skills that will help to ensure a successful program embrace both motivational aspects of the program, as well as methods for maintaining interest (Leitner and Leitner, 1985). A leader should:

1. Be certain that the activity is within the interests and needs of prospective participants.
2. Design and implement the activity for varying ability levels; offer assistance as needed.

3. Use positive reinforcement. Motivate through encouragement to try the activity at least once, but do not force anyone to participate who is not comfortable. In some cases, observing an activity is a form of passive participation and is within the comfort zone of more shy people.
4. Beware of boredom! Implementing new challenges within the program or activity is an important strategy for maintaining interest.
5. Be sure that the group meets on a regular schedule that neither leaves too much time between meetings nor meets so frequently that participants become bored or disinterested because novelty wears off.

It is very important in intergenerational programming to be attentive to both the younger and older participants. Considering both age groups requires that the activity staff be aware of the needs, interests, and capabilities of each when planning and leading the program.

Activity Area III: *Hobbies, Crafts, and Games*

Target Goal

Participants will have available to them hobby and craft classes, materials, and facilities, as well as a calendar of regular times when popular games will be played at various community-based locations (e.g., schools, community and senior centers, community organizations).

Enabling Objectives

• To assess the hobby and craft skills and interests of the senior adults in the community as well as those in long-term care facilities.
• To assess and evaluate the availability of community resources, facilities, and expertise in order to make optimal use of these in planning and implementing the hobby and craft program.
• To plan a regular calendar of board and table games.

Activity Suggestions: *Special-Interest Clubs*

Hobbies, crafts, and games are immensely popular activities among most senior citizens. Items that older persons typically collect or pursue as hobbies include: albums, scrapbooks, coins, medals, toys, dolls, postcards, programs, rocks, flowers, plants, taxidermy, fish, antiques and relics, Indian artifacts, stamps and seals, sculpture, drawing, painting, textile arts, crafts, needlework, rugs, quilts, weaving, woodwork, wood carving, textiles, beadwork, plastic, book binding, jewelry, puppets, pottery, stenciling, iron and metal work, enamel, glass, models (e.g., airplanes, cars, ships, buildings, trains), and photography (Williams, 1962). The list of activities that people pursue as hobbies or collections is endless, and is generally bounded only by the interest of two or more people from the community. Therefore, a wide variety of hobby and collecting clubs can be developed to meet the specific assessed interests of community members.

Clubs in other areas are also very popular. For example, creative writing and publishing have become very exciting activities among seniors. Several popular press books are in print as a result of this kind of program. Educational clubs (including the very popular Elderhostel programs) are growth activities among older persons. Others are literature clubs, birdwatching clubs, silver striders walking clubs, catalog shopping clubs, community service clubs, optimist and public speaking clubs, travel clubs, and game clubs (e.g., bridge, euchre, Scrabble).

A club format is not necessary in order to have informal hours available for games. Games that are popular with older adults include: recreational cards, checkers, chess, darts, shuffleboard, horseshoes, billiards, bingo, board games, and Scrabble. Open hours for games are important in the availability of socialization opportunities for seniors who enjoy meeting at senior centers, churches during nonservice times, or other community center settings.

Crafts provide an activity format that encourages socialization, as well as meeting the need for regular use of fine motor skills and cognitive stimulation. Typical crafts enjoyed by older adults include: weaving, rug making, sewing, pottery, knitting, paper craft, lamp making, stenciling, plastics, woodwork, leather craft, metal craft, textile printing, braiding, knotting, wood carving, crocheting, tatting, jewelry making, embroidery, and making stained glass. It is not uncommon to find craft items for sale at senior centers which attests to the popularity of this kind of activity. Craft classes, clubs, and one time activity sessions may be included in the monthly social calendar with a fairly high success rate to be expected in terms of attendance and outcomes.

Implementation and Materials Suggestions

The success of the hobbies, games, and crafts components of an overall social recreation program rests largely on leadership. Leaders will provide a sound foundation for success if they remember a few important tips about programming in this area (Williams, 1962):

1. Declines in vision, fine motor control, muscle strength, and endurance can affect the older person's work at crafts and some hobbies, or participation in some games. Providing environmental supports (e.g., superior lighting, magnifying glasses, large-print directions, audiotape directions, longer time allowance to complete a project, assistance

with heavy machinery) will be important in order to promote positive experience for all who participate in these activities.

2. Older people need encouragement, just as younger people do, that they have the ability to create beautiful objects. Help older people reach for high standards of workmanship and design.

3. Match skill levels in craft groups and hire skilled leaders. It can be discouraging to be involved in a group whose skills far exceed those of the beginner. Be sure that craft leaders also understand the needs and interests of older persons as well as how to motivate and encourage older participants.

4. The quality of products is commensurate with the quality of the materials, facilities, and tools that are available to the older craftsperson. Program staff need to plan for adequate supplies, facilities, and tools through enlisting donations, sponsorship, and a budgetary planning process that provides adequately in this area. Plan in advance for the (a) rooms and equipment, (b) tools and supplies, and (c) leadership skills that will be needed.

5. Craft sales, hobby shows, and game tournaments are excellent ways to showcase the work of seniors, to raise funds to support the program, and to provide another social event related to these activities. The organization and implementation of sales, shows, and tournaments can be completely managed by the older participants. By organizing themselves into various committees, they can have the opportunity to show off their talents. Essential committees for these events include: general overall program committee, finance and sponsorship, publicity, volunteers, location and equipment, exhibit or game space organization, decorations, hospitality and public relations, transportation, entertainment, cleanup, and (optional) judging and prizes.

Activity Area IV: *Travel and Outdoor Activities*

Target Goal

Participants will have access to a travel and trip program that will include local and long distance trips, travel agency assistance, and staff assistance in planning and implementing an ongoing travel and outdoor activity calendar.

Enabling Objectives

- To plan and implement a varied program of local and distance travel and outdoor activity participation (e.g., birdwatching, day hiking).
- To develop a cooperative agreement with a local travel agency for the purpose of providing special packages for the travel program.
- To train staff in leading trip and travel programs for seniors.

- To assess seniors regarding their travel interests, requirements, and willingness to participate in a travel program annually.

Activity Suggestions: *Day Trips and Group Tours*

Travel and outdoor activities are very popular with older adults, especially persons in the transition years (ages 65–80) who continue to enjoy good health and functional independence. Older adults comprise a large segment of the tourism market for both local, short, day trips, as well as extended travel tours. Activities in the out-of-doors also are increasingly popular among older adults.

Typical outdoor activities that are enjoyed include nature walks, bird-watching, hiking, picnicking, gardening, fishing, walking for pleasure, boating, bicycling, park and nature preserve visiting, and camping. These activities can be enjoyed by most older adults with a few considerations (e.g., available restrooms, proper water and nutrition, proper clothing and shoes, and frequent benches for resting, preferably in the shade). Planning to include some kind of outdoor activity in the monthly social calendar helps to ensure a well-balanced program.

Outings, either local, short, day trips or long, group tours to distant sights and locations, add a measure of excitement to the social calendar. A wide variety of settings can be used to develop a varied and stimulating travel program. Trips to the following destinations can be planned on a regular basis: concerts and theater productions, historic sites, specialty shows (e.g., antique, art, hobby), train excursions, tourist attractions and theme parks (e.g., Disneyland), shopping malls in large cities and local flea markets, festivals and fairs, camps and nature preserves, parks, Elderhostel programs, zoological parks and botanical gardens, museums and galleries, sporting events, cruises, and special tours (Elliott and Sorg-Elliott, 1991). The list is practically endless, based on the curiosity and creativity of the travel program participants. Outings are successful when they are planned carefully with the needs and interests of the older participants in the forefront.

Implementation and Materials Suggestions

The travel and outdoor program requires special planning to ensure its success, including the enjoyment and safety of all participants (Elliott and Sorg-Elliott, 1991). Basic planning includes the following details:

1. Acquiring information about:

   (a) the destination and/or event;
   (b) the location layout and design;

(c) the date and travel times (e.g., departure, arrival at destination, return);

(d) the traveling information (e.g., route, directions);

(e) the kind of transportation and number of available seats; and

(f) the major objective(s) of the trip or outdoor activity.

2. Obtaining detailed information about participants, including:

(a) the number attending;

(b) participants with motor impairment and assistance needs and the number of participants who need an attendant;

(c) information about the health status and any health conditions of participants (with medical release if needed);

(d) special dietary needs; and

(e) a list of supplies and clothing that participants should bring with them on the outing.

3. Contracting or finalizing specific details and arrangements for the outing, including:

(a) transportation arrangements (e.g., number and types of vehicles, drivers, attendants, and time);

(b) dietary arrangements;

(c) securing the necessary staffing, volunteers, and attendants;

(d) budget and participant finances;

(e) advertising the trip or outing;

(f) evaluation plan;

(g) safety plan (e.g., including medical releases, emergency phone numbers, first aid); and

(h) final enrollment figures.

Trip or outing planning also requires that the trip staff conduct a site assessment in order to safeguard accessibility, safety, and a good match between the objectives for the trip, the participants, and the destination choice. Elliott and Sorg-Elliott (1991) recommend that the trip leader or planner conduct a Trip Resources Assessment as presented in Figure 14.1 (page 296). The information obtained from the assessment will help the trip planner to ensure that the safety, accessibility, and comfort needs of older participants are met at each destination included in the travel/outings program.

Figure 14.1

Trip Resources Assessment Form

Assessment Date_____ Trip Date_____

Destination _____

Address _____
          Street, PO Box   City   State   Zip

Contact Person_____ Title_____

Phone Number _____

Size of Group_____ Cost _____ (group, individual)

Preferred Date & Times _____

Directions to Destination _____

_____

Emergency Information _____

_____

Program Title _____ Duration_____

Description _____

Attributes Assessment: Comments:

Type: └─┴─┴─┴─┴─┴─┘
               unstructured   structured

Participation: └─┴─┴─┴─┴─┴─┘
               entertainment   educational

Skill Level:

  Social: └─┴─┴─┴─┴─┴─┘
               low   high

  Physical: └─┴─┴─┴─┴─┴─┘
               low   high

  Cognitive: └─┴─┴─┴─┴─┴─┘
               low   high

Physical Setting:

  Rest Rooms: └─┴─┴─┴─┴─┴─┘
               none   wheelchair accessible

  Eating Area: └─┴─┴─┴─┴─┴─┘
               none   wheelchair accessible

  Steps: └─┴─┴─┴─┴─┴─┘
               many   none   wheelchair ramps

  Seating: └─┴─┴─┴─┴─┴─┘
               none   seats with backs

  Walks/Trails: └─┴─┴─┴─┴─┴─┘
               none   wheelchair accessible

  Terrain: └─┴─┴─┴─┴─┴─┘
               hilly   flat

  Shelter: └─┴─┴─┴─┴─┴─┘
               none   enclosed

  Water Fountains: └─┴─┴─┴─┴─┴─┘
               none   wheelchair accessible

  Lighting: └─┴─┴─┴─┴─┴─┘
               none   adequate

Source: Adapted from Elliott & Sorg-Elliott, 1991.

Activity Area V: *Specific Therapeutic Activities*

Target Goal

Participants will have a variety of community-based, long-term care facility-based, and home-based therapeutic activities provided by trained therapeutic recreation specialists or associated professionals.

Enabling Objectives

- To develop a resource list of trained therapists and professionals who are willing to assist in the provision of a therapeutic activities program that is designed to meet prevention and rehabilitation goals in the psychosocial domain.
- To train staff in therapeutic activity intervention.
- To meet with older clients to plan a program of therapeutic activities, including the provision of the program in various locations (e.g., home, nursing home, community center).
- To implement on a regular basis the offering of one or more specific therapeutic activities (e.g., pet therapy, horticultural therapy, modified exercise, art therapy, music therapy, relaxation therapy).

Activity Suggestions: *Pet and Horticultural Therapy*

Many activities can be planned and implemented as therapeutic intervention. Some of the more common therapeutic activities include pet therapy, horticultural therapy, modified exercise, art therapy, music therapy, and relaxation therapy. Distinguishing attributes of activities that are used as therapy are:

(a) an identified impairment or disability is the target of activity intervention;
(b) rehabilitation, prevention, or maintenance of social interaction skills constitute the goal of intervention;
(c) a specified treatment plan guides activity intervention;
(d) therapeutic activity may be part of an overall treatment plan, and thus, the activity specialist is a member of the treatment team;
(e) activity intervention follows a clinical model;
(f) activity services may be billable and reimbursable;
(g) treatment is provided by a qualified specialist; and
(h) individual client outcomes are documented.

The therapeutic benefits of interacting with pets, growing and caring for plants, engaging in modified exercise, experiencing the creation of art, participating in music, or engaging in relaxation are increasingly recognized by rehabilitation specialists who provide care and treatment to older persons.

Therapeutic recreation specialists either directly provide these therapeutic activity interventions or supervise specialists (e.g., art therapists) in the use of therapeutic activities with specific clients. Older adults who typically benefit from these kinds of activities are those whose social interactions have become impaired through illness (e.g., as in depression caused by medication use), disease (e.g., dementia of the Alzheimer's type), or injury (e.g., stroke). For these individuals, the road to recovery and independent functioning requires the specific application of activities for the purpose of regaining or expressing social interaction skills (e.g., communicating feelings to others as in the use of art therapy).

Implementation and Materials Suggestions

Clinical practice of therapeutic activity intervention is based on the following process: client assessment, activity analysis, intervention planning and implementation, and evaluation. The participant or client will be assessed for his or her general functional status, including degree of independence in the following areas:

(a) physical (e.g., coordination, dexterity, endurance, vision, hearing, strength),

(b) cognitive (e.g., orientation, alertness, perception, attention, comprehension, safety awareness),

(c) social (e.g., interacts socially, helps others, participates, behaves appropriately, relates with others),

(d) emotional (e.g., emotionally stable, confident, appropriate behavior),

(e) initiative (e.g., shows motivation, independent judgment and decision making),

(f) general (e.g., demonstrates interest, completes work, compliant to rules), and

(g) special skills, interests, and capabilities are identified (Hamill and Oliver, 1980).

Activities are selected and analyzed for their specific match in meeting client needs and interests in the treatment process. Activity analysis entails systematically breaking down activities according to the skills and abilities that the client needs to engage in the activities. Activities are usually analyzed across three domains: physical, cognitive, and social or emotional. In the physical domain, the activity is analyzed according to full or partial body involvement, the type of body movement required, mobility and physical fitness requirements, and the demands made by the activity on the senses (e.g., vision, hearing, hot and cold perception). In the cognitive domain, the intellectual requirements of the activity are evaluated—how many rules are involved in the activity and how complex are they, are reading and writing skills involved, what long- and short-term memory skills are required for participation, and what degree of attention is needed? In the social or emotional domain, elements of the activity that are analyzed include: does the activity promote communication of feelings, release of tension or stress, the experience of fun or frustration, self-esteem, and creativity? Also of concern in this area are the elements of cooperation, teamwork, the nature of social interaction and communication with others, whether or not the activity promotes motivation and initiative, and is it done with others or alone?

In planning and implementing the activity, clear client- and treatment-specified goals will guide the final selection of the therapeutic activity intervention. Therefore, the treatment plan should contain treatment goals and enabling objectives as well as target outcomes to evaluate treatment effectiveness. In leading the therapeutic activity intervention, the specialist will pay specific attention to client motivation, interest, and overall functional gains. Evaluation evidence will be needed to assess if the client treatment goals were met, to decide whether the activity was the appropriate treatment strategy, and to demonstrate the efficacy of the activity intervention in the overall care and treatment of the client.

Summary

In this chapter the basic elements of activity programs that are designed to meet the psychosocial needs of older persons are presented. These activities can be implemented in a variety of settings including community-based programs and centers, at home, or in long-term care facilities. The sample program can be used as a guide in the development of a more site-, client- and group-specific psychosocial activity program. Readers are encouraged to consult the additional resources listed in Figure 14.2 and in the References and Resources section at the end of this chapter.

Figure 14.2

Resources for Developing Psychosocial Programs

The *Activity Director's Guide,* published monthly by Eymann Publications (1490 Huntington Circle, Box 3577, Reno, NV 89505, telephone (707) 333-6651), may be helpful in developing additional psychosocial activities, as well as more detailed program plans for the activities described in this chapter.

Additional useful resources are listed in the References and Resources section at the end of this chapter.

Comprehension Questions

1. Discuss the importance of socialization and social activity involvement in older adulthood.
2. What late life developmental challenges are addressed through social programs and activities?
3. Describe appropriate psychosocial activities for older adults in five broad areas or categories.

References and Resources

Elliott, J. E., & Sorg-Elliott, J. A. (1991). *Recreation programming and activities for older adults.* State College, PA: Venture Publishing, Inc.

Flatten, K., Wilhite, B., & Reyes-Watson, E. (1988). *Recreation activities for the elderly.* New York, NY: Springer Publishing Co., Inc.

Hamill, C. M., & Oliver, R. C. (1980). *Therapeutic activities for the handicapped elderly.* Rockville, MD: Aspen Publishers Inc.

Hooyman, N. R., & Kiyak, H. A. (1988). *Social gerontology: A multidisciplinary perspective.* Needham Heights, MA: Allyn & Bacon.

Jones, L. (1987). *Activities for the older mentally retarded/developmentally disabled.* Akron, OH: Exploration Series Press.

Leitner, M. J., & Leitner, S. F. (1985). *Leisure in later life: A sourcebook for the provision of recreational services for elders.* Binghamton, NY: The Haworth Press, Inc.

Powers, P. (1991). *The activity gourmet.* State College, PA: Venture Publishing, Inc.

Rice, W., & Yaconelli, M. (1986). *Play it!* Grand Rapids, MI: Zondervan Publishing House.

Tedford, J. (1958). *The giant book of family fun and games.* Danbury, CT: Franklin Watts, Inc.

Thews, V., Reaves, A. M., & Henry, R. S. (1993). *Now what? A handbook of activities for adult day programs.* Winston-Salem, NC: Bowman Gray School of Medicine, Wake Forest University.

Vickery, F. E. (1972). *Creative programming for older adults: A leadership training guide.* New York, NY: Association Press.

Williams, A. (1962). *Recreation in the senior years.* New York, NY: Association Press.

Zgola, J. M. (1987). *Doing things: A guide to programming activities for persons with Alzheimer's disease and related disorders.* Baltimore, MD: The Johns Hopkins University Press.

Unit V

Professional Practice Considerations

The provision of high quality care and services to older adults relies on a solid base of knowledge about aging, as well as on practical information about specific treatment interventions and professional concerns. Activity specialists are guided by the best practices in treatment and program delivery processes. In this unit several key practice topics are covered. Chapter 15 reviews the importance of documentation and evaluation procedures in care planning. Evaluation tools and documentation processes are discussed. Chapter 16 discusses ethical considerations and standards of practice for activity professionals. The text concludes with a chapter that addresses the basic competencies needed by activity specialists including standard qualifications and recommended hiring practices. The future of therapeutic activity intervention relies upon the commitment of service providers, governmental agencies, and trained professionals to address proactively the needs of the older population. A trained and informed cadre of professionals is a critical cornerstone in the preferred delivery of future service to all older persons.

Key Terms

Accountability
Care Plan
Documentation
Evaluation
Formative Evaluation
Goal Attainment Scaling
Interviews
Merit
Objectives-Oriented Evaluation
Observations

Qualitative Information
Quantitative Information
Questionnaires
Sociometry
Summative Evaluation
Surveys
Task Analysis
Triangulation
Worth

Learning Objectives

1. State the purposes of documentation and evaluation in the care and treatment of elderly persons.
2. Discuss the process of evaluation.
3. Explain formative and summative evaluation in relation to therapeutic activity intervention.
4. Differentiate between qualitative and quantitative evaluation information.
5. Describe task analysis as a planning, documentation, and evaluation tool.
6. Discuss goal attainment scaling as an evaluation tool.
7. Explain sociometry as an evaluation tool.
8. Conduct a case review and recommend a care plan based upon documentation and evaluation information presented in the case.

Chapter 15

Documentation and Evaluation

Introduction

Conscientious documentation and evaluation convey the message that caregivers and staff have a significant investment in the activity program. Documentation and evaluation are instrumental in sustaining programmatic support and funding for individual client treatment and for financial support for the overall program. Because documentation and evaluation are central to good professional practice in therapeutic activity intervention, an entire chapter is devoted to reviewing them.

Evaluation refers to the consistent documentation, measurement, and analysis of client progress in attaining predetermined treatment goals, as well as the constant monitoring of outcomes associated with the overall activity program (Beddall and Kennedy, 1985). Specific client goals and objectives provide standards for determining the merit and worth of both anticipated and unanticipated outcomes. Evaluation also is an ongoing process that enables the determination of the value of various aspects of the activity program in an effort to facilitate improvements in all areas. There is a close relationship between the evaluation of individual client progress and the evaluation of the overall program that is designed to meet identified client needs (Greenblatt, 1988; Wilhite and Keller, 1992). Therefore, the evaluation of programs for elderly persons, as well as the evaluation of individual elderly clients, is considered in this chapter.

The chapter reviews the purposes of evaluation and evaluation methods. Formative and summative evaluation and qualitative and quantitative techniques are presented. Various evaluation tools are discussed, including interviews, observations, and surveys. Task analysis and goal attainment scaling are described as they are applicable in program planning, documentation, and evaluation. The utilization of sociometry as an evaluation tool also is considered. Finally, a case review and recommended plan of care based on the information obtained from documentation and evaluation is described.

The Purposes of Documentation and Evaluation

The documentation of client progress coincides with the evaluation of specific activities and overall program content and process. *Documentation* is at the heart of the evaluation process. The relevance of goals and activities and the determination of progress are ascertained through the use of systematic documentation. The size and type of facility, nature of the participants, program budget, and number of staff members will determine the method of reporting that is necessary and practical (Hamill and Oliver, 1980).

Evaluation information is sought through documentation in order to appraise the merit of planned interventions in regard to specific client goals and objectives. *Merit* refers to the characteristics of the activity intervention or overall program that are valued by clients and staff. Does the program or specific activity produce the desired objectives that are important to the client?

Evaluation also is necessary to verify accountability. *Accountability* refers to determining if clients have received what was approved or promised and if the treatment or services were cost-effective (Bumagin and Hirn, 1990; Wilhite and Keller, 1992). Documentation and evaluation will confirm the efficacy of interventions, justify the program content, and provide evidence of the achievement of desired outcomes in an efficient and effective manner (Wilhite and Keller, 1992).

The attachment of values to facts is a basic component of program evaluation (Teague, 1987). Evaluation results may be used to support funding needs and the apportionment of limited resources. Evaluation data provides evidence for program changes and gives objective feedback to staff members regarding the effectiveness of care plans, specific interventions, and overall treatment programs. Finally, documentation and evaluation produce general information about the quality of care in relationship to established criteria and standards that are associated with various external accrediting groups, such as the Joint Commission on Accreditation of Healthcare Organizations (JCAHO) and the Commission for the Accreditation of Rehabilitation Facilities (CARF) (Theobald, 1979; Wilhite and Keller, 1992). Because of limited resources and increased accountability, systematic evaluation of clients' needs and expectations are of critical importance. Documentation and evaluation of individual activity interventions and overall programs offer explicit information regarding program improvement and the distribution of limited resources (Gillespie, Kennedy, and Soble, 1988-89).

The Evaluation Process

Evaluation can be as simple as desired or as complex as necessary. The evaluation process will be staged or sequenced to serve both formative and summative evaluation goals. *Formative evaluation* is directed by processes that review the strengths and weaknesses of an activity intervention or program in order that improvements may be initiated *during* activity and program development and implementation. The intent of formative evaluation is to use information to modify or revise the activity intervention or program as it is taking place (Schumacher and McMillan, 1993). Typically, the program staff are the users of formative evaluation information. As the data are compiled, information is provided that permits changes throughout the complete program planning process (Greenblatt, 1988).

   Summative evaluation, on the other hand, appraises accomplishments at the completion of the activity intervention or overall program. The utilization of various procedures can substantiate conclusions regarding the effectiveness of the program. Actual outcomes are examined to determine if they correspond to the planned or sought outcomes. The identification of program weaknesses will facilitate changes and the future development of similar activities or programs (Greenblatt, 1988). Those persons who will be most interested in summative evaluation findings are current participants, potential clients, funding sources, policymakers, and program administrators (Schumacher and McMillan, 1993).

   While several approaches to evaluation are available to activity staff, the objectives-oriented approach in this chapter will be reviewed (Schumacher and McMillan, 1993). The focus of an *objectives-oriented evaluation* is how well or to what degree the specific activity intervention or overall program objectives were attained. The first step in the process of an objectives-oriented evaluation is to formulate the measurable objectives which are associated with specific behavioral changes that are expected from the client's participation in the activity or program and specify the criteria for measurement. Sources of data are identified, and the methods for collecting the data are established. The time frame for data collection is confirmed, and the outcomes are measured according to the established criteria for measuring the successful attainment of the objectives. Methods for treatment of the data are selected during the planning phase of an objectives-oriented evaluation. Following the analysis of the data, recommendations are presented, and results of the evaluation are integrated into the planning process (Gunn and Peterson, 1978; Teaff, 1985). The program planning process is cyclic. Thus an objectives-oriented approach can serve both formative and summative evaluation purposes. (See Chapter 7 for a discussion of the therapeutic intervention programming process and evaluation.)

   The preparation of questions to evaluate the specified objectives provides a focus and direction to the objectives-oriented evaluation. Why and for whom is the evaluation being conducted? Audiences for the evaluation may include clients, relatives or guardians of the client, staff and/or treatment team members, accrediting organizations, and funding sources. According to Wilhite and Keller (1992), basic evaluation questions can include the following examples:

1. What were the outcomes of the program?
2. Were activities and interactions appropriate in regard to the stated objectives?
3. Were the objectives valid, realistic, and relevant?
4. Was the program implemented as designed?

Each evaluation question can evolve into several, more discrete subitems that are used to answer the more comprehensive objectives posed in the first phase of the evaluation. Programs may be appraised with a variety of indicators such as calculations of attendance. However, attendance totals do not accurately describe the influence of the activity or program upon individual participants (Rossman, 1989). The identified subitems will guide the selection of pertinent information sources such as attendance records, individual records, files, charts, test results, progress notes, and prior evaluation reports (Wilhite and Keller, 1992).

The evaluation methods used must be considered according to the costs required for implementation. The amount of time, money, specialized training, skills, and experience involved must be anticipated. Either or both qualitative and/or quantitative information can be obtained and analyzed. *Qualitative information* is typically collected through anecdotal records, extensive case notes, interviews, and observations. Qualitative information or data are in the form of words or artifacts which require specific skills and techniques to analyze and interpret in light of the overall goals and objectives of the activity or program. Basic descriptions, analytical accounts, and content appraisal may be included. A qualitative approach generally ensures increased understanding through more personal procedures and presentations such as the exploration of feelings, thoughts, insights, and descriptions in the familiar language of the clients (Reinharz and Rowles, 1988; Wilhite and Keller, 1992).

Quantitative information or data is often derived from records, direct assessments, and surveys or questionnaires. Quantitative data are analyzed and presented as numerical results or in the form of summary statistics such as averages, change measures, or frequency distributions. Both qualitative and quantitative evaluation data are useful in examining how well the activity intervention and program objectives are achieved (Greenblatt, 1988; Wilhite and Keller, 1992). Certain evaluation techniques are inappropriate because of the functional characteristics of the client (e.g., invasive or stressful measures taken on frail clients) or the techniques themselves may impose unnecessary invasions into a client's affairs (e.g., probing sensitive interpersonal information) (Wilhite and Keller, 1992).

The evaluation objectives and specified set of subitems will require distinct times for data collection. Attendance records should be compiled regularly. Evaluations of individual program participants will be gathered as needed and at regular cycles during participation in the program. Data related to program outcomes will be generated at the end of an activity intervention and sometimes at predetermined intervals (Wilhite and Keller, 1992).

Analysis and reporting of the evaluation data involves the determination of how the information will be used and by whom. Formats for the communication of evaluation results often include interim and final reports, case studies, graphs, tables, charts, videotapes, progress notes, care plans, or discharge plans. The formats and methods for relating evaluation information are determined by the purposes of the evaluation and by the intended audience (Wilhite and Keller, 1992). Objectives-oriented evaluations typically are concerned with relating the final information to those parties who are directly concerned about the client who has received the activity intervention or has participated in an ongoing activity program.

Methods of Evaluation

A variety of methods are available for documenting client progress and for evaluating client and program outcomes. *Documentation* plays a significant role in the delivery of activity program services. The format for individual client documentation varies within each facility. Regardless of the method used for client documentation, each individual must be reviewed regularly in order to determine if stated goals are being achieved and plans of care implemented (Greenblatt, 1988).

Several methods used in evaluation are described below including *surveys* or *questionnaires, interviews, observations, task analysis, goal attainment scaling, sociometry,* and *triangulation.* Each method has its own particular advantages and disadvantages. For example, questionnaires and interviews assess variables more directly, while observation is less direct and is likely to yield inaccurate interpretations. Observations are less intrusive and less inclined to prompt biased responses from participants than interviews and surveys (Leitner and Leitner, 1985). Task analysis and goal attainment scaling are more formal techniques for planning and documenting client progress, and sociometry is useful when evaluating group performance and relationships. Triangulation is proposed as a method that blends several methods in order to gain a more complete view of program or activity intervention effectiveness.

Surveys, Questionnaires, and Interviews

Questionnaires and *surveys* completed by program participants can cover a wide variety of issues such as attitudes, beliefs, personal interests, life satisfaction, former and present pursuits, and health. Written questionnaires or surveys are generally less costly, less time consuming, and easier to administer to a large number of persons. Written responses, however, often are not practical or possible with impaired elderly persons. Surveys and questionnaires should be as short and as uncomplicated as possible in order to compensate for any deficiencies in cognitive functioning.

Interviews and *observations,* on the other hand, tend to be more effective with impaired elderly individuals. Interviews also may address beliefs, values, attitudes, needs and interests, life satisfaction, health, and other variables such as family history patterns (Leitner and Leitner, 1985).

The purposes of the interview are clearly stated to the participants. The interviewer will establish rapport with the interviewees. The interviews are conducted in a quiet, isolated area that is free from sensory distractions or interruptions. Predetermined, standardized responses to requests for clarification of questions also can aid in ensuring the validity of the results. The interviewee may intermittently require reorientation to the topic of concern. Negative comments are not dwelled on but may be acknowledged and the interviewee then redirected toward the interview topic. Other data collection methods used in concert with interviews will assist in obtaining more valid results (Leitner and Leitner, 1985).

Observations of Behavior

Observations are one of the most common evaluation procedures used in treatment, and they can be completed with or without the client's awareness of the process. Typical observations might include the number of participants in an activity, the percentage of clients who chose to participate in the activity, the number of participants who arrived or left the activity early, clients who were active versus passive participants in the activity, and the duration and frequency of the activity. Observations of behavior also may include documentation of participants' satisfaction with activities or other areas (Greenblatt, 1988; Leitner and Leitner, 1985).

Direct observation entails the use of specific procedures to record or evaluate various outcomes and behaviors such as tally sheets for target behaviors (e.g., display of social skills and use of motor skills), or observation logs (e.g., detailed descriptions of the participants and environment during the activity). Observations that are conducted by staff who have been trained in the observational technique and associated tools or instruments (e.g., tally sheet or log) will increase the usefulness of the resulting information and will help to control for unwanted bias.

The criteria used for evaluation of the effectiveness of a program will direct the observation of target behaviors. A behavior rating form can be used that lists the specific behaviors to be observed and recorded with added space to indicate the frequency of each behavior and any comments regarding the behaviors (Leitner and Leitner, 1985). Observers should be discreet and should avoid staring at the persons under observation. Observational tools that might distract the attention of the activity participants should not be used (e.g., laptop computers for recording frequency of behaviors). The observer's status as a nonparticipant in the activities should be ensured. The use of observational techniques in evaluation should reflect a trained observer's objective perceptions of an individual's or group's reaction to an activity (Leitner and Leitner, 1985).

Task Analysis

Task analysis is a preparatory phase that is used during planning, documentation, and evaluation of individual treatment plans within rehabilitation and/or developmental programs. Task analysis comprises a basis for the construction of evaluation instruments as well as the design of instructional approaches, supports, and materials. It is a useful method for clarifying the step-by-step approach that is needed for teaching specific activity skills to impaired clients (Greenblatt, 1988; Thiagarajan, Semmel, and Semmel, 1974). (See Chapter 7 for a discussion of the related concept of activity analysis.)

Task analysis is a process that examines the elements of an activity. It involves the study of behavior and the identification of its components. The procedures in task analysis include:

(a) statement of task objectives,
(b) identification of subtasks,
(c) comparable treatment of each subtask by repetition of objective analysis, and
(d) completion of analysis when the subtask results in a logical conclusion or entry level behavior (Thiagarajan, Semmel, and Semmel, 1974).

Initially, the primary task must have relevance to the client's needs. Task analysis should be complete including all the steps needed to engage fully in the activity. The inclusion of trivial tasks, however, is an error of excessive task analysis and should be avoided. Each subtask must be necessary for the performance of the primary task; subtasks should not be excessive or redundant (Thiagarajan, Semmel, and Semmel, 1974).

An activity should be progressive in order to provide for differing physical and mental aptitudes and sequential performance. The achievement of therapeutic goals requires that each functional task be analyzed. An analysis of each individual element provides a greater understanding of how a task may promote successful client participation. A task must permit modification either by simplification or by an extension to include additional challenge. The task also must allow for a conclusion with specified strategies for the verification of performance and competence (Hamill and Oliver, 1980).

Goal Attainment Scaling

Another method for the documentation and evaluation of progress toward established goals and objectives is *goal attainment scaling* (Kiresuk and Sherman, 1968). The predominant aspects of the goal attainment scale are:

(a) establishment of goals;
(b) specification of barriers to goal attainment; and
(c) description of the most favorable, least favorable, and most likely outcomes of intervention (Bumagin and Hirn, 1990).

An advantage of goal attainment scaling is that it provides recognition of partial success. The method is structured yet flexible enough to broaden its applicability. Goals are established with the client, not in the absence of him or her. The design of goal attainment scaling simplifies goals so that they are apportioned and explicitly defined. This process enables practitioners to focus their efforts upon individual goals and to adapt the evaluation to a variety of problems and situations (Bumagin and Hirn, 1990).

Sociometry

The process of sociometry can be used to identify relationships among group members. *Sociometry* is a technique that explores the organization of groups by determining the nature of the structure that is operating within the group. Sociograms are graphic representations of group structure that identify persons who are accepted or popular and those individuals who may be rejected, disliked, or less accepted (Greenblatt, 1988).

Sociometric techniques are valuable for improving the social adjustment of the individual. The identification of acceptance or rejection through sociometric procedures can enable the activity leader to facilitate behavior change for those who require assistance in group formats. Leadership skills also may be presented to individuals who already possess leadership abilities (Danford, 1965).

Sociometric techniques can improve group relations by detecting problem areas within interpersonal relationships, thus allowing the activity leader an opportunity to facilitate more effective social situations. Sociometric approaches also may be used to improve the organization of groups. Sociometric methods identify individuals with similar personalities and preferences, and through the use of cooperative efforts, sociometry can increase the productivity of groups by the promotion of group cohesiveness (Danford, 1965).

Triangulation

Triangulation is a systematic approach that utilizes a variety of evaluation techniques and procedures to compile both qualitative and quantitative information. It encourages the use of a range of evaluative methods and resources to present a more comprehensive description of clients and programs (Howe, 1982).

Triangulation is practical for the analysis of unanticipated outcomes with the emphasis placed upon clients' perspectives and developing a more complete understanding of their needs. The use of triangulation assists in the confirmation of results. Triangulation also yields a more accurate interpretation and application of the results of the activity intervention or program (Howe and Keller, 1988).

Case Review

The specified care plan, documentation process, and evaluation findings collectively play a significant role in the total care of the elderly client. The identification of problem areas and behaviors that determine level of activity participation, individual adjustment to the facility and the activity program, and the development of leisure pursuits will indicate the progress or lack of progress for each client. Awareness of these areas is essential for the generation of effective care plans, including their evaluation and modification (Greenblatt, 1988).

Documentation should include current care plans for clients whose status or classification has been modified. Any client who is reclassified to a different level of care requires a new treatment plan with revisions to the evaluation components as needed. A review of care plans also should be performed for those clients who return to the facility or program from another hospital or agency (Greenblatt, 1988).

The basic considerations in all care plans include factors that relate to the client's medical status and to any physical and/or psychological limitations. Specific attention should be given to the following aspects:

(a) the client's response to the program,
(b) his or her level of participation in the program,
(c) social interactions and relationships with peers and staff members,
(d) staff or agency supports that are provided to the specific client, and
(e) any notable attitudes and patterns of behavior (Greenblatt, 1988).

A combination of these elements, as well as various external factors, appear to influence the thrust of the care plan, and thus, will shape the documentation and evaluation process. Additional components may include standards established by the care facility that are mandated by the various regulatory agencies (Greenblatt, 1988).

Case Review Example

The following case example highlights the use of goal attainment scaling:

> On discharge from the rehabilitation center, Mrs. W and her family established a goal to hire a part-time caregiver or companion for Mrs. W. Mrs. W is 76 years old and prefers to have a companion of her own ethnic background. The companion is expected to assist in the care of Mrs. W who is severely limited in her ability to perform daily routines of self-care. Her limitations are due to severe arthritis and muscular impairment.
>
> After much searching, the family could not locate an individual who fulfilled Mrs. W's and her family's main requirement. At that time, all members of the family agreed with Mrs. W to interview potential caregivers and companions who did not share the same ethnicity with them.
>
> By utilizing goal attainment scaling as the evaluation measure, the most favorable, the least favorable, and the most probable outcomes were predicted in regard to locating an appropriate and satisfactory caregiver or companion for Mrs. W. The best possible outcome would be if the family was able to interview one potential part-time caregiver or companion and to be able to hire him or her. The worst outcome would be that many candidates would be interviewed, but none hired. The most likely result was that several individuals would be interviewed and one would be hired on a trial basis. The result was that the family hired the first person who was interviewed; the most favorable outcome was achieved.
>
> Subsequent goals considered different aspects of the arrangement between Mrs. W and the caregiver. For example, would Mrs. W, her family, and the caregiver be satisfied? Would they be somewhat dissatisfied, but have the ability to resolve their difficulties? Would they be so

dissatisfied that the caregiver would be released within a short period of time? The efforts of the rehabilitation care coordination staff focused on the identification of problems. This provided assistance to Mrs. W, members of her family, and the caregiver to resolve their differences.

If the relationship is eventually rejected, the formation of alternate goals will again be evaluated with Mrs. W and her family. If the caregiver remains for a long enough period of time to enable the family members to obtain the needed release from daily caregiving, partial success will be accomplished. Because of this initial experience, future attempts to hire a part-time caregiver or companion may have a more satisfactory conclusion. Potential resolution of the dilemma also can involve the location of another part-time caregiver or companion or the consideration of an entirely different plan of care for Mrs. W.

Goal attainment scaling, utilized as the method of evaluation in the above case, fostered a team approach to meeting the client's needs (Mrs. W). Members of her family and care coordination staff assumed different responsibilities in working toward the same goal. The structure of goal attainment scaling assisted in reducing criticism and controversy by promoting cooperation and a more comprehensive understanding of the overall purpose and goals of the client's program (Bumagin and Hirn, 1990). Goal attainment scaling proved to be an effective evaluation method for this particular client and her specific treatment goal(s).

Summary

Evaluation is fundamental to the planning process. It enables the determination of the value of various aspects of an activity and/or program in order to influence optimal outcomes in all areas. Methods for evaluation frequently are selected based upon the costs required for their implementation as well as the intended outcome of the evaluation (e.g., client focused versus program or agency focused).

Documentation is an essential component of evaluation. The significance of goals, objectives, activities, and inferences of progress may be determined through documentation. Documentation and evaluation of specific activity interventions and ongoing activity programs provide the necessary information for making immediate and long-range programmatic decisions.

The processes of formative and summative evaluation are discussed, as is qualitative and quantitative evaluation information. Various evaluative methods are discussed including surveys and questionnaires, interviews, observations, task analysis, goal attainment scaling, sociometry, and triangulation.

Surveys, questionnaires, interviews, and observations collect client-specific information from individuals and from groups of participants. These techniques produce both quantitative and qualitative information that can be used in evaluating the effects of an activity intervention or overall activity program.

Task analysis is described as a basis for the development of instruments and approaches to evaluate client-program-activity fit. Task analysis concerns the analysis of a behavior or an activity through the identification of its components. Matching task to client need helps to ensure attainment of the behavioral objective sought through activity intervention.

Goal attainment scaling is emphasized as an additional method for documentation of progress toward affirmed goals and objectives, while sociometric techniques are described as a means to examine the structure within groups. Further, triangulation is defined as a systematic approach focused on the thorough description and characterization of clients and programs. Triangulation often will utilize multiple methods in concert to gain a better understanding of program impact on client progress.

Finally, care plans, documentation, and evaluation are conceived as integral to the comprehensive care of elderly clients. Insight in these areas is considered necessary for the development and implementation of effective care, treatment, and/ or services. A case example is offered as an illustration of these points.

Comprehension Questions

1. What is documentation and why is it important?
2. Describe three different methods that can be used in evaluating a specific activity intervention or overall program. Present the strengths and weaknesses associated with each method.
3. Describe the objectives-oriented evaluation approach.
4. Conduct a case review and provide a description of the evaluation approach and tools that could be used in the care plan.

References

Beddall, T., & Kennedy, D. W. (1985). Attitudes of therapeutic recreators toward evaluation and client assessment. *Therapeutic Recreation Journal, 19*(1), 62-70.

Bumagin, V. E., & Hirn, K. F. (1990). *Helping the aging family: A guide for professionals.* New York, NY: Springer Publishing Co., Inc.

Danford, H. G. (1965). *Creative leadership in recreation.* Boston, MA: Allyn & Bacon.

Gillespie, K. A., Kennedy, D. W., & Soble, K. (1988-89). Utilizing importance-performance analysis in the evaluation and marketing of activity programs in geriatric settings. *Activities, Adaptation, & Aging, 13*(1), 77-89.

Greenblatt, F. S. (1988). *Therapeutic recreation for long-term care facilities.* New York, NY: Human Sciences Press.

Gunn, S. L., & Peterson, C. A. (1978). *Therapeutic recreation program design: Principles and procedures.* Englewood Cliffs, NJ: Prentice Hall.

Hamill, C. M., & Oliver, R. C. (1980). *Therapeutic activities for the handicapped elderly.* Rockville, MD: Aspen Publishers Inc.

Howe, C. Z. (1982). Some uses of multi-modal curriculum evaluation in therapeutic recreation. In L. L. Neal & C. R. Edginton (Eds.), *Extra perspectives: Concepts in therapeutic recreation* (pp. 87-98). Eugene, OR: University of Oregon.

Howe, C. Z., & Keller, M. J. (1988). The use of triangulation as an evaluation technique: Illustrations from regional symposia in therapeutic recreation. *Therapeutic Recreation Journal, 22*(1), 36-45.

Kiresuk, T. J., & Sherman, R. E. (1968). Goal attainment scaling: A general method for evaluating comprehensive community mental health programs. *Community Mental Health Journal, 4*(6), 443-453.

Leitner, M. J., & Leitner, S. F. (1985). *Leisure in later life: A sourcebook for the provision of recreational services for elders.* Binghamton, NY: The Haworth Press, Inc.

Reinharz, S., & Rowles, G. D. (Eds.). (1988). *Qualitative gerontology.* New York, NY: Springer Publishing Co., Inc.

Rossman, B. (1989). *Recreation programming: Designing leisure experiences.* Champaign, IL: Sagamore Publishing, Inc.

Schumacher, S., & McMillan, J. H. (1993). *Research in education: A conceptual introduction* (3rd ed.). New York, NY: HarperCollins College Publishers.

Teaff, J. D. (1985). *Leisure services with the elderly.* St. Louis, MO: Times Mirror/Mosby.

Teague, M. L. (1987). *Health promotion programs: Achieving high-level wellness in the later years.* Indianapolis, IN: Benchmark Press.

Theobald, W. F. (1979). *Evaluation of recreation and park programs.* New York, NY: John Wiley & Sons, Inc.

Thiagarajan, S., Semmel, D. S., & Semmel, M. I. (1974). *Instructional development for training teachers of exceptional children: A sourcebook.* Bloomington, IN: Indiana University.

Wilhite, B. C., & Keller, M. J. (1992). *Therapeutic recreation: Cases and exercises.* State College, PA: Venture Publishing, Inc.

Key Terms

Advocacy Model

Autonomy

Beneficence

Competency

Confidentiality

Dilemma

Ethical Dilemma

Ethics

Informed Consent

Justice

Living Will

Nonmaleficence

Power of Attorney

Privacy

Privileged Communication

Standards of Care

Learning Objectives

1. Describe the relevance and importance of ethics and ethical decision making in activity intervention.
2. Discuss various situations that activity specialists may be confronted with that involve ethical decisions.
3. Identify basic concepts related to ethics and standards of care.
4. Discuss ways in which healthcare professions are dealing with these issues.
5. Describe standards of care in relationship to activity intervention and discuss why they are important to activity specialists working with older adults.

Chapter 16

Ethics and Standards of Care

by Nancy Brattain Rogers and Patricia Ardovino[1]

Introduction

As the number of frail older adults in our population grows, the risk of ethical violations that affect older persons may potentially increase. In order to prevent ethical violations, it is imperative for the practitioner or caregiver to have a basic grasp of ethical concepts and standards of care. Activity specialists, as professionals in the healthcare industry, must be prepared to deal with ethical issues. Preparation is especially crucial for those providing services to older adults. This chapter provides basic information related to ethics, standards of care, and working with older adults in therapeutic activity intervention.

Activity Specialists and Ethical Decisions

There are three reasons why activity specialists working with older adults should be concerned about ethics and ethical decisions. First, older adults are vulnerable to ethical abuse because they are inclined to develop mental and/or physical impairments during the months or years preceding death. Mental impairments such as

---

[1]Patricia Ardovino, CLP, CTRS, has worked in the field of recreation for over 20 years. She worked 10 years for the Memphis Park Commission, Memphis, Tennessee, as the director of a community center serving people with disabilities. The center also provides services to older Americans with disabilities. Presently, she is a student at Indiana University where she is pursuing a Ph.D. in Human Performance/Leisure Behavior with a minor in Criminal Justice. Her area of expertise is the adult offender with mental retardation.

dementia may affect memory, concentration, and judgment. These impairments come at a stage in life when decision making concerning treatment may be critical. Physical and mental impairments that may occur in later life may be responsible for the involvement of a variety of professionals in the delivery of healthcare services. Older adults may find that new faces and personalities suddenly become involved in intimate aspects of their lives. In addition to these concerns, older adults with disabilities are at a high risk of being institutionalized, and institutional living also may provide settings in which ethical problems arise. Further, professional ethics may be violated based on pervasive negative stereotypes that are commonly associated with older adults. These stereotypes typically portray older adults as being unable to understand the particulars of their treatment (Gilhooly, 1986).

The second concern deals with the empowerment of older adults that has occurred in the past few decades. Older people requiring medical treatment have become better consumers who require professionals to be accountable for the decisions they make and the quality of care they provide. They now demand to have their views recognized and respected, and they expect members of the medical profession to be more sensitive and responsive to the needs and interests of the older adult (Gilhooly, 1986).

Finally, the role of caretaker has dramatically changed to one of caregiver. There is a tendency for older adults to stay at or return to their home for care after a debilitating illness or accident. This tendency is the result of a current economic and political climate which discourages expensive nursing home care. As more family members become caregivers, they will be required to make more treatment decisions including end-of-life decisions. Family members may require the assistance of healthcare providers to make ethical decisions that have legal ramifications. Professionals may face dilemmas when family decisions are based on their beliefs regarding the quality of life for their loved one when these decisions are not consistent with social norms codified in the law (Hanks and Settles, 1988-89).

Ethical Dilemmas and Patient Care

Ethics refers to the investigation of what is good and bad in relation to our moral duties and obligations. Our personal ethics are rooted in our character, but they can be refined or developed (Gilhooly, 1986). Activity specialists also must be concerned with professional ethics. Members of professions explore ethical issues to determine a set of moral principles or behaviors that guide professional practice. Many professional organizations have developed Standards of Practice which serve as the code of conduct statement for their members (see Appendix A for the Standards of Practice of the National Association of Activity Professionals). These standards are meant to guide behavior in a general sense and may be open to different interpretations. As a result, it is important for professionals to pursue the question of ethics throughout their professional careers. This section describes some important concepts that are helpful in understanding ethical issues (see Appendix B for the Patient's Bill of Rights as formulated by the American Hospital Association).

A *dilemma* is a situation that requires a decision between alternatives that appear to be equal. People face minor dilemmas every day, such as what movie to see, what telephone call to return first, and what to wear. Most of these dilemmas can be resolved fairly easily because the consequences of the decisions are not severe. It is not so easy to resolve ethical dilemmas. An *ethical dilemma* is a situation in which alternatives are defined by opposing ethical principles (Howell, 1988). For example, a family is facing the decision of institutionalizing an 80-year-old man. He has Alzheimer's disease and the burden of caring for him at home is overwhelming his wife. The two ethical principles his family must confront are: (a) nursing home placement is a sign that the family is not able to adequately care for its members; and (b) if the man is not placed in a nursing home, his wife's health may fail because of the burden of everyday caregiving. The situation may be compounded by other factors such as a promise the couple made 20 years ago never to place each other in an institution. Clearly, resolving this issue will not be an easy task.

Howell (1988) suggested that most ethical dilemmas fall into these categories:

1. Dilemmas arise with regard to the definition, discovery and defense of rights of individuals;
2. Dilemmas arise with regard to competency to make decisions, and consequent needs for protection through guardianship;
3. Dilemmas arise with regard to the process by which decisions can be made on behalf of the person who is deemed to be incompetent;
4. Dilemmas arise with regard to defining and measuring past wrongs or deprivations imposed by social policy, government action, and discrimination, and with regard to questions of restitution or recompense. (p. 444–445)

In their jobs, activity specialists are most likely to deal with the first three categories of ethical dilemmas which deal with patient autonomy. While all healthcare professionals should strive to protect patient autonomy, it is not always possible to ensure autonomous decision making.

Autonomy is an individual's natural right to be self-governing. This means it is the individual's right to determine his or her own destiny. The activity specialist is obliged to assist individuals in coming to this determination by providing appropriate information and helping them to understand that information so an informed decision can be made (Guccione, 1988). Once a decision has been made by the individual, it must be respected, even if it is not judged to be in the client's best interest by the concerned healthcare professionals.

Autonomy can be an ambiguous concept. Although it is not appropriate to coerce a person into making a decision, autonomy does not prevent an individual from deferring decision making to another person. For example, a patient may not want to hear a detailed explanation of the medical treatment a physician has recommended. He or she may simply trust the physician to make the right decision. What is important, however, is that the physician provide the patient the opportunity to make an autonomous decision.

The key to maintaining patient autonomy is *informed consent.* Informed consent is the vehicle by which information is provided to the individual regarding medical treatment and research so that he or she can make an informed decision (Tymchuk and Ouslander, 1990). Levine and Lawlor (1991) identified three components of the informed consent process:

1. Information important to the medical procedure or intervention must be disclosed to the patient. The patient can then refuse or consent to the treatment;
2. The patient must have the capacity to consent to the procedure or intervention;
3. The consent must be obtained voluntarily without any evidence of coercion. (p. 392)

A number of models for achieving informed consent currently exist. Gadow's (1981) Advocacy Model is used to help individuals make their own decisions by promoting the following objectives:

- ensuring the possibility of self-determination;
- enabling the patient to select the information needed to make a decision;
- disclosing personal views;
- assisting the patients to determine their own values; and
- ascertaining how patients comprehend their own individuality.

Activity specialists may feel that informed consent is not as important for therapeutic activity because this kind of intervention is not invasive. The principle of informed consent, however, applies to all types of treatments, and activity specialists must respect the decisions of some individuals to decline to participate in their programs.

Patient *privacy* and *confidentiality* also must be respected in order to preserve client autonomy. Privacy refers to the individual's right to have control over personal information and to be free of invasions into his or her life (Gilhooly, 1986). In certain healthcare settings, such as nursing homes, privacy may be difficult to achieve. Nonetheless, healthcare providers must take available steps to ensure privacy. Activity specialists may help ensure privacy by providing clients the opportunity to socialize with family and friends in an environment where they will not be disturbed. Respect of the client's possessions and living space is important. The public nature of a nursing home may encourage staff to freely walk in and out of clients' rooms. It is important to remember that the room is the client's home and should be treated as such. Confidentiality is the ancient "ethical obligation not to reveal to others anything said by the patients or to acknowledge the existence of a relationship" (Gilhooly, 1996, p. 182). Confidentiality is the key to good communication between the patient and practitioner and provides the ethical foundation for this relationship (Gilhooly, 1996; Guccione, 1988).

Ethical dilemmas often arise when there is concern that an individual is incompetent and no longer able to make decisions. A person is believed to be *incompetent* when his or her impairments limit the understanding and the ability to make or communicate responsible decisions. Competency is not absolute. An individual can be competent in one area such as medical treatment, and not in another such as finances (Guccione, 1988).

When discussing issues of informed consent, the activity specialist should keep in mind factors that can influence consent such as age, values, education, functional status, cognitive function, motivation and previous experience. Different strategies to assess the person's capacity to make an informed decision can be used. For example, Tymchuk and Ouslander (1990) recommend using illustrations in a storybook format and the following seven-step process:

1. Assess physical capacity, especially vision and hearing;
2. Assess mental status to help determine decision-making capacity and potential need for a proxy;
3. Assess reading comprehension;
4. Develop consent material (including how comprehension and application are to be assessed) in format and at difficulty level to match patient/subject abilities;
5. Present information;
6. Assess comprehension and if below criterion, provide some alternative intervention such as the use of repeated trials;
7. Follow up to determine whether comprehension of the information remains at criterion level, and whether they have changed their decision. (p. 250)

Professionals at a long-term care facility in New York City use a three-pronged approach to help resolve dilemmas such as informed consent, confidentiality, privacy, and end-of-life treatment issues. The approach includes education, direct practice, and research. A wide range of educational programs presenting cases involving ethical dilemmas are offered to all families, clients, paraprofessionals and professionals. Special attempts are made to include nurses aides and orderlies because they often know a great deal about the person in treatment, and can be greatly affected by treatment decisions. Monthly ethical rounds are extended which address ethical dilemmas dealing with end-of-life decision making such as tube feedings, restraints, and the impact of religious beliefs on medical decisions. An ethics consultant team evaluates the mental and physical status of the individual including any records of the person's desires and whether or not family or friends would be available to help in the decision-making process. Together with the primary treatment team, the ethics team implements decisions made by the client (Olson et al., 1993).

The appropriate legal procedure to pursue for the family of an incompetent individual is to obtain legal guardianship of that individual. Obtaining guardianship may entail a lengthy process and it is rarely initiated by families. In the situation where the patient is clearly incompetent, but has not been declared incompetent in court and a guardian has not been appointed, it is important to involve the next of kin in the decision-making process. It is not clear whether or not family members can make legally binding decisions for patients who have not been declared incompetent. However, involvement of the next of kin in making decisions for incompetent older adults is widely practiced throughout the healthcare industry.

Problems regarding legal guardianship and incompetence can be avoided by executing a durable power of attorney. This process involves the individual selecting one or more persons to make decisions for him or her when he or she is no longer able to (Levine and Lawlor, 1991). The person who is selected should know the desires of the individual and be trusted to carry them out. A durable power of attorney can be applied to general areas or specific areas, such as medical treatment. This legal procedure is fairly simple and allows the individual assurance that his or her wishes will be respected. It also saves the family the more lengthy legal process of declaring the individual as incompetent. Older adults who worry about retaining autonomy should not be frightened by durable power of attorney. It will be used only in situations where the individual is clearly no longer competent.

An important related concept that ensures personal choice is the *living will*. A living will is a written legal document that establishes how a patient wants to be treated if he or she is terminally ill and can no longer make decisions concerning his or her health (Levine and Lawlor, 1991). Many older adults have living wills that indicate they do not want any extraordinary measures taken to prolong their lives such as the use of life support. Most states honor living wills at this time, but there are still some controversies surrounding their use. The rights of family members to overturn the requests put forth in a living will, for example, have yet to be determined.

The ethical dilemmas related to competency arise when decisions made by caregivers or healthcare providers conflict with the wishes of the client. If the client is deemed incompetent, a legal guardian or healthcare provider may initiate an action to which the client is opposed if the action is deemed to be in the client's best interest. For example, an older adult with Alzheimer's disease may wish to live alone in an apartment. If that older adult has started fires by not remembering the stove is on, legal action may be taken to remove that individual from an independent living situation. This type of action is called *beneficence*. Beneficence is the basis of doing good acts or deeds in an effort to promote the well-being of the individual. It is founded on the principle that caregivers are committed to do as much good as they can (Guccione, 1988; Shank, 1985). In addition to acting in the client's best interest, the healthcare provider also is obliged not to harm an individual. *Non-maleficence* is the principle that the healthcare provider will do no harm (Guccione, 1988).

The process of determining the best decision for an incompetent individual should be consistent for each case. Hanks and Settles (1988-89) suggested a model for decision making to be used with involuntary clients in a case management setting. Treatment planning would:

1. Explicitly state value premises that influence assessments;
2. Explicitly construct, based on available information, the client's views of his or her situation and wishes;
3. Acknowledge data regarding the client's past coping strategies and how these are likely to influence response to dependency and frailty;

4. Explicitly state beliefs and professional judgments regarding risks inherent in the current situation;
5. Explicitly state beliefs and judgments about risks inherent in available alternative options;
6. Elicit input from panel members regarding alternative value premises, ethical choices, and risk assessments;
7. Weigh risks and decide on the action which the professional, the team, and the agency will support on behalf of the client. (Hanks and Settles, 1988-89, p. 47)

Decisions made on behalf of the client can best be achieved with the assistance of family members who are most likely to know the client's wishes, values, and beliefs.

Ethics and Aging Research

As the older population grows, more research is being conducted with older adults. While most research is positively viewed by older adults and their families, care should be taken to be sure that older adults know that their participation is voluntary and that their privacy is not invaded (Williams, 1993). When reviewing research proposals, the role of ethical committees should be:

1. To protect the right of subjects and associated staff in terms of confidentiality and privacy by emphasizing the voluntary aspects of participation via appropriate informed consent mechanisms; and
2. To evaluate the scientific merit of the research proposal and the qualifications of the investigators in order to assess the appropriateness of the risk-benefit relationship of subjects. (Gilhooly, 1986, p. 189)

Educators and trainers of healthcare professionals need to help their students develop ethical sensitivities. The combination of a core curriculum based on the essential body of knowledge coupled with the case study method provides a solid approach to teaching ethics (Gilhooly, 1986).

Standards of Care

Standards are established for two reasons. First, they guarantee that a minimum level of service is provided. Second, they protect the consumer. Activity specialists should be familiar with external standards set by agencies outside of the facility providing direct service (e.g., Joint Commission on Accreditation of Healthcare Organizations, the Commission for the Accreditation of Rehabilitation Facilities). Activity specialists also need to know internal standards set by professionals providing direct service (e.g., National Association of Activity Professionals, the National Therapeutic Recreation Society) (Smith and Land, 1989).

Standards of care for practitioners working with older adults provide the necessary framework for describing problems so that all professionals have a common understanding. Standards of care also suggest strategies to use when problems surface and recommend protocols to apply in care management (Janicki, Heller,

Seltzer, and Hoge, 1995). Standards of care are based on the premise that the practitioner needs to understand what changes take place during normal aging, what risk factors are involved for the older client, and what changes may be indicative of an onset of physical or mental impairments. Standards suggest to the practitioner that assessments and evaluations should be conducted in order to confirm a suspicion of impairment. Finally, standards recommend the establishment of care management (Janicki, Heller, Seltzer, and Hoge, 1995).

Care management seeks to help the person maintain and maximize his or her function, to use appropriate treatment interventions, and to use the resources from many disciplines when planning care management. The level of care, support, attention and sensitivity may increase as the mental or physical impairment progresses (Janicki, Heller, Seltzer, and Hoge, 1995). Training practitioners in standards of care is essential. Necessary elements of this training include learning about the normal aging process and changes that might indicate impairment. Training and educational materials also should be available to families and caregivers (Janicki, Heller, Seltzer, and Hoge, 1995).

Summary

Activity specialists working with older adults need to have an understanding of ethical concepts and standards of care because older adults are vulnerable to ethical abuse. In recent years, older adults have become more informed consumers of medical care and issues related to their own care. In addition, the changing role of the caregiver has further underscored the importance of high standards of care and solid ethical practices. This chapter helps the activity specialist recognize and resolve ethical dilemmas faced by older adults. Activity specialists should possess a basic understanding of privacy, confidentiality, incompetence, autonomy, beneficence, and nonmaleficence. The process of informed consent, the decision making required for creating a living will, and the responsibility needed when research is being conducted with older adults are also important considerations. Finally, standards of care used by activity specialists when working with older adults will help to ensure client well-being. Activity therapists will apply these concepts as they develop sensitivity to the delicate ethical situations often faced by older people and their caregivers.

Comprehension Questions

1. Identify four key concepts related to professional ethics. Define them and discuss why they are important in the process of activity intervention.
2. Describe a situation in which the activity specialist may be confronted with an ethical dilemma. Discuss different strategies for dealing with the situation.
3. Discuss why standards are important in the delivery of professional services to older adults.

References

Gadow, S. (1981). A model for ethical decision-making. *Oncology Nursing Forum, 7*(4), 44-47.

Gilhooly, M. L. M. (1986). Ethical and legal issues in therapy with the elderly. In I. Hanley, & M. L. M. Gilhooly, *Psychological therapies for the elderly* (pp. 173-197). New York, NY: New York University Press.

Guccione, A. A. (1988). Compliance and patient autonomy: Ethical and legal limits to professional dominance. *Topics in Geriatric Rehabilitation, 3*(3), 62-73.

Hanks, R. S., & Settles, B. H. (1988-89). Theoretical questions and ethical issues in a family caregiving relationship. *The Journal of Applied Social Sciences, 13*(1), 9-39.

Howell, M. C. (1988). Ethical dilemmas encountered in the care of those who are disabled and also old. *Educational Gerontology, 14,* 439-449.

Janicki, M. P., Heller, T., Seltzer, G. B., & Hoge, J. (1995). *Practice guidelines for the clinical assessment and care management of Alzheimer and other dementias among adults with mental retardation.* Washington, DC: American Association on Mental Retardation.

Levine, J., & Lawlor, B. A. (1991). Family counseling and legal issues in Alzheimer's disease. *The Psychiatric Clinics of North America, 14*(2), 385-396.

Olson, E., Chichin, E. R., Libow, L. S., Martico-Greenfield, T., Neufeld, R. R., & Mulvihill, M. (1993). A center on ethics in long-term care. *The Gerontologist, 33*(2), 269-274.

Shank, J. W. (1985). Bioethical principles and the practice of therapeutic recreation in clinical settings. *Therapeutic Recreation Journal, 19*(4), 31-40.

Smith, S. H., & Land, C. (1989). Playing the standards game: Considerations for the 1990s. In D. M. Compton (Ed.), *Issues in therapeutic recreation: A profession in transition* (pp. 271-288). Champaign, IL: Sagamore Publishing, Inc.

Tymchuk, A. J., & Ouslander, J. G. (1990). Optimizing the informed consent process with elderly people. *Educational Gerontology, 16,* 245-257.

Williams, S. G. (1993). How do the elderly and their families feel about research participation? *Geriatric Nursing, 14*(1), 11-14.

Key Terms

Ageism
Aging in Place
Certified Therapeutic Recreation
    Specialist
Demographic Trends
Functional Impairment
Intergenerational Relationships
Life Expectancy

Long-Term Care
Maximum Life Span
Medicaid
Medicare
Normal Aging
Retirement Age
Social Security
Therapeutic Activity Intervention

Learning Objectives

1. Identify the basic competencies needed by activity specialists who provide therapeutic activity intervention to older adults.
2. Identify professional preparation and standard qualifications that activity specialists should possess in order to provide therapeutic activity intervention to older adults.
3. Provide examples of current and future trends that influence the delivery of therapeutic activity intervention to elderly persons.
4. Discuss hiring policies and practices as they pertain to the provision of therapeutic activity intervention.

Chapter 17

The Future of Therapeutic Activity Intervention

Introduction

In this text the reader has been introduced to the older adult population from a variety of perspectives. Unit I provides background information about the population, as well as discusses healthcare for older persons. Unit II describes the normal aging process and introduces the reader to some of the more common illnesses, diseases, and disabilities experienced by older persons. Units III and IV provide detailed information about the intervention process, as well as activity strategies that are commonly used by activity specialists in the therapeutic care and treatment of older adults. Last, in Unit V, the importance of documentation, evaluation, ethics, and standards of care is reemphasized. In this final chapter of the text, issues related to the future of therapeutic activity intervention services are addressed.

By now, most readers of this text recognize that the life course for most adults tends not to follow a straight, linear pathway but rather weaves itself along a zigzag route (Kelly, 1993). The journey of life brings some losses and some gains. With most losses, lifestyles will be affected; personal resources and social resources will be impacted, and they may even dwindle. Maintaining meaningful activity involvement is one way in which older adults can keep in touch with each other, thus improving the quality of their lives.

The future quality of life for older persons and the role of professionals that provide therapeutic care to them are dependent on many factors. Professional and service developments that are achieved or rejected now will surely influence the future, just as the past has inspired the present. Public responsibility for services to an aging population is of vital concern. The need for service coordination, the acknowledgment of manpower shortages, and a recognition of the limits of professionalism are critical issues affecting services to the senior population—now and into the future (Morris, 1989). This chapter provides a discussion of two broad areas of concern affecting the future of therapeutic activity intervention services for older adults: (a) the basic professional qualifications for activity specialists, and (b) current and future trends influencing therapeutic activity intervention services.

Professional Qualifications of Activity Specialists

In 1987 the U.S. Department of Health and Human Services expressed concern over the lack of a broad array of trained professionals to provide care and treatment services to the growing older adult population. Recreation therapists, or activity specialists, were included as an area in which manpower was needed and will continue to be needed well into the twenty-first century. In spite of many federally-sponsored projects to increase the availability of trained personnel, there remains slow growth in the availability of trained activity specialists (or therapeutic recreation professionals with specialization in gerontology) (Hawkins, MacNeil, Hamilton, and Eklund, 1990). The recreation and leisure services field is just entering the arena of specialized efforts to assess personnel needs, standardize professional preparation curricula, and to track the placement of graduates into jobs that service older adults. The overall goal of specialized training for activity specialists is to improve the delivery of appropriate services to elderly persons in the community, institutions, and home settings (Hawkins and Eklund, 1990).

Specific Knowledge Competencies of Activity Specialists

Hawkins and her associates (Hawkins and Austin, 1990; Hawkins and Eklund, 1990) identified the basic competencies needed by activity specialists who provide *therapeutic activity intervention* to older people. The identified competencies were grouped under general education in gerontology and content areas specific to the practice of therapeutic recreation with frail, vulnerable, and impaired elderly adults. The most important knowledge competencies listed under the broad topic of leisure and aging were as follows:

- understanding of the role of physical, mental, emotional, and social activity in the promotion of wellness for older adults;
- understanding the changing role of leisure across the life cycle;
- knowledge of how exercise and physical activity can improve the health status of older adults;
- understanding the role of leisure services in preserving optimal personal independence and well-being;
- understanding the impact of social leisure involvement on cognitive, psychological, and physical functioning of older adults;

- awareness of the importance of leisure in later adulthood;
- knowledge of the importance of common areas of activity programming for older adults including, but not limited to, the following: outdoor recreation, physical activities, adult and leisure education, and social activities;
- awareness of the major findings from leisure research that address the needs of the older adult population;
- understanding the social, economic, and emotional significance of retirement, the use of preretirement planning, and the role of postretirement activities; and
- knowledge of current public policies and policy issues regarding the older adult population.

The most important knowledge competencies that were identified as necessary for the specific area of therapeutic activity intervention were as follows:

- knowledge of common physical illnesses and disabilities that are typical among older adult populations;
- knowledge of psychological and cognitive functions common to *normal aging* and the discrimination of these capacities from psychopathological and cognitive changes, diseases, and dysfunction;
- understanding of the physical, psychological, emotional, and social areas that increase vulnerability to disability and infirmity for older adults;
- understanding of and ability to use, with proficiency, recreation activity as a therapeutic intervention that promotes the greatest benefit to older adults;
- knowledge of and ability to implement therapeutic activity intervention methods and procedures;
- ability to assess the leisure needs, interests, and abilities of specific older adult populations, including insight into the diversity of gerontologic and geriatric assessment instruments;
- awareness of major research findings that apply to the efficacy of activity intervention with older adults; and
- understanding of the benefits received by participating in therapeutic activity intervention.

While a specific program of education for training activity specialists who intend to work with the aged in a variety of treatment settings is not widely available, numerous options exist for receiving some of the aforementioned knowledge competencies. One option is to enroll in special courses established for training activity directors who work in skilled nursing facilities—an Activity Directors Training Course commonly offered by State Departments of Health or Aging Services. Another avenue is to take specialized courses that are offered in conjunction with degree programs in therapeutic recreation or general recreation. Additionally, certificate programs in gerontology at postsecondary educational institutions also present another option for obtaining training in normal aging processes. Either a certificate or a minor course of study can be added to a degree program in recreation to accomplish the overall basic level of knowledge competency needed by activity specialists. Most accredited curricula in therapeutic recreation also require practicum hours which can be completed in activity centers that serve older adults. A good approach for individuals who are interested in acquiring the necessary background training is to review courses and training programs in light of the competencies listed above.

Specific Practice Skills Needed by Activity Specialists

Federal and state agencies periodically review and improve the regulations that specify a level of professional qualification for personnel who provide therapeutic activity intervention to elderly persons. A minimum of a certificate or a minor in gerontology or aging studies appended to a degree in recreation or therapeutic recreation is the preferred approach. Program accrediting groups (i.e., the Joint Commission on Accreditation of Healthcare Organizations and the Commission for the Accreditation of Rehabilitation Facilities) typically review and improve regulations that specify the level of professional qualifications for personnel who provide therapeutic activity intervention to elderly clients (Hawkins, MacNeil, Hamilton, and Eklund, 1990). Within these guidelines, a set number of internship hours are usually required to develop the skill competencies for professional practice.

It also is desirable that a commitment be made by employing agencies which give preference to job candidates who have basic knowledge and skill competence in gerontology and therapeutic recreation when hiring for positions related to therapeutic activity intervention with elderly persons. Under optimal conditions, employing agencies will require minimum qualifications for activity specialists including an academic major, minor, or certificate in gerontology or aging studies, and certification as a *Certified Therapeutic Recreation Specialist*. These qualifications will help to ensure a high quality of care for older adult clients (Hawkins, MacNeil, Hamilton, and Eklund, 1990).

General Standards in Therapeutic Recreation and Gerontology

The National Recreation and Park Association/American Association on Leisure and Recreation Council on Accreditation (1990) has established guidelines and standards for the professional skills that are necessary to attain the status of *Certified Therapeutic Recreation Specialist*. These standards include the following:

- ability to analyze and to apply the theories and concepts of therapeutic recreation;
- ability to facilitate the concepts of mainstreaming, integration, and normalization in all programming;
- ability to apply activity and task analysis in all programming;
- ability to apply programming concepts including conceptualization, planning, implementation, and evaluation of comprehensive and specific therapeutic recreation services;
- ability to select, conduct, analyze, and utilize a variety of assessment techniques and procedures in therapeutic recreation programs;
- understanding of and the ability to design individual program and/or treatment plans;

- understanding of the impact of social attitudes toward illness and disability;
- understanding of the conceptualizations and attitudes of individuals with illnesses and/or disabilities toward leisure programs;
- ability to implement a variety of individual and group techniques including therapeutic intervention, instruction, leadership, and supervision;
- ability to apply management techniques in the areas of finance, personnel, and reimbursement for therapeutic recreation services;
- understanding of interagency and intraagency client referral processes;
- ability to use and understand the nature and function of various forms of documentation including those related to staff, programs, management, and quality assurance in therapeutic recreation;
- understanding of and the ability to use a variety of assistive techniques and adaptive devices related to specific illnesses and disabilities in therapeutic recreation services;
- ability to analyze professional and ethical behavior related to therapeutic recreation services;
- understanding of the role of the therapeutic recreation professional as an advocate for leisure, human rights, and services for individuals with illnesses and disabilities;
- understanding of the use of legal tools and processes to improve therapeutic recreation services;
- understanding of and the ability to apply local, state, and federal regulations and standards to therapeutic recreation services;
- understanding of the nature and implications of professional accreditation standards and the ability to comply with accreditation standards in therapeutic recreation services;
- understanding of credentialing processes and the ability to comply with credentialing standards in therapeutic recreation services;
- understanding of the resources for professional development;
- ability to promote, advocate, interpret, and articulate therapeutic recreation concerns; and
- ability to apply leisure education content and techniques.

The promotion of minimum qualifications for therapeutic recreation and activity specialists who work with elderly populations by employing agencies is desired. These minimum qualifications include certification and academic preparation in therapeutic recreation and gerontology/aging studies. In general, gerontology education programs typically consist of a standard set of requirements that are fundamental to the knowledge and practice background needed by individuals who work with older adults. An undergraduate certificate will include coursework in the following program areas:

- introduction to gerontology,
- biological aspects of aging,
- psychological aspects of aging,
- social aspects of aging,

- integration of gerontological course content with a major area,
- elective course in gerontology, and
- practicum. (Association for Gerontology in Higher Education, 1989, p. 41)

A graduate certificate will include the following requirements:

- biology of aging,
- psychology of aging,
- sociology of aging or social gerontology,
- basic or applied research,
- two elective courses in gerontology, and
- practicum or supervised research. (Association for Gerontology in Higher Education, 1989, p. 28)

Through a program of studies that combines the knowledge and practice competencies outlined above, the activity specialist can obtain the comprehensive professional preparation needed to provide high quality services and care to older adult populations. The combination of substantive gerontology education and professional preparation in therapeutic recreation provides the most advanced state-of-the-art in training for activity specialists. Quality intervention and treatment for at-risk, frail, infirm, impaired, and disabled older adults will be significantly advanced if activity specialists receive this level of professional preparation. In addition, hiring practices used should show preference for job candidates with these skills.

Prevailing and Future Trends Influencing Therapeutic Activity Intervention

The American population is aging rapidly, as measured by the escalating numbers of older individuals, the expansion of the proportion of older persons in the total population, and the general increase in average age. *Demographic trends* indicate that persons age 65 and over comprise about one-fifth of the population and will constitute about two-fifths of the population by the year 2040. In 1991 the U.S. had the world's fourth largest elderly population after China, India, and the Soviet Union. The projected increase in the U.S. population aged 60 and over is 69% from 1991 through 2020 (Hess, 1991; Lumsdaine and Wise, 1990; U.S. Department of Commerce, 1991). However, the labor force participation of older Americans has decreased dramatically in recent years, thus associated trends have occurred in Social Security and other retirement pension plan coverage (Lumsdaine and Wise, 1990).

While the trends in demographic change are well-publicized and addressed on a daily basis in the media, a number of significant issues will undoubtedly affect activity services to the aging population. The following selected areas that will continue to have implications for the provision of activity programs and services to older adults are:

(a) aging in place,
(b) retirement trends,
(c) healthcare issues,
(d) personnel shortages, and
(e) program/service proliferation.

Aging in Place

Aging in place is a term used to describe the ideal condition of not having to move from one's home when there is a change in the need for personal assistance and support services. Many older adults are becoming increasingly vocal about their desire to receive in-home services rather than to be relocated to a nursing home. Aging in place also has come to mean the idea of remaining within a familiar home or a community that was established in later maturity such as a retirement community. In this regard, aging in place refers to long-term care settings that are designed to accommodate clients within the same environment throughout various stages of disease or decline (Cohen and Day, 1993).

Aging in place can become a process that results in older persons becoming concentrated in certain communities and neighborhoods over a period of time. As aging in place becomes the norm, significant numbers of older persons will remain in their residences, living independently for as long as possible (Morrison, 1992).

Future elderly persons who age in place will want to have the necessary supports to have their needs met within their residences, which has implications for how services will be configured and delivered. The needs of older adults will be served through various forms of assistance such as continuum of care retirement communities, assisted living programs, or home delivered care. Aging in place presents a national and global challenge to envision additional possibilities and responses to aging adults in the future (Morrison, 1992).

A major deficiency of national healthcare policy is the lack of a structured and comprehensive system of long-term care that uses various delivery approaches. Currently, substantial resources are expended through existing federal programs for meeting the care needs of the elderly. Under the present system, program structures and requirements tend to be slanted toward a "medical model" of care with less attention being given to in-home and community-based services. Institutional management is sustained partly because of the lack of a willingness to consider alternatives or because there does not appear to be a better model that is widely available. There is little agreement among policymakers on how to address this problem; consequently, the prospects for fundamental reform appear uncertain at this time (Cohen and Day, 1993; Somers, 1991).

Individuals who age in conventional housing that is not designed to monitor needs or to provide support services are at risk for either inappropriate transfer or segregation. When these individuals are transferred inappropriately to long-term institutions, care is provided that is enormously expensive and often results in noticeable functional loss and precipitous decline of the individual. The most desirable situation would be one in which long-term care institutions provide care for persons who are truly in need of dependent nursing care. Frail but basically well persons require a variety of assisted independent living environments and programs that will permit aging in place (Heumann and Boldy, 1993).

Aging in place as a trend holds multiple implications for the range of service environments in which activity specialists need to be prepared to deliver services and programs. Traditionally, activity specialists have considered the skilled nursing home and adult day activity center as the two primary service delivery sites. With the trend toward supporting people to age in place, outreach service delivery may well become the more typical service modality for the activity specialist.

Life Expectancy and Retirement

In addition to the general increase in individual life expectancy, the overall change in the distribution of the population to a generally older profile among adults is a significant policy area for the country. The oldest age groups (people over 85) are growing the fastest, thus an increasingly large proportion of the population is older than the typical *retirement age* (65). From an individual perspective, increasing life expectancy encourages people to think about taking later retirement. Longer life expectancy generally means that retirement pensions, Social Security entitlement, and personal savings must be used to support consumption over an increasing number of retirement years. From a societal standpoint, a much larger older population means that a smaller labor force must think about supporting a growing number of retirees (Lumsdaine and Wise, 1990).

A majority of families rely heavily upon Social Security benefits for support after retirement and, to a more limited extent, on retirement pension plans. About 95% of persons over the age of 65 receive Social Security benefits and about 50% collect pensions. The expansion of Social Security and improving company pension plans have allowed and encouraged the consideration of earlier retirement (Grad, 1990; Lumsdaine and Wise, 1990).

There is evidence of a general decline in real wages across all age groups in the U.S. since 1972. Therefore, the decline in real wage earnings has contributed to earlier retirement in recent years. Personal savings also have declined to less than 1% of disposable private income (Lumsdaine and Wise, 1990; Summers and Carroll, 1987). There is a large range in personal savings rates, with a large proportion of the elderly population saving almost nothing except in the form of housing equity. Older persons experience a decline in their incomes for several reasons including the loss of pension income when a spouse dies and the erosion of savings over a life time (U.S. Senate Special Committee on Aging, American Association of Retired Persons, Federal Council on the Aging, and U.S. Administration on Aging, 1991; Venti and Wise, 1989).

Trends that continue to affect and shape retirement practices will ultimately have an impact on the activity specialist. Early retirees may need less direct activity intervention and more service delivery facilitation, whereas retirees who are disabled may fit more closely with the aging in place model of outreach and in-home service delivery. Retiree income and health status, as well as chronological age, are important trends to watch for the implications they have on the need for and nature of therapeutic activity intervention services.

Health Status and Health Services Utilization

Our present knowledge that has resulted from the various theoretical views on aging may one day merge to form a more complete explanation of human aging. Even if this occurs, however, few researchers expect that there will be a significant change in what is believed to be the maximum life span of the human organism. For human beings, maximum life span is estimated to be between 110 and 120 years. Life expectancy is the average age that a person in a given time and place can expect to reach. While the human life span may not be extended, lengthening of life expectancy can continue to be realized (Can you live longer? What works and what doesn't, 1992).

Gerontologists predict that the next 10 to 20 years will bring technological advances that will enable individuals to meet the challenges and the oddities of aging. For the present, however, longevity can be maximized by following familiar risk-reduction strategies such as consuming a healthy diet, exercising regularly, and by avoiding smoking, alcohol abuse, and obesity (Can you live longer? What works and what doesn't, 1992).

The majority of today's younger elderly persons are relatively healthy and not especially limited in activity even if they have chronic health problems. However, health and mobility do decline with advancing age. By the time that most people reach their 80s or 90s, they can expect to have limitations in their daily activities and/or have an increased need for health and social services (U.S. Senate Special Committee on Aging, American Association of Retired Persons, Federal Council on the Aging, and U.S. Administration on Aging, 1991).

In spite of the increasing propensity for health and functional limitations with age, older persons tend to regard their health positively. Nearly 71% of elderly persons living in the community described their health as excellent, very good, or good. Only 29% reported their health to be fair or poor. Income would appear to be directly related. Approximately 41% of those elderly persons who assessed their health status as fair or poor had annual incomes below $10,000. Impaired older persons are more likely than other elderly individuals to have limited incomes or assets. However, over 83% of those older individuals with incomes of $35,000 and over characterized their health status as excellent, very good, or good (National Center for Health Statistics, 1990; U.S. Senate Special Committee on Aging, American Association of Retired Persons, Federal Council on the Aging, and U.S. Administration on Aging, 1991).

The link between health status and income is significant. Around 3.5 million older people live with incomes below the poverty level. An additional 8.2 million older citizens live with near-poor incomes which lie between 100% and 199% of the poverty level. Older women—particularly older minority women—are the most likely to be poor or near-poor (Rowland, 1990).

Older people who are living with low incomes must rely on social programs such as Medicare for their health insurance coverage. Living without health insurance is a reality for 3% of the poor elderly. To the uninsured, as well as older individuals without Medicaid or supplemental health insurance, out-of-pocket medical expenditures are an ongoing concern. Although Medicaid was designed to protect the poor and medically indigent, a low proportion of the poor (33%) and near-poor (10%) actually utilize or have the benefit of Medicaid protection (Rowland, 1990).

By the year 2000, approximately 2 million persons age 65 and over will require long-term care and by 2040, roughly four million elderly persons will be in need of long-term care and/or services (Manton and Soldo, 1985). Most elderly persons with *functional impairment* acquire long-term care services in the community. Community services include senior centers, special transportation, meals provided at home or other community locations, adult daycare, and home visitations by nurses or health aides (National Center for Health Statistics, 1987).

Most older persons have little or no protection against the excessive costs of long-term care. The funding of long-term care is derived principally from individual or family payments and public payments by Medicaid. Long-term care insurance covered approximately 2% of expenditures in 1990, and by the year 2020, long-term care insurance is expected to pay for nearly 7% of total long-term care expenses. In 1990 the expenditures for long-term nursing home care were $37.6 billion (Levit, Freedland, and Waldo, 1990; U.S. Senate Special Committee on Aging, American Association of Retired Persons, Federal Council on the Aging, and U.S. Administration on Aging, 1991).

By the year 2005, long-term care expenditures are projected to be $64 billion, and by 2020, total nursing home payments are expected to surpass $112.6 billion. Home healthcare expenditures also will increase; total costs for home healthcare in 1990 were nearly $8 billion and are projected to be approximately $20 billion by the year 2020. In general, future predictions suggest that the number of older persons requiring nursing home and home healthcare will increase significantly, as will the expenses for these efforts (Levit, Freedland, and Waldo, 1990; U.S. Senate Special Committee on Aging, American Association of Retired Persons, Federal Council on the Aging, and U.S. Administration on Aging, 1991).

The solvency of Social Security Trust Funds is jeopardized in the next 75 years with Disability Insurance funds predicted to become exhausted possibly by 1998. Medicare also will encounter a deficit by the turn of the century. Escalating healthcare costs rather than disbursements for retirement incomes account for the majority of public expenditures for the elderly. Social Security retirement and disability benefits and healthcare programs are expected to comprise over 41% of the total Federal budget in 1995. By the year 2040, over 60% of the Federal budget is projected to include Social Security programs and a healthcare agenda (Palmer and Torrey, 1983).

Because of separate goals and priorities, public policies in disability and aging have evolved along different paths. Care for the elderly is oriented toward hospitalization and institutionalization rather than rehabilitation. However, the number of persons living to old age requires a closer examination of the structure of public policy. As these individuals reach advanced age, the potential for disabling conditions increases (Galvin and La Buda, 1991).

The current healthcare policy for the nation is ineffective, unresponsive, and exceedingly expensive. With increasing needs and decreasing assets, the necessity to maximize the resources of both disability and aging policies for the benefit of everyone is essential. However, as long as there is a fragmented system that focuses on acute medical intervention instead of prevention, the current problems will persist. Reform of healthcare policies and systems is not only needed but also critical in order for service sectors and professions to develop new strategies for ensuring adequate service delivery to a growing elderly population. Such reform would assure access for all persons and would establish a priority for quality care at a reasonable cost (Galvin and La Buda, 1991).

Personnel Shortages

There are currently only 1.32 geriatricians per 10,000 individuals age 65 and over. Unless there is a collective effort to increase the number of geriatricians in the U.S., the severe shortage will worsen. A substantial increase in the number of geriatricians is required in order to maintain the health, independence, and productivity of older persons (U.S. House of Representatives, 1992).

The severity of the shortage of healthcare providers with training to serve older adults, combined with the ongoing shift in the nation's demographic profile, make it critical that physicians, scientists, and faculty members use their influence to encourage students to enter the fields of gerontology and geriatrics (U.S. House of Representatives, 1992). Activity specialists with specific preparation in gerontology and therapeutic recreation are considered to be allied healthcare professionals. Therefore, specialized training programs are needed in order to ensure an adequate supply of activity specialists as the demand for services continues to rise.

Crucial to any solution to the manpower shortage problem is the recognition of the need for physicians and other allied health professionals to be trained in all areas of gerontology. Without such teachers, the problem of manpower shortages will continue to exist. The supply of general physicians, specialists, and allied healthcare professionals will never satisfy the demand for care of the rapidly expanding elderly population (Small, Fong, and Beck, 1988).

Program and Service Proliferation

Since the middle of the present century, remarkable growth has occurred in the service delivery structure and in the cadre of professions that provide support and care to the elderly. This growth has not occurred without some serious side effects according to Morris (1989). The proliferation of organizational structures and bureaucratic procedures has created additional burdens and barriers for older persons as well as for the service providers who genuinely wish to meet their clients' needs. Elaborate systems for obtaining information and referral, gate-keeping systems like case management, and a never-ending process of rule changing and rule generation can make seeking assistance from government sponsored programs a formidable nightmare. These management elaborations (information, referral, and case management) add substantial expenditures to an already cost-burdened system. While the functions of specialization, fragmentation, and organizational management might appear justifiable, the results have often not provided direct benefits to older consumers.

Service and program proliferation, while offering more options to meet varying needs, is costly. Each agency or system requires its own infrastructure, documentation and evaluation systems, fundraising, etc. (Morris, 1989). The growing industry of aging service providers, both public and private, adds to the cost of care for the elderly while adding to class separation (e.g. near-poor, poor, well-to-do) among this segment of the population. This proliferation actually increases the volume of unmet needs and thus aggravates an already critical problem in the human services area.

Morris (1989) noted that fundamental change is necessary in order to meet more effectively, efficiently, and professionally the needs of the elderly population—now and into the future. This change must address the primary question of how the general well-being of the older adult population is to be secured while meeting the whole-person needs of each individual. Technology has not protected the wholeness of the individual with dignity and respect, and the resulting megasystem has tended to mirror this same problem. Activity specialists will need to view themselves as part of a more simplified but responsive system serving the whole person. Therefore, the training and preparation that activity specialists receive will become more important as the service system meets this challenge.

Prospects for the Future

The value placed on youth and appearance continues to be a pervasive theme in modern American life. Often, youth and appearance seem more important than productivity and usefulness. Also, Americans tend to focus upon individualism and independence which often act against the ideas of interdependence and community. As a consequence, the idea of requesting assistance from others continues to be difficult for most people. When assistance can be regarded as an instrument for autonomy rather than as a threatening technique or as a substitute for personal independence, society can concentrate upon the creation of community rather than continuing to promote intense individualism. One strategy that can be used is to promote a greater sense of community—*intergenerational programs to build relationships across the ages.* Through the building of these relationships and connections across the age groups, older persons may then have the opportunity to function in the more productive roles of teachers or counselors as is customary in other cultures (Erikson, Erikson, and Kivnick, 1986; Shimp, 1990).

The problems and prospects of older adults in the U.S. seem to point to the need to rethink our fundamental values and beliefs about people. When individualism is replaced by interdependence, self by a sense of community, and worth as measured by who one is and not what one looks like, then there may be hope for an emerging society that is prepared for an elongated life span, not just an improved life expectancy. In this future scenario, older persons transform their traits and characteristics into resources. They are empowered because of who they are and no longer forgotten just because they have lived long enough to be conveniently excused from the mainstream activities of the society.

Choices are created by the restructuring of society and by the new conceptualizations of the aging condition. Choices in the aging process are not isolated variables; they are personal and situational. *Ageism* is rejected. Individual and community choices that inspire higher levels of human consciousness are conceived within the design of a society as responsible to its elderly population, as it is to all other members of its nation (Kannady, 1993).

Summary

Basic knowledge and practice skills are desired of activity specialists in order to qualify them for providing activity interventions to older adults. In addition to these basic qualifications, certification as a therapeutic recreation specialist coupled with training in gerontology is important in the developmental hiring policies and practices of agencies that provide therapeutic activity intervention to elderly individuals. Current trends and issues that are affecting services to the aging population may be expected to provide new challenges to agencies in the future. Especially notable are the following trends: sustained population growth, the need for additional trained manpower to meet the demand for services, and prospective changes in healthcare policies. A sense of community and the importance of building intergenerational relationships continue to be desired goals for the older generations.

"Being human is being responsible—[truly] responsible for one's . . . existence" (Frankl, 1975, p. 26). Individuals cannot survive in an environment void of other responsive and caring beings. Activity specialists are entrusted with the task of creating humanistic programs and environments for all aging individuals, whether they be younger or older, in the future society to which all aspire.

Comprehension Questions

1. Select six knowledge competencies needed by activity specialists who provide services to older adults and explain why they are important.
2. Discuss the importance of developing practice skills for working with elders.
3. Why is it important to have established qualifications for working with older adults in activity intervention?
4. What impact do the following trends have on activity specialists and what they do: retirement practices, healthcare services, aging in place, service proliferation, and manpower shortages?

References

Association for Gerontology in Higher Education. (1989). *Standards and guidelines for gerontology programs*. Washington, DC: Author.

Can you live longer? What works and what doesn't. (1992, January). *Consumer Reports, 57*(1), 7.

Cohen, U., & Day, K. (1993). *Contemporary environments for people with dementia*. Baltimore, MD: The Johns Hopkins University Press.

Erikson, E. H., Erikson, J. M., & Kivnick, H. Q. (1986). *Vital involvement in old age*. New York, NY: W. W. Norton & Company Inc.

Frankl, V. (1975). *The unconscious God*. New York, NY: Washington Square.

Galvin, J. C., & La Buda, D. R. (1991). United States health policy issues into the next century. *International Journal of Technology and Aging, 4*(2), 115-127.

Grad, S. (1990). *Income of the population 55 or over, 1988* (Pub. No. 13-11871). Washington, DC: U.S. Social Security Administration.

Hawkins, B. A., & Austin, D. R. (1990). Identification of competencies needed in gerontological recreation courses: An application of the Delphi technique. *Annual in Therapeutic Recreation, 1*, 21-27.

Hawkins, B. A., & Eklund, S. J. (1990). *Professional preparation in gerontology therapeutic recreation curriculum guide*. Bloomington, IN: Indiana University.

Hawkins, B. A., MacNeil, R. D., Hamilton, E. J., & Eklund, S. J. (1990). *Professional preparation and practice in gerontological therapeutic recreation: Status and recommendations*. Bloomington, IN: Indiana University.

Hess, B. B. (1991). Growing old in America in the 1990s. In B. B. Hess & E. W. Markson (Eds.), *Growing old in America* (4th ed.) (pp. 5-22). New Brunswick, NJ: Transaction Publishers.

Heumann, L. F., & Boldy, D. P. (1993). *Aging in place with dignity: International solutions relating to the low-income and frail elderly*. Westport, CT: Praeger Publishers.

Kannady, G. (1993). Meaning amidst chaos: The challenge of the 21st century. *International Forum for Logotherapy, 16*, 43-50.

Kelly, J. R. (1993). Problems and prospects: Looking to the future. In J. R. Kelly (Ed.), *Activity and aging: Staying involved in later life* (pp. 264-265). Newbury Park, CA: Sage Publications, Inc.

Levit, K. R., Freedland, M. S., & Waldo, D. R. (1990). National health care spending trends: 1988. *Health Affairs, 9*(2), 171.

Lumsdaine, R. L., & Wise, D. A. (1990). *Aging and labor force participation: A review of trends and explanations*. Cambridge, MA: National Bureau of Economic Research.

Manton, K. G., & Soldo, B. J. (1985). Dynamics of health changes in the oldest old: New perspectives and evidence. *Milbank Memorial Fund Quarterly/Health and Society, 63*(2), 206-285.

Morris, R. (1989). Challenges of aging in tomorrow's world: Will gerontology grow, stagnate, or change? *Gerontologist, 29*(4), 494-501.

Morrison, P. A. (1992). *Is aging in place a blueprint for the future?* Santa Monica, CA: Rand.

National Center for Health Statistics. (1990, October). Current estimates from the National Health Interview Survey, 1989. *Vital and Health Statistics, 10*(176).

National Center for Health Statistics. (1987). *Health interview survey: Supplement on Aging, 1984.* Baltimore, MD: The Johns Hopkins University Press.

National Recreation and Park Association/American Association on Leisure and Recreation Council on Accreditation. (1990). *Standards for accrediting postsecondary professional preparation programs.* Alexandria, VA: National Recreation and Park Association.

Palmer, J. L., & Torrey, B. (1983). Health care financing and pension programs. *Urban Institute Conference on Federal Budget Policy in the 1980s.* Washington, DC: U.S. Government Printing Office.

Rowland, D. (1990, May). Fewer resources, greater burdens: Medical care coverage for low-income elderly people. *Bipartisan Commission on Comprehensive Health Care.* Washington, DC: U.S. Government Printing Office.

Shimp, S. (1990). Debunking the myths of aging. *Occupational Therapy in Mental Health, 10*(3), 101-111.

Small, G. W., Fong, K., & Beck, J. C. (1988). Training in geriatric psychiatry: Will the supply meet the demand? *American Journal of Psychiatry, 145*(4), 476-477.

Somers, F. P. (1991). Long-term care and federal policy. *American Journal of Occupational Therapy, 45*(7), 628-635.

Summers, L., & Carroll, C. (1987). Why is U.S. national saving so low? *Brookings Papers on Economic Activity, 2*, 607-642.

U.S. Department of Commerce. (1991). *Global aging: Comparative indicators and future trends.* Washington, DC: U.S. Bureau of the Census.

U.S. House of Representatives. (1992). *Geriatricians and the senior boom: Precarious present, uncertain future.* Washington, DC: U.S. Government Printing Office.

U.S. Senate Special Committee on Aging, American Association of Retired Persons, Federal Council on the Aging, & U.S. Administration on Aging. (1991). *Aging America.* Washington, DC: U.S. Department of Health and Human Services.

Venti, S. F., & Wise, D. A. (1989). *Aging and the income value of housing wealth.* Cambridge, MA: National Bureau of Economic Research.

Appendix A

National Association of Activity Professional's Standards of Practice[2]

Standard 1

The collection of information about the past, present, and future interests as well as the values, characteristics, traits, and individuality of the client is systematic and continuous. The information is recorded, communicated, and accessible.

Rationale

To be meaningful and realistic, programs must be based on a person's past and present lifestyle, interests, values, and capabilities. The client must be the primary source of information to the extent possible.

Criteria

1. Activities information should include:
   - family history,
   - ethnic and cultural background,
   - educational background,
   - social habits (large and small groups, alone),
   - vocational background,
   - recreational interests and hobbies (talents, sports, games, travel, reading, television, and fine arts),

[2]Reprinted with permission of the National Association of Activity Professionals.

- membership in clubs and organizations (leadership positions),
- volunteer activities,
- political involvement (voting habits),
- spiritual activities (church attendance, roles, scripture study),
- past profile of typical day and week,
- future profile (what client wants within the facility),
- life goals, aspirations, and dreams, and
- levels of participation; supportive, maintenance, and empowerment activity programs.
2. Information is collected by the activity professional from:
    - client,
    - records and reports,
    - other professionals directly involved in the care of the client, and
    - family and significant others.
3. Information is obtained through:
    - interviews,
    - observations, and
    - reading records and reports.
4. There is a format for the collection of information which is:
    - systematic,
    - coordinated with information or data from all other professionals directly involved with the care of the client, and
    - continuous as evidenced by recording of changes in participation in daily programs.
5. The information is:
    - accessible for all disciplines in the client record and
    - retrievable from record-keeping systems.

The National Association of Activity Professionals has developed three categories of activities which reflect the essential philosophy of basing programming on individual clients needs rather than specific types of activities. These categories are referred to as supportive, maintenance, and empowerment activities.

Supportive activities promote a comfortable environment while providing stimulation or solace to clients who cannot benefit from either maintenance or empowerment activities. These activities are generally provided to clients who may be severely physically or cognitively impaired and/or are unable to tolerate the stimulation of a group program. Examples are: playing soft music, placing colorful objects in a client's room, and providing tactile or olfactory stimulation.

Maintenance activities will vary from one facility to another, but their primary function is to provide clients with a schedule of events that promotes the maintenance of physical, cognitive, social, spiritual, and emotional health. These activities are provided to clients with a variety of functioning levels. Examples include: exercise groups, sports, etc., to improve physical functioning; discussion groups, current events, etc., to improve cognitive functioning; pet therapy, volunteer service, etc., to improve emotional functioning; and participation in life review, religious services, etc., to enhance spiritual functioning.

Empowerment activities emphasize the promotion of self-respect by providing opportunities for self-expression, choice, and social and personal responsibility. These programs differ from maintenance activities in that they assist clients directly in redeveloping a sense of purpose in their lives. Examples include: self-government, cooking, gardening, client volunteer programs, and creative activities.

In addition, activities are classified into two types: passive and active.

Passive activities require no participation or response from clients; almost all supportive activities would be passive.

Active activities require participation and response from the clients. This might be an oral response, some physical action or movement, or it might involve some action over a period of time. Most maintenance and empowerment activities would be active.

Standard 2

The analysis of the client's needs and strengths are derived from the activity assessment.

Rationale

The data collected for the analysis is used as the baseline for determining the needs that can be filled through activities that enable each client to attain or maintain the high(est) practicable level of physical, mental or psychological well-being.

Criteria

1. The client's past, present and future activity interests and levels are identified.
2. The client's present and past health status is identified.
3. The client's capabilities and limitations are identified.
4. The client's needs are formulated from the completed Activity Assessment.

Standard 3

The activity plan is developed based on the client's strengths and needs.

Rationale

The client's strengths and needs are used to develop goals and objectives.

Criteria

1. Goals are mutually set with the client whenever possible.
2. Goals are set to maximize life satisfaction of the client.
3. Goals are incorporated into the interdisciplinary care plans.
4. Goals and objectives are measurable and realistic.

Standard 4

The client's individual activity program is designed to facilitate the accomplishment of his or her goals.

Rationale

The client needs an opportunity to accomplish goals through independent individual and group activities.

Criteria

1. The client's interests are reflected in the activity programs.
2. The program is consistent with the plan of care.
3. The program allows for changes in the client's health status.
4. The program is consistent with the facility's mission statement.
5. The client is involved in the planning and implementation of activities, if possible.
6. The program is evaluated and monitored to ensure safety of the client and of the environment.
7. Community resources are utilized in the implementation of the program.

Standard 5

The client's status, or any change in the client's status in goals of achievement, is reviewed on a regular basis. The goal is reviewed on an ongoing basis.

Rationale

Goal achievement is a process that must be continually monitored throughout for maximum effectiveness.

Criteria

1. Current data is issued to evaluate progress toward goal achievement including data collected from activity documents and from other members of the interdisciplinary team.
2. Client evaluation of progress includes information related to:
    * progress toward goal,
    * appropriateness of activity plan,
    * effectiveness of program development,
    * goal achievement,
    * resources used (within facility, department and the community),
    * client involvement, and
    * staff and volunteers used.
3. Client is involved in setting new goals.

Appendix B

American Hospital Association's Patient's Bill of Rights[3]

1. The patient has the right to considerate and respectful care.
2. The patient has the right to and is encouraged to obtain from physicians and other direct caregivers relevant, current, and understandable information concerning diagnosis, treatment, and prognosis.

   Except in emergencies when the patient lacks decision-making capacity and the need for treatment is urgent, the patient is entitled to the opportunity to discuss and request information related to the specific procedures and/or treatments, the risks involved, the possible length of recuperation, and the medically reasonable alternatives and their accompanying risks and benefits.

   Patients have the right to know the identity of physicians, nurses, and others involved in their care, as well as when those involved are students, residents, or other trainees. The patient also has the right to know the immediate and long-term financial implications of treatment choices, insofar as they are known.
3. The patient has the right to make decisions about the plan of care prior to and during the course of treatment and to refuse a recommended treatment or plan of care to the extent permitted by law and hospital policy and to be informed of the medical consequences of this action. In case of such refusal, the patient is entitled to other appropriate care and services that the hospital provides or

Note: These rights can be exercised on the patient's behalf by a designated surrogate or proxy decision maker if the patient lacks decision-making capacity, is legally incompetent, or is a minor.

[3]Reprinted with permission of the American Hospital Association, © 1992.

transfer to another hospital. The hospital should notify patients of any policy that might affect patient choice within the institution.

4. The patient has the right to have an advance directive (such as a living will, healthcare proxy, or durable power of attorney for healthcare) concerning treatment or designating a surrogate decision maker with the expectation that the hospital will honor the intent of the directive to the extent permitted by law and hospital policy.

   Healthcare institutions must advise patients of their rights under state law and hospital policy to make informed medical choices, ask if the patient has an advance directive, and include that information in patient records. The patient has the right to timely information about hospital policy that may limit its ability to implement fully a legally valid advance directive.

5. The patient has the right to every consideration of privacy. Case discussion, consultation, examination, and treatment should be conducted so as to protect each patient's privacy.

6. The patient has the right to expect that all communications and records pertaining to his or her care will be treated as confidential by the hospital, except in cases such as suspected abuse and public health hazards when reporting is permitted or required by law. The patient has the right to expect that the hospital will emphasize the confidentiality of this information when it releases it to any other parties entitled to review information in these records.

7. The patient has the right to review the records pertaining to his or her medical care and to have the information explained or interpreted as necessary, except when restricted by law.

8. The patient has the right to expect that, within its capacity and policies, a hospital will make reasonable response to the request of a patient for appropriate and medically indicated care and services. The hospital must provide evaluation, service, and/or referral as indicated by the urgency of the case. When medically appropriate and legally permissible, or when a patient has so requested, a patient may be transferred to another facility. The institution to which the patient is to be transferred must first have accepted the patient for transfer. The patient must also have the benefit of complete information and explanation concerning the need for, risks of, benefits of, and alternatives to such a transfer.

9. The patient has the right to ask and be informed of the existence of business relationships among the hospital, educational institutions, other healthcare providers, or payers that may influence the patient's treatment and care.

10. The patient has the right to consent or decline to participate in proposed research studies or human experimentation affecting care and treatment or requiring direct patient involvement, and to have those studies fully explained prior to consent. A patient who declines to participate in research or experimentation is entitled to the most effective care that the hospital can otherwise provide.

11. The patient has the right to expect reasonable continuity of care when appropriate and to be informed by physicians and other caregivers of available and realistic patient care options when hospital care is no longer appropriate.

12. The patient has the right to be informed of hospital policies and practices that relate to patient care, treatment, and responsibilities. The patient has the right to be informed of available resources for resolving disputes, grievances, and conflicts, such as ethics committees, patient representatives, or other mechanisms available in the institution. The patient has the right to be informed of the hospital's charges for services and available payment methods.

Appendix C
Glossary

Accident: A happening or event that takes place without foresight or expectation such as falls, pedestrian accidents, or motor vehicle accidents; seventh leading cause of death in older adults.

Accountability: Determination of whether approved or promised treatment was received by the client and if treatment and services were cost-effective.

Active Listening: Attending to the feelings of others and to one's own feelings or reactions.

Active Rehabilitation Program: Intervention approach which involves the performance of skilled therapy.

Activities of Daily Living (ADLs): Essential tasks associated with basic daily functioning such as bathing, dressing, grooming, getting out of bed and/or chairs, and toileting.

Activity Analysis: Systematic evaluation of activities for appropriateness and utility in attaining individual treatment goals.

Activity Theory: Based on the premise that high levels of activity are associated with perceptions of high life satisfaction in old age.

Acute Disease: Episodic, short-term disease caused by bacterial or viral infection, characterized by rapid onset; usually curable through medical treatment.

Adaptation: To change so that one's behavior, attitudes, etc. conform to new or changed circumstances.

Adjustment: Bringing into harmony or agreement; acclimation.

Adult Daycare: A community-based service designed to assist individuals with functional impairments who otherwise would be at risk for institutionalization to remain at home while receiving social, health, emotional, and medical care.

Advocacy Model: Conceived by Gadow to assist individuals in choosing their own actions; ensures the possibility of self-determination; enables the client to select information in order to make a decision; discloses personal views; assists clients in determining their own values; and establishes how clients perceive their own individuality.

Aerobic Activity: Any exercise that increases oxygen uptake and elevates the heart rate over a sustained period of time.

Age Discrimination Employment Act: Legislation passed in 1967 that restricts employers from failing to hire a person because of age, discharging an employee because of age, or discriminating in pay because of age.

Ageism: Stereotypical attitudes and behaviors that result when society attributes certain characteristics (usually negative) to all older persons based solely on chronological age.

Age Stratification Theory: Based upon the concept that people are assigned into categories by society according to age.

Aging in Place: Term used to describe the condition of not having to move from one's home when there is a change in the need for personal assistance and support services.

Alcoholism: Diseased condition caused by excessive or continuous use of alcoholic liquors.

Alzheimer's Disease: Primary degenerative or senile dementia; the most common form of dementia in the U.S.

Amotivation: Nonmotivated behaviors in which individuals perceive a lack of connection between their behaviors and outcomes.

Anosognosia: Apparent unawareness of or failure to recognize one's own functional defect.

Antecedents of Behavior: Events and circumstances that immediately precede and influence an individual's action or reaction.

Antidepressant Drug: Medication used to treat the symptoms of depressive illness.

Anxiety Disorder: State of inner distress comprised of dread, fear, or anticipation of imagined harm that is accompanied by various symptoms including shortness of breath, dry mouth, dizziness, increased heart rate, trembling, sweating, and/or chills.

Apportioned Grandparent: Views social norms and personal needs as important in the achievement of satisfaction in the grandparent role.

Arthritis: A class of over 100 inflammatory and degenerative conditions of the joints and bones of the skeletal system.

Assessment: Specific techniques and procedures used to construct a precise picture of the individual and his or her environment; a systematic approach to identifying and describing client problems.

Autonomy: Refers to self-rule or self-determination; includes liberty, independence, and choice.

Beneficence: The concept of doing good in an effort to promote the well-being of the individual.

Bereavement: Universal human experience and normal response to deprivation and loss of a loved one, a job, economic security, or one's home.

Biomedical Model of Aging: Relating the social construction of aging and the practice of aging as medical problems.

Bipolar Disorder: Characterized by severe mood swings from depression to euphoria; often termed manic-depressive illness.

Blocks to Communication: Hindrances to the effective exchange of information such as ordering, commanding, warning, threatening, preaching, lecturing, judging, criticizing, blaming, diagnosing, and providing solutions.

Cancer: A malignant growth anywhere in the body; a malignant tumor.

Cardiovascular Disease: Heart and circulatory conditions such as atherosclerosis, coronary artery disease, hypertension, congestive heart failure, and stroke.

Cardiovascular System: The system of the body that is instrumental in transporting oxygen rich blood throughout the body and returning carbon dioxide laden blood to the lungs for the exchange with fresh oxygen.

Caregiving: The provision of emotional support and physical services to a dependent older adult.

Care Plan: Plan of treatment for client that includes factors that relate to medical status, physical and/or psychological limitations, client's response to the program, level of participation, social interactions, relationships, staff or agency supports, and notable attitudes or patterns of behavior.

Certified Therapeutic Recreation Specialist: Professional credentialed by the National Council on Therapeutic Recreation Certification, having met the minimum qualifications for an entry-level therapeutic recreation practitioner.

Chronic Disease: Ongoing disease characterized by progressively deteriorative effects and which usually is irreversible or incurable.

Chronological Age: The number of years a person has lived.

Classic Aging Pattern: Describes cognitive performance in old age; verbal intelligence scores will remain stable while performance scores of intelligence will decline with age.

Cohort Effect: Reflects the impact of historical times upon a specific age group and distinguishes that age group from persons of other eras.

Comorbidity: The circumstance of having more than one chronic disease or disability at a time.

Competency: The ability to make and communicate responsible decisions.

Compliance: Yielding to a request, wish, desire, demand, or proposal of another person.

Confidentiality: The ethical obligation not to reveal to others anything said by clients or to acknowledge the existence of a relationship.

Consequence of Behavior: Result, either good or bad, of a person's actions.

Continuing Care Retirement Community (CCRC): Retirement community that offers in-home assistance and social support in addition to short-term and long-term nursing care in a CCRC-based health pavilion; also referred to as a life-care community.

Continuity Theory: Suggests that personality remains stable over the life span.

Control: Regulate or exercise authority over behavior of self or others.

COPD: Chronic obstructive pulmonary disease characterized by seriously damaged lung tissues that result from other conditions such as chronic bronchitis, emphysema, fibrosis, and asthma.

Counseling: Providing information, advice, resources, and referrals to "normal individuals" in order to realize concrete goals.

Creativity: Artistic or intellectual resourcefulness.

Deconditioning: Added and accelerated loss in functioning beyond that which is associated with normal aging-related change.

Deep Friendship: Intimate relationships that have a lesser focus upon mutual interests and that tend to last throughout life with the individuals who are involved, usually unconcerned with equity.

Delirium: An organic, psychiatric syndrome characterized by acute onset and impairment in cognition, perception, and behavior; also termed transient cognitive disorder or acute confusional state.

Delusion: False personal belief that is firmly sustained despite external reality.

Dementia: Loss of intellectual abilities to the degree that it interferes with social or occupational functioning; memory impairment; and at least one of the following: impairment in abstract thinking, judgment, higher cortical function, or personality change.

Demographic: Pertaining to vital statistics such as births, deaths, and marriages of particular populations.

Dependency Ratio: The number of adults under age 65 in comparison to the number of adults over age 65; ratio currently is 8 to 1.

Depression: An emotional condition characterized by discouragement, feelings of inadequacy, sadness, low spirits, dejection, etc.; viewed as a function of genetic and biological factors, environmental stresses, and habitual ways of thinking and acting.

Designated Autonomy: Conceding to others the authority to make decisions or act.

Diabetes: Elevated levels of glucose in the blood and urine caused by a lack of production or utilization of insulin in the metabolic processes of the cells of the body.

Dilemma: A situation that requires a decision between alternatives that appear to be equal.

Direct Autonomy: Making decisions and acting on one's own.

Disability: Functional limitation in role or task performance due to impairment arising from a health problem and determined by the social and physical environment in which one lives.

Disengagement Theory: Based on the idea that a mutual withdrawal of the elderly and society from each other results in higher life satisfaction among the elderly.

Disruptive Behavior: Actions such as angry outbursts or throwing objects that interfere with the established routine or current activities.

Documentation: Supplying supportive references or evidence related to the treatment of a client.

Drug Abuse: Habitual use of narcotics or any medicinal substance.

Education: The process of training and developing knowledge, skill, mind, and character, especially by schooling and teaching.

Ego Integrity: Resolution of conflicts from earlier stages of life and integration of past experiences into the present; successful completion of Erikson's final stage of psychosocial development.

Elderly Mystique: The myth that disability in old age indicates inevitable decline and disintegration, including a significant termination of skill and mastery.

Electroconvulsive Therapy: A treatment option for depressed individuals that involves causing a series of seizures with electrical stimulation.

Empty Nest Syndrome: Children leaving the parents' home, mistakenly perceived to create a crisis for most older adults, especially women.

Endocrine System: The group of glands responsible for the production and secretion of chemical messengers that regulate bodily functions.

Environment: The conditions, circumstances, and influences surrounding and affecting developmental functions.

Environmental Assessment: Evaluation of community resources.

Environmental Press: The demands placed on an individual by the environment both socially and physically.

Erikson's Psychosocial Model: A stage theory of personality which states the individual moves through eight stages of development during the life course. The final four stages are completed in adulthood.

Ethical Dilemma: Situation in which alternatives are defined by opposing ethical principles.

Ethics: Refers to the investigation of what is good and what is bad; the way in which choices are contemplated.

Ethnocentric: Having the attitude that one's own race, nation, or culture is superior to all others.

Evaluation: Appraisal of appropriateness, effectiveness, acceptability, efficiency, adequacy, efficacy, and impact of a program or intervention.

Excess Disability: Increased cognitive impairment due to the impact of depression compounded with dementia.

Exchange Theory: Based on the premise that the status of older adults is based largely on the balance between contributions to society made by older people and the cost of supporting elderly individuals.

Extrinsic Motivation: When extraneous or extrinsic factors or rewards guide behavior.

Family Therapy: Intervention to improve the functioning of the family system.

Feminization of Poverty: Theory of society to lock women in poverty through social institutions and economic structure.

Flexibility: The ability to move joints through the entire range of motion.

Formal Functional Assessment: Determines health status eligibility for insurance, social services, and living arrangements.

Formative Evaluation: Review of the strengths and weaknesses of an activity intervention or program in order to pursue improvements in activity or program development and implementation.

Functional Age: Determined by an individual's ability to accomplish activities of daily living (ADLs) and to live independently.

Functional Assessment: Evaluation of the capacity to function independently or with assistance.

Functional Competence: Ability to perform activities and tasks in relation to degree of impairment involved.

Functional Impairment: Debilitation or weakening with no apparent degeneration, damage, or structural change in the body.

Functional Independence: Ability to maintain autonomous functioning; an important indicator of overall quality of life.

Functional Limitation: Describes the effects that are present in a person's capacity to perform as a whole entity either independently or with assistance.

Functional Mental Disorders: Diseases in which behavioral problems or distress are not due to physical disease processes.

Gastrointestinal System: The network responsible for receiving and processing food into nutrients for the body; also called the digestive system.

Genetic Theories of Aging: Biological theories of aging that describe the influences of human genes on the cell division and replacement process as it causes systemic change across the life span.

Geriatrics: The area of medicine that specializes in the care and management of disease in elderly persons.

Gerontology: The multidisciplinary field in which the biological, psychological, and social aspects of the aging process are studied.

Goal Attainment Scaling: A method of evaluation involving the establishment of goals, specification of barriers, and a description of the most favorable, the least favorable, and the most likely outcomes of an intervention.

Group Therapy: Treatment intervention in psychological problems that presents opportunities for socialization and learning from peers.

Hallucination: Psychotic symptom involving sensory perceptions of sights and sounds that are not actually present.

Health Promotion: Expands healthcare beyond the medical technologies of surgery, medications, comfort, and consideration to include a quality of life dimension.

Health Status: Measured on the basis of key vital statistics such as life expectancy, mortality rates, incidence of morbidity, and occurrences of infectious disease; affects individual functional independence and limitations.

Health/Wellness Status Assessment: Identification of strengths and weaknesses in the following areas: general health, physical fitness, nutrition, and stress/emotional adjustment.

Heart Disease: Disease of the cardiovascular system; the leading cause of death among older persons.

Home-Bound: Unable to leave one's home to obtain needed health services.

Iatrogenic Disorder: Pathological brain condition that results from incorrect use of medications, diagnostic procedures, or therapies and not from any physical dysfunction.

Impairment: Damage, injury, or deterioration of an organ or organ system that results in loss in mental or physical function.

Independence: Freedom from the influence, control, or determination of others; self-maintenance; includes the right to flourish.

Individual Competence: The upper level of a person's ability to function includes physical health status, sensory and perceptual capacities, motor skills, cognitive capacities, and ego strength.

Individualized Grandparent: Views the personal benefits of grandparenting as rewarding and generally is unconcerned with social norms.

Individual Treatment Plan: Match of specific treatment goals and objectives with selected activities for the individual client.

Influenza: An acute, contagious, infectious disease caused by any of several viruses and characterized by inflammation of the respiratory tract, fever, muscular pain, and often intestinal disorders.

Informal Functional Assessment: Involves collection of data concerning survival skills, support systems, barriers, problems, and other issues.

Informed Consent: The concept of providing information to the individual regarding proposed medical treatment and research.

In-Home Care: Therapeutic intervention and health services that are provided to individuals within their homes.

Instrumental Activities of Daily Living (IADLs): Complex tasks that are concerned with the integral responsibilities of everyday life such as meal preparation, management of one's finances, shopping, utilizing community services, etc.

Integumentary System: The largest system of the body; it comprises the skin and related structures such as the hair and nails.

Intelligence: The ability to deal with information, new situations, symbols, abstractions, and ideas.

Interest-Related Friendship: Developed on the basis of common lifestyles and interests between two individuals.

Intergenerational Relationship: Association between or among people of varying ages.

Intervention: Activity used for inducing, facilitating, and maintaining independent functioning.

Interview: Face-to-face meeting of individuals to confer or to provide information related to a client's treatment.

Intrinsic Motivation: Belonging to the real nature of a thing; not dependent upon external circumstances; results in behaviors that are engaged in for their own sake.

Justice: Fair allocation of goods, services, and general resources; individuals without relevant differences between them are treated equally.

Learning: Cognitive process that involves the processing and storing of new information.

Leisure: That part of life that comes nearest to allowing freedom from a regimented and conforming world, and enables the pursuit of self-expression, intellectual, physical, and spiritual development.

Leisure Activity Assessment: Involves data on activities, interests, preferences, desires, and skills that support independent functioning.

Leisure Education: Focuses on the development of knowledge, attitudes, and beliefs about the value of leisure for enhancing quality of life.

Life-Care Community: Residence in which elderly individuals may receive in-home assistance and social support and the assurance of short-term and long-term nursing care in a health facility.

Life Expectancy: The projected number of years an individual born in a particular year is expected to live; the life expectancy of a child born in 1993 is 75.5 years.

Life Review: The process of reviewing, organizing, and evaluating one's life.

Lifestyle: Factors such as exercise, eating, and health habits that have a significant impact on the rate of aging decline and the quality and longevity of life.

Living Will: A written legal document that establishes the manner in which a client wants to be treated if he or she is terminally ill and can no longer make decisions concerning his or her health; someone is appointed by the individual to make decisions for the client when he or she is unable to do so.

Long-Term Care: Community or institutional services designed for persons with functional impairments.

Lymphatic System: The immune system; it protects the body from infections and is responsible for the collection of excess fluids from cells.

Maintenance: Treatment or interventions designed to maintain the client's current level of functional ability.

Maximal Oxygen Consumption: Amount of oxygen taken in and distributed to working muscles during exercise at maximum rate.

Maximum Life Span: Estimated to be between 110 and 120 years for human beings; the maximum number of years any member of a species can live.

Medicaid: Public medical protection payment plan implemented by state and county governments for those who meet certain criteria and are unable to afford medical treatment.

Medical Assessment: Involves the examination and evaluation of all body systems.

Medicare: Social program providing health insurance administered by the U.S. federal government for those who meet the age-based requirements.

Memory: Cognitive process that involves the process of retrieving learned information.

Merit: Refers to characteristics that are valued.

Metabolic Disease: Disorders involving the continuous chemical and physical processes of living organisms and cells.

Metabolism: Chemical and physiological operations that occur in living organisms and cells; food is converted to protoplasm and the protoplasm is used and reduced into simpler substances or waste matter, producing a concurrent release of energy for all vital processes of the body.

Modernization Theory: Based on the premise that the status of older adults declines as a society increasingly modernizes.

Morbidity: Rate of disease or proportion of persons with diseases in a given locality.

Motivation: Sources that energize behavior in general and in particular situations.

Multidimensional Assessment: Includes assessment of mental status and affect, functional status, social and economic circumstances, values, and preventive strategies including a traditional medical assessment.

Multidisciplinary Team: A treatment group that includes professional representatives with various individual approaches and talents.

Multi-Infarct Dementia: Dementia that results as a consequence of multiple small strokes throughout the brain.

Muscular Endurance: Ability of a muscle to sustain work over a period of time.

Musculoskeletal System: The network that provides the support structure for the body; it is composed of bones, muscles, ligaments, cartilage, and tendons.

Near Poor: Individuals who exist between the poverty level and 125% of this level.

Nervous System: The communications network for the body responsible for coordinating and organizing the functions of all body systems.

Nonmaleficence: Principle that the practitioner does no harm.

Nonverbal Technique: Method for motivation such as touch, hugs, smiles, and laughter.

Normal Aging: Common and usual changes associated with maturation and growing older.

Nursing Facility: A general term for facilities that provide long-term residential care for individuals with disabilities.

Nursing Home Care: Provision of a protective environment and assistance with basic daily living skills; more intense medical and critical care also are offered.

Objective Autonomy: Freedom from barriers; i.e., choices in clothing, bed times, types of food.

Objectives-Oriented Evaluation: Focuses on how well or to what degree a specific activity intervention or overall program objectives were realized.

Observation: The act or practice of noting and recording facts and events; one of the most common evaluative procedures used in treatment using specific procedures to record or appraise various outcomes and behaviors.

Older Adult: Person who is 65 years of age or older.

Oldest Old: Individual above 85 years of age.

Old Old: Person who is between 75 and 84 years of age.

Oral Disease: Conditions of the mouth involving loss of teeth, gum disorders, dental caries, or ailments of the tooth roots.

Organic Cognitive Disorder: Designation for a variety of organic mental syndromes for which the cause has been identified.

Osteoporosis: Accelerated aging-related loss of bone mass that causes serious structural weakness and vulnerability to fractures.

Paranoia: Pathological suspiciousness or the sense of being treated unfairly.

Paraphrenia: Schizophrenia with a late life onset.

Pathology: Changes in the tissues and cells of the human organism that are produced by injury, infection, disease, birth defects, and other means.

Perseveration: The tendency to continually emit the same verbal or motor response.

Physical Restraint: Actual control of a person's movements.

Planning: Determination of what and how therapeutic interventions will be provided; involves stating treatment goals and objectives, selecting activities, identifying resources and problems, and writing a treatment plan.

Pneumonia: A disease of the lungs in which the tissues become inflamed, hardened, and watery.

Polypharmacy: Concurrent use of two or more medications, particularly in excessive doses or inappropriate combinations.

Poverty Level: The amount of income, determined by the federal government, below which an individual is judged to have inadequate resources.

Power of Attorney: Written statement legally authorizing a person to act for another.

Presbyopia: Condition in which the older adult has difficulty focusing on near objects because the lens and pupil of the eye are unable to adjust quickly.

Prevention: Actions that prevent or minimize disease or disability; type of healthcare that focuses on maintenance of health rather than on cure of disease.

Preventive/Maintenance Program: Utilizes interventions that are integrated into the everyday life of the client to maintain current level of functional ability.

Privacy: A place of seclusion from company or observation; withdrawal from public view; retreat; solitude; an individual's right to have control over his or her own personal information free of invasions into his or her life.

Privileged Communication: Legal protection provided for patients and clients by statute or by the courts in legal matters relating to the client.

Promotion: Therapeutic activity intervention designed to facilitate optimal functioning with minimal support.

Prosthetic Approach: Assumes that a disability cannot be modified, and therefore, prosthetic supports (such as a walker) are required to allow the individual to negotiate the environment.

Pseudodementia: Term used to describe reversible depression-related cognitive disorders.

Psychiatric Assessment: Evaluation of the potential for delirium, functional disorders, and depression.

Psychosis: Psychiatric disorder that involves major distortions in reality.

Psychosocial: Pertaining to or concerning the mental factors or activities that determine the social relations of an individual.

Psychotherapy: The application of various forms of treatment to maladjusted nervous and mental behaviors, problems, and disorders.

Qualitative Information: Collected through anecdotal records, case notes, interviews, and observations in the form of words or artifacts.

Quality of Life: Desired attributes of one's existence including optimal health and well-being, growth, physical fitness, functional abilities, intellectual stimulation, social inclusion, equal rights, dignity, respect, and good fortune.

Quantitative Information: Data that is capable of being measured in extent, size, greatness, or magnitude.

Questionnaire: Written or printed form used in gathering information on some subject or subjects, consisting of a list of questions to be submitted to one or more persons.

Range of Motion: The space or expanse taken or passed over by moving the body or any of its parts.

Rapport: Relationship, especially a close or sympathetic relationship; agreement; harmony.

Reality Orientation: A treatment approach focused upon daily routines and behavior and principles of reinforcement to assist clients in maintaining a sense of self, time and place.

Recreation: Any form of play, amusement, or relaxation used to renew the body or mind; i.e., games, sports, hobbies, reading, walking.

Rehabilitation: Restoration to a state of physical, mental, and/or moral health through treatment and training; facilitating, causing, and/or maintaining the client's control over his or her physical, cognitive, emotional, and social capacities.

Relaxation: A corrective, adaptive, enrichment, or preventive intervention that is focused upon the self-control of internal feelings such as anxiety and anger.

Reminiscence: The vocal or silent recall of events in one's life.

Remote Grandparent: Views the grandparenting role as unsatisfactory and unrewarding.

Remotivation: A treatment approach focused upon helping older adults regain a sense of dignity and raise self-esteem through participation in group activities that utilize verbal and cognitive skills and memory.

Reproductive System: Network of hormones and reproductive organs.

Resocialization: A treatment approach focused upon helping confused or withdrawn clients by providing opportunities to develop new relationships and maintain long-term friendships.

Respiratory System: The system of the body responsible for providing oxygen from inhaled air to the bloodstream and the removal of carbon dioxide from the blood, transporting it back into the environment through exhaled air.

Retirement: Withdrawal from work or service typically near the age of 65 in the U.S.

Schizophrenia: Psychiatric disturbances in several of the following areas: content and form of thought, perception, affect, sense of self, behavior, and relationship to the external world.

Screening: To interview or test in order to separate according to skills, personality, attitudes; used to identify individuals who require a more complete assessment.

Self-Determination: Permits the individual to attempt new activities to explore unfamiliar regions or establishments and to receive satisfaction from one's endeavors.

Sensory Stimulation: A treatment approach for cognitively impaired older adults focused upon providing concrete, sensory cues that enable clients to appropriately respond to their environment.

Sensory System: Network that governs the body's interactions with the environment through vision, hearing, touch, pain, temperature sensation, taste, smell, and equilibrium.

Skill Performance: Involves tasks concerned with intellectual, motor, and personality traits.

Social Breakdown: Refers to the spiral that occurs when criticism and negative feedback of older persons leads to lowered self-esteem and decline in performance which then leads to further criticism.

Social Gerontology: The branch of gerontology that concerns itself with the social and cultural factors that influence both older adults and how an aging population impacts upon society.

Socialization: Adapting to the common needs of a social group.

Social Network: Persons on whom one relies for daily social exchange and support.

Social-Role Performance: Execution of roles within society and interpersonal functioning.

Social Security: An age-based entitlement program administered by the federal government to ensure a minimum level of income in retirement.

Sociocultural/Socioeconomic Assessment: Includes data on family structure, housing, work and retirement, friendships, economic circumstances, social roles, activities, and interests.

Sociometry: A technique that explores the organization of groups by determining the nature of the structure that is functioning within the group.

Spirituality: Individual beliefs regarding religion or the existence of a higher power.

Stage Theories of Personality: Define personality development as a process of phases or intervals. Individuals progress through a series of developmental stages during the life course.

Standards of Care: A framework that establishes minimal guidelines of service affecting the scope and methods of care provided and parameters for the role of service providers.

Stochastic Theories of Aging: Biological theories that describe the influence of random attacks on the body by accumulated external forces and internal factors.

Strength: Ability of an individual to apply force by muscle contraction.

Stress Test: Method for assessing baseline fitness.

Subculture Theory: Based on the premise that older adults primarily interact with each other, forming a subculture.

Subjective Autonomy: A sense of freedom of choice that can involve independent relationships with other persons.

Summative Evaluation: Appraises accomplishments at the conclusion of an activity intervention or overall program.

Sundowning: Agitated and confused behaviors of clients with delirium that often occur in the evening and night.

Survey: General view, comprehensive study, examination, or inspection.

Symbolic Grandparent: Views the status of being a grandparent as more important than the personal relationship with grandchildren.

Symbolic Interactionism: Views the interaction of the environment, the individual, and various situations as central to the aging process.

Tardive Dyskinesia: A side effect of antipsychotic drugs that involves involuntary movement that may appear after three to six months of treatment with antipsychotic medications.

Task Analysis: A process that examines the elements of an activity involving the study of behavior and the identification of its component parts.

Therapeutic: Intended to stimulate change; serving to cure or heal.

Therapeutic Activity Intervention: Specific treatment action or pursuit that ameliorates, restores, and/or rehabilitates various illnesses, injuries, and disabilities.

Therapeutic Approach: An approach to therapeutic intervention in which the environment is adapted to fit the ability of the client.

Therapeutic Humor: A therapeutic approach that focuses upon the restorative qualities of amusement and laughter.

Thyroid Disease: Dysfunction of the thyroid gland characterized by either an excess or a deficiency of thyroid hormone.

Triangulation: A systematic approach that uses a variety of evaluation techniques and resources to present a more comprehensive description of clients and programs.

Triggers: Stimuli that prompt recall of life events.

Urinary System: The network responsible for cleansing the blood of waste products produced by body cell use of nutrients.

Validation Therapy: A therapeutic approach that focuses upon the well-being of clients with severe disorientation through acceptance of the client's thought and beliefs, rather than emphasis on reality orientation.

Wandering Behavior: Problem associated with persons with Alzheimer's disease; roaming or roving caused by physical discomfort, disorientation, restlessness, or agitation.

Weight Bearing: Exercises such as walking, aerobic dance, or weightlifting that increase large bone mineral content and strength.

Wellness: High level of vitality and elevated quality of life.

Worth: Quality of a thing that renders it useful.

Young Old: The 65 to 74 age group.

About the Authors

BARBARA A. HAWKINS is an Associate Professor in the Department of Recreation and Park Administration at Indiana University. She holds a Doctorate in Recreation from Indiana University. Dr. Hawkins holds a Master of Science degree from the University of Montana and a Bachelor of Science degree from the University of New Hampshire in Recreation and Park Administration. Dr. Hawkins has professional experience in activity programming for older adults with disabilities, especially in health promotion, fitness, and leisure education. She specializes in life span development, developmental disabilities, and leisure behavior. She has received numerous federal and state grants to study the special concerns of aging adults with mental retardation and other developmental disabilities. She has served as President of the Leisure and Recreation Division and member of the Board of Directors in the American Association on Mental Retardation, President of the Society of Park and Recreation Educators, and Vice Chair of the Special Interest Group on Aging/Mental Retardation in the Gerontological Society of America.

MARTI E. MAY holds a Bachelor of Science degree with a dual major in Psychology and Health and Physical Education, as well as a Master of Arts in Health Science from Ball State University. She also holds a Master of Science in Therapeutic Recreation from Indiana University. Ms. May is currently a doctoral candidate at Indiana University majoring in Recreation/Leisure Studies with a minor in Gerontology. She has worked as a rehabilitation and behavioral therapist at several hospitals and as a recreation director at a sheltered workshop. Ms. May also has professional experience in several community recreation facilities.

NANCY BRATTAIN ROGERS is an Assistant Professor in the Department of Recreation and Sport Management at Indiana State University, Terre Haute, Indiana. In 1995 she completed her Ph.D. in Human Performance with an emphasis in Leisure Behavior and a minor in Gerontology at Indiana University. She holds a Bachelor of Science degree in Recreation Administration from Western Illinois University and a Master of Science degree in Recreation Administration from Indiana University. Dr. Roger's research interests include the development of leisure services for older adults and issues related to women and leisure. She has expertise in the study of leisure behavior utilizing naturalistic methodologies. Dr. Rogers has previously worked as Project Director for the Foster Grandparent Program in Omaha, Nebraska.

Other Books from Venture Publishing

Interpretation of Cultural and Natural Resources
    by Douglas M. Knudson, Ted T. Cable and Larry Beck
Introduction to Leisure Services—7th Edition
    by H. Douglas Sessoms and Karla A. Henderson
Leadership and Administration of Outdoor Pursuits, Second Edition
    by Phyllis Ford and James Blanchard
Leisure And Family Fun (LAFF)
    by Mary Atteberry-Rogers
Leisure Diagnostic Battery Computer Software
    by Gary Ellis and Peter A. Witt
The Leisure Diagnostic Battery: Users Manual and Sample Forms
    by Peter A. Witt and Gary Ellis
Leisure Education: A Manual of Activities and Resources
    by Norma J. Stumbo and Steven R. Thompson
Leisure Education II: More Activities and Resources
    by Norma J. Stumbo
Leisure Education Program Planning: A Systematic Approach
    by John Dattilo and William D. Murphy
Leisure in Your Life: An Exploration, Fourth Edition
    by Geoffrey Godbey
Leisure Services in Canada: An Introduction
    by Mark S. Searle and Russell E. Brayley
Marketing for Parks, Recreation, and Leisure
    by Ellen L. O'Sullivan
Models of Change in Municipal Parks and Recreation: A Book of Innovative Case Studies
    edited by Mark E. Havitz
Outdoor Recreation Management: Theory and Application, Third Edition
    by Alan Jubenville and Ben Twight
Planning Parks for People
    by John Hultsman, Richard L. Cottrell and Wendy Zales Hultsman
Private and Commercial Recreation
    edited by Arlin Epperson
The Process of Recreation Programming Theory and Technique, Third Edition
    by Patricia Farrell and Herberta M. Lundegren
Protocols for Recreation Therapy Programs
    edited by Jill Kelland, along with the Recreation Therapy Staff at Alberta Hospital
    Edmonton
Quality Management: Applications for Therapeutic Recreation
    edited by Bob Riley
Recreation and Leisure: Issues in an Era of Change, Third Edition
    edited by Thomas Goodale and Peter A. Witt
Recreation Programming and Activities for Older Adults
    by Jerold E. Elliott and Judith A. Sorg-Elliott
Recreation Programs that Work for At-Risk Youth: The Challenge of Shaping the Future
    by Peter A. Witt and John L. Crompton
Reference Manual for Writing Rehabilitation Therapy Treatment Plans
    by Penny Hogberg and Mary Johnson
Research in Therapeutic Recreation: Concepts and Methods
    edited by Marjorie J. Malkin and Christine Z. Howe

Risk Management in Therapeutic Recreation: A Component of Quality Assurance
    by Judith Voelkl
A Social History of Leisure Since 1600
    by Gary Cross
The Sociology of Leisure
    by John R. Kelly and Geoffrey Godbey
A Study Guide for National Certification in Therapeutic Recreation
    by Gerald O'Morrow and Ron Reynolds
Therapeutic Recreation: Cases and Exercises
    by Barbara C. Wilhite and M. Jean Keller
Therapeutic Recreation in the Nursing Home
    by Linda Buettner and Shelley L. Martin
Therapeutic Recreation Protocol for Treatment of Substance Addictions
    by Rozanne W. Faulkner
A Training Manual for Americans With Disabilities Act Compliance in Parks and Recreation Settings
    by Carol Stensrud
Understanding Leisure and Recreation: Mapping the Past, Charting the Future
    edited by Edgar L. Jackson and Thomas L. Burton

    Venture Publishing, Inc.
1999 Cato Avenue
State College, PA 16801

Phone: (814) 234-4561; FAX: (814) 234-1651